The Eating Disorders

A. James Giannini   Andrew E. Slaby
Editors

The Eating Disorders

With 11 Illustrations

Springer-Verlag
New York Berlin Heidelberg London Paris
Tokyo Hong Kong Barcelona Budapest

A. James Giannini, M.D.
Clinical Professor, Psychiatry
Ohio State University
Columbus, OH 43210, USA
and
P.O. Box 2169
Youngstown, OH 44504, USA

Andrew E. Slaby, M.D., Ph.D., M.P.H.
Medical Director
Regent Hospital
425 E. 61th Street
New York, NY 10021, USA

Library of Congress Cataloging-in-Publication Data

The eating disorders / [edited by] A. James Giannini, Andrew E. Slaby.
p. cm.
Includes bibliographical references and index.
ISBN 0-387-94002-2. — ISBN 3-540-94002-2
1. Eating disorders. I. Giannini, A. James, 1947–
II. Slaby, Andrew Edmund.
[DNLM: 1. Eating Disorders. WM 175 E14612 1993]
RC552.E18E282 1993
616.85′26—dc20
DNLM/DLC
for Library of Congress 93-20481

Printed on acid-free paper.

Production coordinated by Chernow Editorial Services. Inc. and managed by Christin R. Ciresi; Manufacturing supervised by Jacqui Ashri.
Typeset by Best-set Typesetter Ltd., Hong Kong
Printed and bound by Edwards Brothers, Inc., Ann Arbor, MI, USA.
Printed in the United States of America.

9 8 7 6 5 4 3 2 1

ISBN 0-387-94002-2 Springer-Verlag New York Berlin Heidelberg
ISBN 3-540-94002-2 Springer-Verlag Berlin Heidelberg New York

To
Juliette Nicole Giannini
and
Jocelyn Danielle Giannini

Always there when needed most.

Preface

As fish must swim
so must man drink and eat

Titus Petronius Arbiter

Examine thy customs of diet

Francis Bacon

For John eat & drank to drive away Loves pain
But all he could do he grew thinner & thinner
Tho he eat & drank as much as Ten men for dinner

Some said he had a Wolf in his stomach day and night

William Blake

To paraphrase and cast in contemporary speech observations of the Gothic-era monk Bernard of Clairvaux, the eating disorders may be viewed as a corruption of the social process, a distortion of the body image, and a perversion of bodily processes. It is this multifactorial etiology that makes the diagnosis and treatment of dietary disorders so difficult and frustrating. Because of social demands and a distorted (body) image, men and women have perverted the simple act of eating into always painful, sometimes tragic, and occasionally deadly outcomes.

The eating disorders fall into three categories. There is obesity—the overconsumption of food, and its antithesis, anorexia—the act of voluntary starvation. In true Hegelian fashion, there follows the synthesis, bulimia—the voluntary purging of overconsumed amounts of food to produce an anorectic-like countenance. As the contributing authors emphasize in their chapters, these diseases are not unique to contemporary culture. Rather they are cultural artifacts, created by both men and women, since classical antiquity.

The recognition of these diseases is dependent upon recognizing a disease actually exists: that there is a distortion of the eating process. Both medical and psychiatric etiologies are explored. The use of the clinical laboratory and neurological examination as an adjunct to medical and pediatric treatment is explored. Special groups such as the male, the addict, and the geriatric patient receive attention. In addition to general medical management, the authors have dealt with ancillary treatment approaches from a dietary and occupational therapeutic perspective. The internationally acclaimed BASH approach is also reviewed. For the physician-manager, there is a chapter describing the initiation and administration of an eating disorders unit.

This book is intended to be both an introductory clinical text for the treatment of the eating disorders and a reference guide to clinical practice. It is the editors' intention that the reader will extract as much from the chapters as did they.

Acknowledgments

The editors would like to thank all of those individuals who assisted in the production of *The Eating Disorders*. Our senior research assistant, Marian Flaviani and her staff members, Ann Nakoneczie RN and Ann Watkins, helped to coordinate the content of the chapters and to conduct the library search. A special category of gratitude is due to Dr. Louis Zona, director of the Butler Institute of American Art, for permitting us to reproduce the paintings and sketches from the Institute's collection. Also acknowledged is the assistance of Philip José Farmer, master science-fiction writer who taught us something of the craft of writing, and the editorial and production staff at Springer-Verlag. Crisis intervention was given p.r.n. by Amy Dyer, Denise Stavana, and Angela DeCapua.

The understanding of different cultural approaches to food and eating was most useful in framing this book. The editors hereby acknowledge the advice and wisdom given in this area. These were given in generous measure by Dr. Ivan Tulevski of Skopje, Macedonia; Dr. Vassos Pyrghos of Nicosea, Cyprus; Prof. Enrico Tempesta of Rome, Italy; Mr. James Biwott of Nairobi, Kenya; Dr. Mohammed El-Masry of Cairo, Egypt; and Dr. Jorg Beyer of Bonn, Germany. Gratitude is also expressed to editor, Dr. Carmelo Nicolosi, for continuously furnishing us with copies of *Ricerca e Salute*, a most invaluable resource.

Finally, the senior editor wishes to note his personal debts to Drs. Henry Nasrallah, A.L. Carter Pottash, Mark Gold, and Carlton Turner.

Contents

the flesh and fasting repeatedly reported in Christian times to heighten spirituality represented religiocultural self-constraint or illness.[2] The absence of a delusional fear of being fat suggests the former. There is a report, however, in the fifth century[7] of a Christian girl refusing food for 70 days pursuant to a vision of an obscure image while bathing. She confessed that the devil in the form of a bird fed her by night. She was cured when the devil left her after she received Holy Communion. Comparable occasions of refusal of food obstensibly due to possession by the devil or divine intervention were reported in the eighth, ninth, and thirteenth centuries.[7]

Early Arabian physicians were recorded to employ a number of psychological techniques in their practice.[8] In one such instance in the ninth century, behavioral modification was used by Bukhtishu ibn Jibrad, a noble Syrian physician to a number of the Khalifah, the supreme political and religious leaders in the Islamic period of the time.[8] Jibrad successfully treated a teenage Prince who refused food and drink by offering rewards for intake of food and drink. While the exact nature of the disease is lost in history, we do have an example of an eating disorder that responded to behavioral modification techniques.

About the same time in Europe a religious cult emerged that suggested that the clinical features, psychopathology, and treatment of anorexia nervosa were understood by ecclesiastical authorities.[9] Saint Wilgefortis of Uncumber, the seventh daughter of the King of Portugal, after pledging herself to a life of virginity for God, learned that her cruel father intended to marry her off to the Saracen King of Sicily. In order to preserve her body for God she prayed with an intensity that impressed observers. She became ascetic and overcame appetite. She petitioned God's help to lose any beauty she possesed. God granted her wish, giving her bodily hair including a beard. The King of Sicily on hearing of her physical change withdrew his suit. Enraged, her father had her crucified. She died somewhere between 700 and 1000 A.D.[9]

About 200 years after her death her legend had spread throughout Europe. Her name varied at a time of limited communication by country. She was Saint Ont Kommena in the Netherlands, Saint Kummernis in Germany, Saint Liberata in Spain, and Saint Livrade in Gascony. It is possible that Wilgefortis is not one saint but rather several girls with similar clinical histories. She was applauded by the pious of Medieval times as one who preserved herself from sex by self-induced starvation (with obvious attendant endocrine changes). She was a saint who to preserve her virginity lost the shape of a woman and appeared a man. She became the protectress of women with sexual problems. In England where she was called Saint Uncumber she was prayed to, according to contemporary sources, exclusively by women to the derision of men.[9]

Other forms of asceticism described in pre-Renaissance times do not comport to what we today deem anorexia. Men and women heaven-bent on achieving a heightened sense of spirituality sought to detach themselves by a constellation of annedonic practices only one of which was limitation of food intake.[2] Other forms of self-immolation included isolation from others, sleeping on stones, wearing sack cloth, and shaving off their hair—none of which are common to what we refer to as anorexia nervosa. This is not to imply that there were not many cases of anorexia among the ascetics, but rather that all religious self-mortification leading to thinness does not represent an eating disorder. When it does there are as with St. Wilgefortis the associated symptoms.

The life of Saint Catherine of Siena for instance does suggest she suffered the disorder.[10] Data from her *Dialogue* and *Letters* and from a medieval hagiographer, Raymond of Capus (her confessor in her adulthood and a friend of her earlier confesser), provided much detail concerning her life. Catherine, the twenty-third of twenty-five children born to her mother, was the only one of the lot to be breastfed. Her mother stated she loved Catherine more than her siblings and the saint of Siena strove for autonomy from her mother. Her mother wished her from age 12 always to appear attractive to men. Only briefly did she comply, as she wished not to be an object of sexual desire. She was said to suffer more from taking food than a starving man did from being deprived of it. To further this end she induced vomiting daily unto death, despite her confessors' attempts to dissuade her. She had vowed from early childhood to maintain virginity and fought through asceticism certain thoughts or acts that would compromise this posture. She exhibited other anorexia traits: abhorrence of sexual intimacy, hyperkinetic involvement in work, and removal of her hair. She sustained herself at times alone on the Holy Eucharist.[10]

Chlorosis

In 1554, Lange[11] described a disease of young women, most often virgins, but also found in the unmarried and married who were childless. A few other authors of the time maintained the disease could occur in men—"the young and delicate of the male sex." No reference was made in the original description by Lange of a green color of the skin reported by others, nor was this illness referred to as chlorosis, the term by which it eventually became known. A professor at Montpellier in 1615 first described an abnormal color, change of skin to patients who were virgins—from white to green—contending these patients had capricious or depraved appetites[11] associated with decreased food intake and at times nausea and vomiting. Pica (eating indigestable materials such as wax, chalk, and egg shells) was also seen. The relatively constant feature of pica led early observers to conclude that chlorosis was a form of iron deficiency anemia. Death from self-starvation and increased susceptibility to phthisis were also reported.[11]

Clifford Allbutt believed that an actual panic fear of obesity existed and Layrcock described examples of bulimia alternating with anorexia.[11] Lauden Lange's cure for the illness he described was that women so afflicted live with men and copulate, as conception was to bring recovery.[12] Richard Napier,[12] a famous healer and Anglican rector of Great Linford in Buckinghamshire in the early seventeenth century, described a number of women with the green-sickness of ages ranging from 17 to 22, all of whom were unmarried, pale, and amenorrheic. A number of other early descriptions of psychogenic malnutrition were published in the seventeenth century.[13] The German surgeon, Fabricius Hildanus[7] reported a girl, Appolonia Schreyer, from Gals in the Bern district who fasted from age 17 (1601) to 27 (1611) and was amenorrheic throughout her fast. The physician to Cardinal Richelieu, Francois Citesius from Poitiers, described a girl who became anorexic at age 11 in 1599 and had no menarche. She remained so for three years.[7] Other cases were reported by Hildanus and by van der Wiel[7] but the most celebrated were those of Richard Morton, physician to James II, who described anorexia due to nervous causes, so called *phthisis nervosa*, in 1689[7] and distinguished the condition from "chlorosis."

Morton[6,14,15] described cases of nervous consumption were patients presented as skeletons "only clad with skin" and where a woman "fell into a total suppression of her monthly course from a multitude of cares and passions of her mind."[3,14,15,16] The course was distinguished from tuberculosis, a common malady of the time, by absence of fever, cough, and shortness of breath. Morton[14] concluded that the illness ended with swelling of the body, particularly of the lower and dependent parts.

The current observation that the illness is most frequently seen in women of middle class status appears also to have existed in the seventeenth century, as those afflicted were often reported to be particularly interested in books and reading. Morton's magnum opus, *Phthisiologia, seu Exercitationes de Phthisi*, first published in 1689, was translated into English five years later and subtitled "A Treatise of Consumptions;" describing a number of diseases that resulted in wasting of the body tissues[16] in addition to "nervous consumption."[14]

The most celebrated case of the eighteenth century was that of Christina Kratzer from Aeschi near Bern.[7] Blind from childhood, she founded a religious sect. She terminated a three-year fast when accused of cheating with an enema of beef tea. A number of other cases were reported during the century,[7] but it is difficult to ascertain from the descriptions which would truly comport to what we call anorexia nervosa today and what were other disorders in the differential diagnosis (e.g., pituitary disease, major depression, schizophrenia). For instance, a case is described of Marie-Joseph Dahl of Disonguin, France,[7] who in 1773 fell in love with a farmer's son who stated he would give her a son if she reaped a field in three days without assistance of anyone. He deceived her and after she indeed completed her task without fulfillment of the assumed contract, she crouched in a posture for eleven years, at which time she died. Her only nourishment for the decade was watered honey fed to her through a gap in her teeth created by breaking three of her teeth in her locked jaw.[7] This case obviously is more likely schizophrenia or profound depression than it is an uncomplicated eating disorder.

Between 1750 and 1850, the terms chlorosis and amenorrhea were frequently used interchangeably because they so frequently occurred together.[11] It was generally believed that there was an actual obstruction of the menses resulting in reabsorption of the menses, and circulation of crude humors resulting in the symptoms of chlorosis. The appetite disturbance, however, was so constant in chlorosis that Boissier de Savvages in 1763 used it as an index symptom in the classification of chlorosis. Anorexia, partial rather than complete, was reported prior to 1850 and was usually accompanied by pica.[12] Hall in 1830 noted that a chlorotic girl likes those substances in her mouth particularly when anxious or agitated.[12] A commonly held belief at the time was that the illness was due at least in part to the habit of tight corseting, a habit interestingly enough also noted to be espoused by dandified young men of the time who, if any men were afflicted, were the group most likely.[12]

Prior to the nineteenth century, chlorosis was felt on the whole to be a disease of the affluent.[11] The basis for the social class distinction was believed to be due to the perceived value placed on sexual restraint in this group. A full, sensuous body could only lead to the attention of men, which could result in capitulation to carnal desire. To make one's body like that of a man reduced interest and temptation. Fascinatingly, in Victorian times the disease began to be reported in all social classes as the Puritanical mores proclaimed by the privileged became societal norms.[11] In the 1800s it was fairly consistently held that chlorosis had its onset most typically in puberty and adolescence. The disease continued to increase in Victorian times to nearly epidemic proportions and then "mysteriously" disappeared in the 1920s[12] with the advent of markedly changed sexual mores for women.

Early Treatment

Long before the consideration of anemia as a critical factor in the genesis of chlorosis and before it was understood iron was important in blood formation, iron or "steel" was recommended as a treatment of choice.[12] Other remedies included a bland diet, exercise, aspirin, fresh air, electricity, spa waters, and bark.[12] The fact that an eating disorder is usually self-limited led to the perception that many concurrent therapies were beneficial including the exhortation for consummated sex. When death occurred, it was either due to the result of unremitting starvation or due to intercurrent infection.

The implications of an element of sexual frustration in chlorosis as indicated by its early appellations "febris amatoria" and "morbus virgineo" disturbed physicians from the seventeenth century to Victorian times.[12] The awareness that the disorder was rare among men save the very delicate and effeminate[12] because of societal acceptance of open expression of traditional male sexuality and high among women, particularly the well bred, because of the demand for sexual abstinence unto marriage served to direct the critical observer to the inequities of the double standard. In some ways, anorexia nervosa may have been a gender hazard of women, given the demands placed on them by people around them. It should come as no surprise then that the illness nearly disappeared in the "roaring twenties" when sex role stereotypes began to tumble. Why it tended to reemerge in the sixties and seventies at a time when new pressures emerged for early sexual expression should be apparent. Both sexual frustration and demand for performance when one is not yet prepared seem to play a role.

Anorexia in Victorian Times

While numerous references were made to chlorosis or the "virgin's disease" since the sixteenth century, it was not until the middle of the nineteenth century that there was some consensus as to the etiology of the disease. Early reports (prior to 1750) attributed it to unrequited love. During the ensuing century, it appeared to be due to a disorder of menstruation, given its cardinal symptom: amenorrhea. With the advent of hematology as a science in the mid-nineteenth century, hypochromatic anemia was felt to be at its pathogenesis. And then the illness all but—disappeared, or did it?[11] The suggestion that the disorder was due to a blood disorder was particularly attractive to the constrained Victorian physician who was uncomfortable discussing menses and sexual fulfillment with female patients. The relief from such a potentially embarrassing discussion for the women he saw, of course, was equal to or greater than that felt by their consulting physicians. It was a time when masturbation and erotomania were seen as pathogenic in a number of disorders and assumed in excess could be fatal.[11] The problem with hypochromatic anemia as the etiological variable is that it is not limited to one sex and is not associated with pica, extreme changes in appetite, and amenorrhea. Psychological changes obviously would not precede an anemia if the anemia is assumed to be responsible for the mental status.[12]

Certain subtypes of chlorosis may not have compared to what we today call anorexia nervosa, but there was a comparable group in the nineteenth century. These chlorotics were predominently of middle or upper class origin; had insidious onset of the symptoms with depressed affect; disturbance of appetite with anorexia, bulimia, vomiting, and pica; amenorrhea, onset at puberty, and weight change with perhaps binging.[11] These features are most like the illness described independently by Laseque and Gull later in the century which we have come to know as anorexia nervosa. The other subgroups of chlorosis did not include marked disturbance of appetite nor were they preceded by psychiatric symptoms. Often these other types included physical signs suggestive of other medical illnesses, such as melana or hematosis, that could lead to a hypochromatic anemia. Amenorrhea was not a consistent finding and this group was more of working or lower class origin. Loudon[12] has referred to the former group as "chloro-anorexia" and the latter group as "chloro-anemia." It is possible that some of the so-called chloro-anemics were servant girls who did truly develop anorexia in observing their charges do so.

Nineteenth century literature includes a number of other interesting and, in some instances, humorous allusions to what we today see as anorexia nervosa. Louis-Victor Marce in 1859 reported instances of dyspepsia where young girls obstinately refused food. He saw this not of gastrointestinal origin but rather a hypochondriacal delirium. Fin de siecle physicians continued in the assumption that tight corseting may contribute, but there is no evidence that this somewhat barbaric practice did more than induce an occasional hiatus hernia.[12] Janet noted that self-induced vomiting may occur with anorexia as well as with bulimia as an associated symptom.[2] Although as reported here, not all chlorotics were anorexic, the peculiar loss of energy, amenorrhea, and diminished form seen with that subgroup that were probably anorexic nervotics were perhaps iatrogenically induced to some degree by Victorian physicians' preoccupation with sexuality and sex role stereotypes. Mothers were cautioned to be on the alert for the "master vice" (masturbation) and to observe their daughters unobtrusively and minimize time allotted them alone. In addition, in the 1870s an eminent Harvard Professor of Medicine named Dr. E. Owens Clarke cautioned that too much education of women may lead to disturbance of the complicated process of their development as women.[17] It is noteworthy that another subgroup of chlorotics also presented with wasting and shortness of breath which may have been tubercular. Masturbation was also felt to contribute to development of this disease. It is surprising given the Victorians' preoccupation with sex that more women (and "sensitive" men) did not develop this illness more often.

Nearly a decade before Gull's and Laseque's seminal descriptions of anorexia nervosa, Dr. Louis-Victor Marce read a paper at the October 31, 1859 convening of the Societe Medico-Psychologique in Paris entitled "Nate sur une forme de delire hypochondriaque consecutive aux dyspepsies et caracterisee principalement par le refus d'aliments."[18] In it he described the condition so well that both Gull and Laseque acknowledged his contribution. His untimely passing at the age of 36 may have played a role in his recession into oblivion.[18] Other causes of anorexia nervosa were described at this time under a number of appellations: hysterical vomiting, anorexia melancholica, dyspepsia uterina, asthenic insanity, visceral nervosis, and nervous atrophy.[7] Support for the last notion has been provided by Katz and Weiner in 1975 who postulated hypothalamic immaturity as the pathogenesis of the disorder.

Gull and Laseque

Sir William Withey Gull is credited with first using the term anorexia nervosa in 1874 for a disease he first described in 1868 as apepsia hysteria.[11] Gull considered it a "central" rather than "peripheral" condition in which the "want of appetite" was attributed to "a morbid mental state."[11] He commented that women at the age of onset were particularly prone to psychological harm. Gull noted both the hyperactivity and the disparity between the accelerating emaciation and the capacity for physical exercise.[11] Gull ostensibly abandoned the term apepsia hysteria for anorexia nervosa both because of his dislike of the term "hysteria" and to distinguish his report from that of Ernest Charles Laseque, a French neuropsychiatrist who published a similar report in April of 1873 entitled "De l'anorexic hysterique" with eight cases clinically consistent with our current concept of anorexia nervosa.[19]

Gull at the time was renowned in England as an excellent clinician and keen observer. Laseque was more of a philosopher opposed to medical dogmatian who championed empirical observation as the basis of medical investigation. He published only one paper on the subject and never competed with Gull for a place of primacy.[19] The descriptions of both somewhat resembled each other and included reference to the fact that patients so afflicted could not be relied upon to cooperate in treatment. Gull was more alert to the presence of amenorrhea and the dangers of self-starvation; Laseque, to the role of denial. Neither mentioned the dread of fatness nor the preoccupation will body weight.[20] The German word for the illness "Magersucht" reflects the longing of the patient to be thin.[20] The reports of Gull and Laseque stimulated many other reports in the ensuing decades of the nineteenth century[13,15] in the English and French literature and ultimately in the American.

Gull's report, although seminal, in retrospect was more remarkable than perhaps often noted. In frail health due to a paralysis suffered in 1887, Gull was forced to retire. The paper published on March 17, 1888 describing the illness and recovery of a 14 year old girl with anorexia nervosa indicated that the clinical acumen for which he was renowned did not fail him, nor did his etiological considerations. He attributed a major role to psychological factors in his assumption that it was caused by "perversions of the 'ego.'[21] Gull was more popular among patients than colleagues. Those who worked with him deemed him too self-assertive and sarcastic. This paper, however, brought widespread praise. Gull abandoned the popularly held beliefs that the primary psychology was failure of the nerves to the stomach by seeking a more psychological explanation. In addition, his suggested treatment was clear: warmth, rest, separation from family, and frequent introduction of food without regard to the anorexia.[21,23] The further abandonment of the use of the word "hysteria" from "nervosa" allowed that men like women may suffer the malady. Following a brief debate in *The Lancet* involving Hovell, a prominent physician who with Gull was soon to pass into the annals of history, no more articles on the subject appeared in the journal for years.[21]

Gull, Laseque, and other notables of the time clearly delineated a number of corollary symptoms of the disorder. Gull spoke of the restless activity despite the degree of emaciation[22] and of the features of the cachectic state attributable to malnutrition: anemia, hypotension, bradycardia, and constipation.

By 1895 the illness was included in standard textbooks such as the ones by Charcot and by Gilles de Tourette.[23] Charcot[2] included in his writing a description of a case that included discussion of the power struggle between himself and a patient's family where, like contemporary anorexia, the patient reluctantly acknowledged need for help and the family attempted to keep the patient in the family as long as possible. In the 1913 American translation from the French of Dejerine and Gauckler's *Psychoneuroses and Their Treatment by Psychotherapy* the illness was said to have two subtypes: "true" or "primary" anorexia and "secondary" mental anorexia. Primary mental anorexia entailed an actual loss of the "psychic idea of appetite."[23] Prerre Janet, yet another prominent neuropsychiatrist of the period, described in 1903 a subgroup of patients as "obsessionals" who entertained ruminative thoughts centered on food, intense loathing of the body, and appetite control.[24] Both Charcot and Janet mentioned the secret eating of anorexics.

At the turn of the century of concept of chlorosis was on the decline when looking at new cases reported and by the 1930s nearly nonexistent.[17] Dr. Richard C. Cabot, a prominent Boston physician, stated in 1915 that he did not believe that the decrease was merely due to the fact that the cases were being subsumed into another category.[17] History, however, does not support his view, as it appears that as our sophistication in both diagnosis and differential diagnosis improved many illnesses including senility, depression, seizures, and mental subnormality have been found to be due to a wide variety of etiologic agents with multiple contributing factors. Chlorosis probably included what today we know as true or primary anorexia nervosa and a number of illnesses that would present with some

introduce chlorosis

of the symptoms but are predominantly of another nature. Obviously metrorrhagia with menses would have led to those cases where anemia was a prominent finding. Early identification and treatment with iron supplementation would reduce the incidence of this subtype. Other cases may have been infectious in origin such as tuberculosis with wasting, neoplastic disease with cachexia, affective illness with weight loss, schizophrenia with delusions regarding oral intake, and the various endocrinopathies. The change in societal attitudes regarding female sexual actualization without social disapprobation in the 1920s and 1930s would certainly play a role in reduction of the anxiety that may have occurred in pubescent women who wished to have a close relationship with a man prior to marriage without ostracism.

The Biological Era

Simmonds, a pathologist at the University of Hamburg, described in 1914 death from emaciation associated with microscopic evidence of infarction of the pituitary.[3,15] Pituitary cachexia (Simmond's disease) provided a facile biological explanation for many cases of unexplained extreme weight loss and led to many years of uncritically attributing this disease to cases of anorexia even in the absence of other signs of pituitary failure.[15] Many true anorexic nervotics were treated for nearly a generation ineffectively with pituitary extract.[3] The use of the diagnosis of Simmond's cachexia was supported by the widely held adage of the father of modern pathology, Virchow which stated that there were no general diseases, only diseases of cells and organs.[13,23] The Germans, intrigued by the concept of panhypopituitarism proffered by a national authority and by the frequency of the symptoms of cachexia and amenorrhea with anorexia nervosa, were the last to revert their attention to psychological forces.[2]

Although Calder at Johns Hopkins raised questions regarding the potency of pituitary extract in all cases of anorexia nervosa,[23] it was not until Sheehan's work was published in 1949 that this fallacy was laid to rest.[6] Sheehan and his co-workers in Scotland[23] delineated the difference between the relatively rare condition of pituitary insufficiency and the more common anorexia nervosa. A review of the world literature on Simmond's disease published in 1942[23] indicated that only 101 of 595 cases reported to be Simmond's disease were indeed so on pathologic examination.

The abuse of thyroid medication and laxatives for weight control was first reported in 1913 by Nogues.[2,25] Actually, although not specifically marketed as a cathartic, nineteenth century anorectic were reported to drink vinegar, which had for centuries been used as a laxative.[2] Overeating was reported in 1916 by Atraham[24] to be related in women to repression of the libido. The process itself was said to resemble addictive disorders.

Although overeating and vomiting were reported for centuries, bulimic attacks to control weight were not reported until the 1930s.[2]

On April 12, 1932, Moshe Wulff presented a paper before the German Psychoanalytic Society entitled "An Interesting Oral Symptom Complex and Its Relationship to Addiction."[26] In it were described five cases of eating and sleeping mania that he perceived as an obsession between addiction and melancholia.[24] The four women and one man reported shared an eating disorder characterized by apathetic depression, hypersomnolence, compulsive greedy eating, and disparagement of the body image.[2,26] Although somewhat different from contemporary descriptions these patients alternated binge eating with periods of prolonged fasting. They preferred starchy food and sweets when binging and when fasting, milk and fruit. They experienced a strong disgust of their bodies. Wulff's paper is important not only in its description of how bulimia relates to anorexia but also in making us aware that instances of anorexia may have been described centuries prior to bulimia. Bulimia itself is also not of recent vintage.[26] It in reality was less common than anorexia but also underreported. Today reports of the incidence of bulimia are as great at 19 percent although more careful studies indicate clinically significant bulimia in less than 2 percent of college women.[26]

By the 1930s, the clinical features of anorexia were well understood.[13] While the disorder could occur at all ages, the majority were clustered in late teens or early twenties. The disease was rare among males. Weight loss was due to restriction of caloric intake. Food tastes were eccentric (e.g., dry toast and evaporated milk). Some lost their appetites. Others would binge with food like a substance abuser may with alcohol only to feel remorseful later, which would lead to semistarvation. Laxatives and cathartic use was frequent. Those so affected hid their food and disposed of it surreptitiously.[13] The excessive concern over thinness did not appear common until 1960.[25] Bliss and Brunch[23] suggested that a 25 pound weight loss due to psychological causes be the sole criterion for the condition.[23]

Widespread interest in the disease did not reemerge until the 1930s when John Berkman, brother-in-law and student of Henry Plummer at the Mayo Clinic, published a report of 117 cases in which the physiologic disorder was deemed a manifestation of a psychic disturbance.[3,23] Berkman felt that these patients suffered a reversible insufficiency of anterior pituitary gland secretion as a feature of their starvation. Other reports emerged from Canada, England, and elsewhere in the United States[3] on the diagnoses, classification, and treatment of the disease. Subsequent to these reports and an understanding of the evolving clinical presentation, the reported incidence of the disease increased remarkably. A fivefold increase was reported in Malmo, Sweden, between the 1930s and 1950s; incidence doubled in Monroe County, New York, between 1960 and 1976, and incidence rose from 1.6 to 4.1 per 100,000 in Scotland from

1966/69 to 1978/82.[20] In addition to increased diagnostic acumen, the increase in social pressure in women during the past several decades has probably played a role in increasing prevalence.

The Psychoanalytic Era

From the earliest descriptions of illness that retrospectively appear to comport with current clinical features of anorexia, the syndrome was seen as a defense against sexuality[22] including, according to Waller, a defense against unconscious fantasies of oral insemination.[3] Anorexics were conceptualized as young girls refusing to grow up and develop into sexually mature women. Even after recovery many such patients were noted to continue to exhibit problems fulfilling themselves sexually. The earlier psychoanalytic explorations focused on Sigmund Freud's impression that nutritional deprivation is related to an individual's failure to master sexual excitation.[22] The conflict with food was deemed symbolic of a deeper sexual struggle. Nemiah in 1950 posited anorexia and excessive dependency to be an outgrowth of an overprotective mother.[22] Helene Deutsch (1981), another prominent analyst in the middle of this century, wrote in a paper delivered to the Boston Psychoanalytic Society in the 1940s of a patient with a central conflict over a compulsion to starve and another to overeat. In her description of the case Deutsch sympathetically described the patient in the context of her family history without overemphasis of infantile variables. Deutsch, although a traditional analyst, included periodic weighings in a contract to manage the patient. Deutch would not mention eating if the patient complied. It was Hilda Bruch in 1961 who was first to consider the essential psychodynamic disturbance in the disorder to be a disturbance in body image and of recognition of bodily states and a sense of ineffectiveness. Bruch, the psychoanalyst whose name is most frequently associated with anorexia nervosa, also introduced the need for differential diagnosis. She distinguished the disorder not only from organic conditions but also from similar manifestations of schizophrenia and neurotic disorders.[22] Perhaps Bruch's greatest contribution was elaboration of the fact that in anorexia there is not a true loss of appetite but rather a preoccupation with food and eating.[22] It is the "relentless pursuit of thinness that appears to be the driving motive."[22] She deemed a need to establish a sense of identity and control the most fundamental characteristic of primary or true anorexia nervosa. In cases of other illnesses such as depression or schizoaffective disorder there is a true loss of appetite which may be misconstrued as anorexia and diagnosed atypical anorexia nervosa.

Bruch, in a series of contributions commencing in 1961, described a number of cases[15] in which there was a pervasive sense of ineffectiveness, a disturbance of body image, and a failure to recognize nutritional needs.

Pilazzoli in 1963 subsequently added the patients' attempts to gain independence and Crisp in 1967 added a weight phobia coupled with a fear of normal pubertal development.[15] Russell in 1969 posited that the cause was hypothalamic dysfunction disturbing mechanisms of regulation control of food intake.[15]

Bruch felt that many of the postmedieval women who became famous for starving themselves were suffering a gross hysterical paralysis in which food had great symbolic value. She saw the hyperactivity of true anorexics as an attempt to deny as long as possible the state of emaciation.[2] The patients she studied appeared locked in a desperate fight against feeling exploited and enslaved, unable to lead a life of their own. In their search for an identity and development of selfhood of their own they refused anything their parents offered. Rather than accommodate they would starve.[20,23,27]

The misperceptions of body width and weight were confirmed by several studies[20] subsequent to Bruch's initial dynamic formations.

Anorexia Today

Research in the past two decades has explored biological, epidemiologic, genetic, and psychological variables that help delineate anorexia nervosa as a specific disease in order to objectively evaluate the cost-efficient-effectiveness of various therapeutic interventions. While the fact that the relatively rare illness has a fairly predictable age of onset (adolescence and young adulthood), impacts a particular subpopulation (middle and upper-middle class women), and course (hyperactivity, fear of overweight, sexual and identity conflicts, struggles with autonomy and individualization), it does not consistently respond to one therapeutic intervention. Some champion behavioral interventions; others, psychopharmacotherapy; and most, a combination of both. It is possible that the phenomenology may represent the clinical manifestations of a number of different illnesses. The clinical picture may simply be the manner in which a number of illnesses are set off by a stress (perhaps that of burgeoning sexuality and an ambivalent desire for autonomy and individualization) in certain personality types.

There is some evidence of anorexia nervosa occurring in more than one member of the family and presence of unusual attitudes toward food in several family members.[3,28] It is, however, difficult to separate nature and nurture unless there were a sufficient number of adopted away cases to ascertain how in absence of parental and other familial models the illness emerged. Genetic evidence would help to confirm Hilda Bruch's impression that this drive for thinness is an independent disorder and not a unique cultural manifestation of many illnesses.

Epidemiologists in recent years[15,29] have characterized the period of greatest risk from late adolescence to the early 30s with those up to 28 at greatest risk. The disease is most common in females particularly, those of middle and upper class origin and particularly actresses, models, ballet dancers, jockeys, and flight attendants. Current incidence is given as 0.37 per 100,000.[15] Prevalence is about 1 percent of middle class adolescent girls. About 30 years ago as many as 15 percent of the patients died while today the figure is only one in thirty with full recovery in over half in six years.[29] Death occurs from not only malnutrition but suicide.

The relationship between affective illness, substance abuse, anorexia nervosa, and bulimia nervosa has been another avenue of recent interest.[30] Comparison of young females with affective illness and anorexia[30] indicates little difference in birth order or social class but significant differences in marital status, educational attainment, and age of onset, suggesting the two disorders are distinct.[30] Other areas of recent concern are family dynamics and family therapy,[31] personality factors,[32] and the role of culture in determining how the illness may manifest itself.[3,27,33,34,35] The latter emphasizes the pressure on young middle class women today not to repress sexuality as in early times but to be thin[3], and with the growing liberation of women to do something that makes them outstanding.[27] These standards are reflected in art, in advertising, and in the media.[33,35] Men contribute to the problem by placing as a critical variable in their choice of a sexual partner greater emphasis on physical attractiveness than do women on men. Social opportunities for women are limited to the relative conformance to arbitrary cultural parameters of pulchritude.[35] In this century alone the standard has ranged from the fragility of the fin de siecle Gibson girl to the bosom mania of the 1950s to the quest for thinness today.

Summary

A review of the history of anorexia nervosa has much to teach us in how medicine has over the centuries struggled to understand what an aberration in human behavior means, what may explain the deviation, what is illness and what is not, and how an understanding of etiology is necessary for diagnostic-specific therapy. It is humbling to know that even the most prominent physicians of their day fell prone to errors wedded to their cultural and temporal context and how quickly their conclusions were accepted by others as dogma. Review of the history of anorexia also makes us acutely aware of the role of culture in creating stresses that give genesis to disease as well as to the manifestation of illness in adolescents and young adults who are particularly prone to the impact of external forces on their evolving identities.

References

1. Laxenaire M, Marchand P. Has anorexia nervosa changed? *Med Psychol* (Paris) 1982; 448–453.
2. Habermas T. The psychiatric history of anorexia nervosa and bulimia nervosa: weight concerns and bulimic symptoms in early case reports. *Int J Eating Disord* 1989; 8:259–273.
3. Lucas AR. Anorexia nervosa; historical background and biopsychosocial determinants. *Seminars in Adolescent Medicine* 1986; 2:1–9.
4. Fichter MM. Franz Kafkas Magersucht. *Fortsch Neurol Psychiat* 1988; 56: 231–238.
5. Dally P. The illnesses of Elizabeth Barrett Browning. *Br Med J* 1989; 298:963.
6. Parry-Jones WL. Archival exploration of anorexia nervosa. *J Psychiat Res* 1985; 19:95–100.
7. Skrabanek P. Notes towards the history of anorexia nervosa. *Janus* 1983; 70:109–128.
9. Lacey JH. Anorexia nervosa and a bearded female saint. *Br Med J* 1982; 285:1816–1817.
10. Rampling D. Ascetic ideals and anorexia nervosa. *J Psychiat Res* 1985; 19:89–94.
11. Laudon I. Chlorosis, anaemia, and anorexia nervosa. *Br Med J* 1980; 281: 20–27.
12. Laudon I. The diseases called chlorosis. *Psychological Medicine* 1984; 14: 27–36.
13. Bliss EL. History of anorexia nervosa. In Gross M (ed): Anorexia Nervosa: A Comprehensive Approach. Lexington, DC, Collamore Press, 1982.
14. Morton R. Of a nervous consumption. In Anderson AE (ed): Practical Comprehensive Treatment of Anorexia Nervosa and Bulimia. Baltimore, MD, Johns Hopkins Univ, 1985.
15. Waltos DL. Historical perspectives and diagnostic considerations. In The Evaluation and Treatment of Eating Disorders. New York, Hayworth Press, 1986.
16. Silverman JA. Richard Morton, 1637–1698: Limner of anorexia nervosa: His life and times. *J Psychiat Res* 1985; 19:83–88.
17. Brumberg JJ. Chlorotic girls, 1870–1920: A historical perspective on female adolescence. *Child Development* 1982; 53:1468–1477.
18. Silverman JA. Louis-Victor Marie 1828–1864: Anorexia nervosa's forgotten man. *Psychological Medicine* 1989; 19:833–835.
19. Vandereycken W, van Deth R. Who was the first to describe anorexia nervosa: Gull or Laseque? *Psychological Medicine* 1989; 19:837–845.
20. Russell GFM. The changing nature of anorexia nervosa: An introduction to the conference. *J Psychiat Res* 1985; 19:101–109.
21. Silverman JA. Anorexia nervosa in 1888. *Lancet* April 23, 1988; 928–930.
22. Bruch H. Anorexia nervosa. In Arieto S (ed): American Handbook of Psychiatry, Vol 4 (second edition). New York, Basic Books, 1975.
23. Giannini, AJ: Drug abuse and depression: Possible models for geriatric anorexia. *Neurobiology of Aging*. 9(1):26, 1988.
24. Blinder BJ, Cadenhead K. Bulimia: A historical overview. *Adolesc Psych* 1986; 13:231–241.

25. Casper RC. On the emergence of bulimia nervosa as a syndrome. *Int J Eating Disord* 1983; 2:3–16.
26. Stunkard A. A description of eating disorders in 1932. *Am J Psychiatry* 1990; 147:263–268.
27. Bruch H. The Golden Cage: The Enigma of Anorexia Nervosa. Cambridge, Massachusetts, Harvard University Press, 1978.
28. Kassett JA, Gerbon ES, Maxwell ME, et al. Psychiatric disorders in the first-degree relatives of probands with bulimia nervosa. *Am J Psychiatry* 1989; 146:147–148.
29. Patton G. The course of anorexia nervosa: About one in 30 die, and half recover fully after six years. *Br Med J* 1989; 299:139–140.
30. Eagles JM, Wilson AM, Hunter D, et al. A comparison of anorexia nervosa and affective psychosis in young females. *Psychological Medicine* 1990; 20: 119–123.
31. Neal JH, Herzog D. Family dynamics and treatment of anorexia nervosa and bulimia. *Pediatrician* 1983–1985; 12:139–147.
32. Strober M. Personality factors in anorexia nervosa. *Pediatrician* 1985; 12: 134–138.
33. Appels A. Culture and disease. *Soc Sci & Med* 1986; 23:477–483.
34. Bemporad JR, Ratey JJ, O'Driscoll G, et al. Hysteria, anorexia and the culture of self-denial. *Psychiatry* 1988; 51:96–103.
35. Mazur A. US trends in feminine beauty and overadaptation. *J Sex Research* 1986; 22:281–303.

Bibliography

Brumberg JJ. Fasting girls: Reflection on writing the history of anorexia nervosa. *Monogr Soc Res Child Dev* 1985; 50:93–104.

Gull WW. Anorexia nervosa (Anorexia hysterica). In Anderson AE (ed): Practical Comprehensive Treatment of Anorexia Nervosa and Bulimia. Baltimore, Johns Hopkins University Press, 1985.

Hajal F. Psychological treatment of anorexia: A case from the ninth century. *J History Med Allied Sci* 1982; 37:325–328.

Lucas AR. Toward the understanding of anorexia nervosa as a disease entity. *Mayo Clin Pro* 1984; 56:254–264.

Roazen P. Introduction to Helene Deutsch's paper on anorexia nervosa. *Bulletin of the Menninger Clinic*. 1981; 45:499–501.

2
A History of Bulimia

A. JAMES GIANNINI

The first written description of bulimia in Western culture was recorded in Xenophon's *Anabasis*.[1] This account, written about 970 B.C., recorded bulimia among Greek soldiers retreating to the mountains of Asia Minor. It is not clear however if purging was associated with the engorgement. Self-purging was evidently noted by later Greek authors in both social and religious circumstances. The cult of Addis and Cybele notably included anorexia, bulimia, and self-castration.[2] In this cult, an upwardly mobile man, loved by the goddess Cybele, offers the only gift he has, his body.

The upper and middle classes of the Roman Empire institutionalized bulimia in their social rituals, as well as their domestic archiecture. As the boundaries of the Empire expanded, the wealth of Rome also expanded. As a form of conspicuous consumption, wealthy citizens would give great banquets. During these all-day affairs, guests would consume twenty or more courses. To handle this alimentary load, the men and women would be escorted between courses to a small room adjacent to the dining area. Equipped with fountains, scented water, and flowers, this then-novel addition to the Roman home provided a pleasant environment for the guests to purge themselves of previous courses. Once their stomachs had been sufficiently emptied, slaves would clean their faces and clothing so that they could return and gorge themselves anew. This "vomitarium," which was graphically described in Petronius's *Satyricon*, became an integral part of Neronian life.[3]

During the late Middle Ages forced emesis again emerged though its role again changed. It was used by religious penitents to ritualistically purge themselves of their sins. It would also be used to sharpen one's wit and reduce sexual desire especially by scholar monks. Professors at the great medieval medical schools—Naples, Salerno, Bologna, Paris, Montpelier, and Oxford all prescribed powerful emetics, sometimes on a chronic basis. On occasion the patient learned to abuse the emetics he received from his physician, his pharmacist, and his barber.[4]

The twelfth century troubadour poet Marcabru of Gascon wrote many chansons describing gluttons and drunkards who used forced emesis to continue their revels.[5] His contemporary, the nobleman, warrior, and poet Bertran de Born also scathingly described bulimic ladies of court who would purge themselves to maintain a youthful silhouette.[6] Ironically, the poet Dante Alighieri placed gluttons in Hell, submerged in vomit and feces. They were thus doomed to spend eternity while the digested products of their gluttony rained down upon them. This punishment which he visited upon them expressed the shared communal disgust with the practice of forced engorgement.[7]

During the Renaissance, the medical practice of prescribing emetics continued to spawn the more than occasional chronic bulimic. The earlier causes of bulimia as described by Marcabru and de Born were repeated in the poetry of Villon and the prose of Boccaccio.[8,9] Mustard and "nux vomica" (a nut containing strychnine and brucine) were often employed.

The word "bulimia" was first used by Trevisa in 1398.[10] Its initial meaning included only immoderate appetite. Specifically not mentioned was emesis or other means of purgation. The Tudor court of King Henry VIII, aping its master, was known for compulsive overeating. As a trencherman, Henry knew not moderation. Eating at banquets became affairs of engorgement. Though there seemed to be some not uncommon incidents of emesis, these were most likely due to the effects of ale and malmsey rather than of intent.[11] As Henry's eating practices began to be copied further down the social ladder, English fashion and physique reflected an everexpanding girth. Power also begat immoderation farther South in Italy. When Allessandro Borgia left his native Spain for employment as a Vatican secretary, he was, for his time, a man of relative moderation. Later, as Pope Alexander, his efforts to reprise Imperial Roman glory also apparently included gluttony. His infamous dinner the "Ballet of the Oranges" faithfully reproduced the Neronian banquet. It combined the elements of gluttony, sensuality, and emesis sans vomitarium.[12] Engorgement, while never common, became accepted by all strata and clines of European society. The great astronomer, Tycho Brahe, was contemporaneously known for his bulimic banquets as well as his scientific observation. The Flemish peasants painted by the Bruegels depict the social institutionalization of engorgement at the lower levels of society.[13] A darker side of this practice was demonstrated in the paintings of Hieronymous Bosch. A lack of resistance and fortitude was seen in the depicted peasants who lived a life without an inner faith to guide them.[14]

While a large dietary intake persisted over the centuries, at least among the upper and middle classes, the incidence of enforced engorgement seems to have been reduced. This was probably due to the effects of abstemious Protestantism, the Catholic Counter-Reformation and the reemergence of a powerful warrior class. As the middle class expanded in size and influence, leisure time also expanded. Due to the great explorations of the time, as well as technological and social ferment, new diversions were developed. The dining board thus had to compete with a variety of attractions. There were notable exceptions, however. The great eighteenth century dictionarist, Samuel Johnson was noted by his biographer, James Boswell, to be "bulimous." His bulimia included engorgement to the point that"... his looks seemed rivetted to the plate... nor would he... say one word... till he had satisfied his appetite which was so fierce... that while in the act of eating, the veins of his forehead swelled and generally a strong perspiration was visible.[15]

It was during Johnson's lifetime in 1743, that James wrote the first clinical description of "boulimos" and "caninus appetitus."[16] Both involved short hyperphagic periods that were followed by syncopal episodes in the former condition and induced emesis in the latter. Forty-two years later Motherby expanded this definition to include bulimia associated with hunger.[17] Blachez, in 1869, then systemized the concept of bulimia.[18]

Associated with the medicalization of bulimic engorgement was a decreased tolerance for the practice. Apparently, the French King Louis Phillippe was so sensitive to Daumier's cartoons of his gluttony that he had the satirist imprisoned.

In the twentieth century, an extremely voracious appetite was associated with the person and persona of King Edward in England and President William Howard Taft in the United States. The silhouette of the American President had expanded considerably in girth from the lanky frame of Lincoln through the potbelly of McKinley and his Golden Age contemporaries to the substantial girth of Taft. The definition of bulimia had, however, been altered and expanded to encompass emesis as well as engorgement. In 1903, Janet published his classic work on neurosis and included bulimia.[19] By 1928, Binswager published the first detailed case history of a bulimic—Ellen West.[20] Since then, bulimia has been recognized as a clinical entity occurring at all socioeconomic levels. Though as many as 20 percent of all private-university women are thought to be bulimic, both sexes are at risk.

References

1. Xenophon. Memorabilia and Works. London, MacMillan, 1914.
2. Petronius Arbiter G. Satyricon. New York, Gilette, 1953.
3. Harrison JE. Prolegemia to the Study of Greek Religion. Cambridge, Cambridge Press, 1922.
4. LaCroix P. Manners, Customs and Dress During the Middle Ages. New York, Oxford Press, 1876.
5. Roncaglia L. Venticinque poesie dei primi trovatori. Modena, Cantoni SPR, 1949.
6. Hill RT, Bergin TG. Anthology of the Provencal Troubadours. New Haven, Yale, 1944.

7. Alighieri D. Commedia: Inferno: Canto VI. (Tr. Carlyle-Okey-Wicksteed). New York, Modern Library, 1932.
8. Villon F. The Legacy, The Testament and Other Poems. (Tr. P. Dale). New York, St. Martins, 1973.
9. Boccaccio G. Decameron (Tr. R. Addington). New York, Doubleday, 1930.
10. Oxford English Dictionary. Oxford, Oxford University Press, 1983.
11. Baker JA (ed). The Reports of Sir John Spelman. London, Selden Society, 1977.
12. Burchard J. Diarum 1478. Paris, Thuame, 1886.
13. Janson JW. History of Art. New York, Abrams, 1986.
14. Detolney C. Heironymous Bosch. Baden-Baden, Germany, Holle Verlag, 1965.
15. Boswell J. The Life of Johnson. New York, Penguin, 1970.
16. James R. A Medical Dictionary. London, Osborne, 1743.
17. Motherby G. New Medical Dictionary or a General Repository of Physic. London, Johnson & Robinson, 1785.
18. Blachex PF. Boulimie. In Dechandre A (ed): Dictionaire Encyclopedie des Sciences Medicales. Paris, Victor, 1864.
19. Janet P. Les Obsessions et la Psychasthenie. Paris, Alcan, 1903.
20. Binswanger R. The Case of Ellen West. May R, Angela E, Ellenberger HF (eds). New York, Baser Books, 1957.

3
The History of Obesity

Deirdre K. Kocjan and A. James Giannini

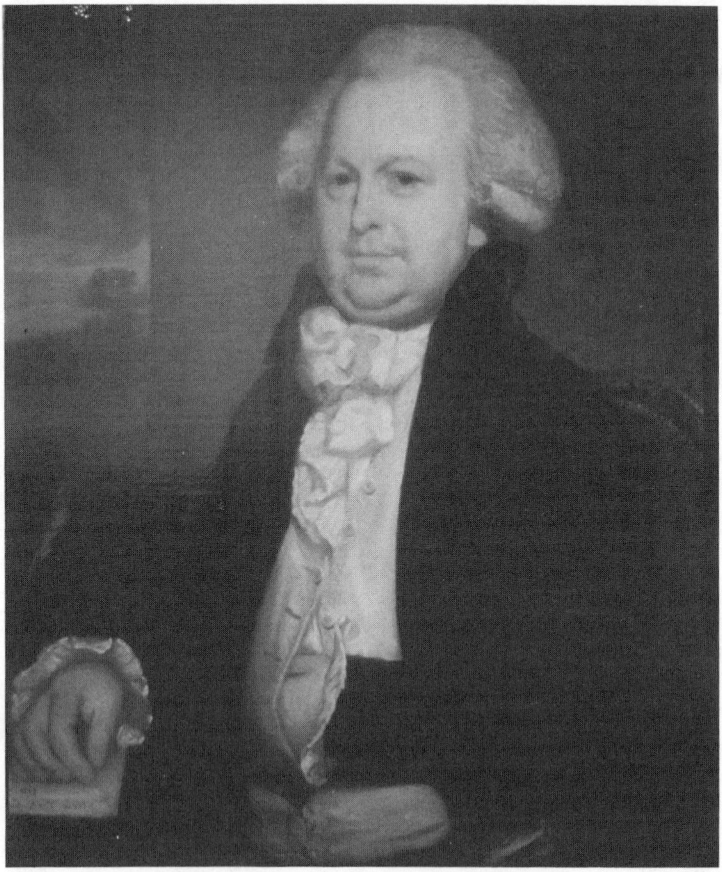

Brown, Mather—*Mr. Miles of New York*—(Private collection of A. James Giannini)

Obesity has been a component of Western culture since prehistory. Paleolithic statuary such as the Laussel "Venus" revealed steoptygian attributes, large pendulous breasts, great overflowing bellies, and massive thighs.[1] In ancient times, the rotund female body was considered healthy, fertile, and prosperous in affairs of the heart. The "fattening room" in Nigeria has been used for two millenia to create a fat and culturally defined "beautiful" girl. This room was located in the father's compound. Here his prepubescent daughters were kept for a period that ranged from three months to seven years, depending on the father's wealth. The sole purpose of this place was the creation of plump women. It was thought that a surplus of flesh would ensure greater chances of fertility and a healthy baby. This custom is still maintained in those parts of Nigeria where food is scarce and obesity is viewed as a status symbol.[2] Notably the foods consumed by this culture are expensive and consist of primarily lean meats and whatever small amounts of vegetables the family is able to grow. Historically, obesity in women has not been considered undesirable but rather beauteous especially in cultures where there is a shortage of food.

The Golden Age in Greece personified the goal of perfection in many forms. The Greek mathematician Polycleitus hypothesized "perfect human dimensions" using mathematics. His ratio idealized women who were short and stocky. The Polycleitian canon called for a round head, broad shoulders, stocky torso, wide hips, and short legs. This produced a figure of strength rather than of grace. It was conceptualized that the dimensions of any one part of a perfect body should bear a given ratio to dimensions of another part[3] (e.g., the length of the index finger compared to the length of the leg). In Polycleitus's "Doryphorus," the body is viewed through the use of an imposed system of proportions. This powerful body with its broad shoulders, thick torso, and muscular limbs strikes us as the embodiment of the Spartan ideal of the warrior physique.[4]

The alternative representation of sensuous beauty and grace was perfected by the classical Greek sculptor, Praxiteles. His prototypical "Aphrodite of Cnidus" depicted a women with short legs and a protruding abdomen. While she would not be considered "well proportioned" by today's standards, she was widely regarded in antiquity as the most beautiful of all statues and the pride of Cnidus, the city that housed it. A descendant of the Proxitelean ideal was the "Aphrodite of Melos" (i.e., the Venus deMilo). She was the final personification of the Greek ideal of beauty; rounded hips, smooth stomach, and firm breasts.[4]

The Roman Emperor Augustus believed that too many Roman citizens were devoting their lives exclusively to the unbridled and degrading pursuit of wealth and luxury. A lavish dinner party in an aristocratic Roman household would consist of such delicacies as leek-a-mint hors d'oeuvres, followed by olives, snails, crabs, and oysters. Then came perhaps a Trojan pig (stuffed with black pudding, almonds, or sausage) young kid, peacock, whole boar, roast goose, lamprey, sows' udders, fattened pheasants, or the day's catch of home grown pike from the Tiber River.[5] After the guests had stuffed themselves with such rich dishes, they might recline on the sofas or engage in a drinking contest. Lastly, they might intentionally vomit in order to drink or eat anew.[6]

The evolving Greek ideal was then accepted throughout the Hellenistic period and Roman Republic. Modifications did not occur until the Roman Imperium. Emperor Claudius (born 10 B.C.) developed a reputation in his youth as an irrepressible glutton and incorrigible womanizer. He loved to eat: the smell of roast beef could send him into a frenzy and he seldom left a dining hall except when gorged and sodden. Typical of upper class Roman dietary behavior, he would fall asleep on his back so that servants could push a feather down his throat. This would induce emesis allowing him to engorge himself once again. Another option would be to retire to the 'vomitorium' where one could purge the ingested food and later indulge with more dining.

"Men eat to vomit, and vomit to eat," complained the Stoic philosopher, Seneca, who disparaged such excesses partly because he suffered from chronic gastric distress and could not partake of them himself. "Their dishes are fetched from every corner of the earth and then they do not even deign to digest them." Emperor Augustus was appalled by this hedonistic behavior. He pushed a program of patriotic and pro-family legislation through the Senate and exercised his personal influence to pressure the patrician class into compliance.[5]

Whereas the Greeks projected more idealistic impressions of beauty, the Romans illuminated a realistic view. The "Girl Athlete" (detail of a pavement) of about 400 A.D. displays a modern looking maiden. Her torso is elongated and taunt with muscular arms and heavy thighs. She appears, however, to fit the general ancient proportion of 8 heads high, instead of our modern 9 heads high.[7]

Later, during the Medieval period, the most popular feminine ideal in art was the "Madonna." In Giovanni Pisano's "Madonna," we view a woman of grace and middling stature. She is not bound to the convention of pronounced hips and large breasts but appears lithe and graceful.[7] A new mental climate originated in fourteenth-century Florence, Italy. The new "humanist period" began here and later spread throughout Europe. Artists and poets were promoted during this time and were seen as important men of ideas not just craftsmen. This was a very modern view of art and artists and was easily adopted in its Florentine milieu.[8]

One of the favored painters of the Renaissance period was Sandro Botticelli. His famous "Birth of Venus" was completed in about 1480 and represents the climax of a peculiar style of line and movement. His figure of Venus does not appear earthlike or human, but more as an intangible spirit or angel. Her form is elegant and slim with an aura of delicacy and paleness, not strength. "Venus" is unlike the earlier Greco-Roman ideal body: it appears mor elongated and graceful rather than short and stocky.[7]

In counterpoint, Leonardo DaVinci projected a synthesis of Classical and Botticellian women. The forms seen in "Virgin and Child" and "Virgin of the Rocks" are majestic, robust, and monumental but still possess grace. Another Renaissance artist, Michelangelo Buonarroti further developed the Renaissance ideal. His scupture of "David" is his earliest statement of the heroic male physique of this period. "David" appears muscular, taut, and agile without bulging abdomen or heavy thighs. He is slim and graceful but with power rather than unearthliness.

In the sixteenth-century court of Henry VIII, there were many idiosyncratic examples of the differences in beauty and size. Henry VIII was indeed renown for his "roaming eye" and prowess with women. Although he did have affairs with ladies of the court who were conventional beauties, his choices of wives were not considered beautiful by his English subjects or foreign diplomats.[9]

Depicted in a portrait by an unknown artist, Anne Boleyn, Henry's second wife, was described by a contemporary as "not one of the handsomest women in the world, she is of middling stature, swarthy complexion, long neck, wide mouth, bosom not much raised and dark beautiful eyes." Although Anne's 'middling stature' and 'unraised bosom' are addressed, it is not mentioned that Henry himself, who was once quite athletic, was quite obese.[10] This was because of a new dichotomy in attractiveness. Men were judged by their sexual prowess, intelligence, and power; women were discussed according to their physical attributes, a view that persisted in some degree to the writing of this chapter. Incidentally, all of Henry VIII's wives were considered to be rather plump and plain except Anne Boleyn, and his fifth wife, Catherine Howard, who was also Anne's cousin. Howard was painted by the English artist, Holbein, and was said to be beautiful and graceful. Graceful was a word used to describe only Anne and Catherine, not the other four wives who were even by their contemporaries considered plump.[11]

Tiziano Vecellio (Titian), a Venetian artist, further refined and depicted the evolving ideal of feminine beauty. In his "Sacred and Profane Love" and "Venus and Adonis" his focus was on women of moderate girth but large breast. While not thin by today's standards, his models are considerably more slender than the Greco-Roman ideal.[4]

Although the term "Baroque" originally meant contorted or grotesque and was thought to be an insulting term, we use the word today to capsulize the seventeenth century as a whole. Gianlorenzo Bernini was the greatest sculptor of that century. His "David" can be compared with Michelangelo's. Although both drew spirit from the ancient styles, they reflected differing contemporary views of the ideal male form. Bernini's "David" is more energized and less classically statured. His forearms and legs are very muscular with an unviewed face bringing about his body's deployed motion.

A term used today to identify a shapely, robust women is "Rubenesque."[4] Peter Paul Rubens developed this mode in paintings such as "Marie de' Medici, Queen of France." His romantic art depicted women who were more rotund, with the stomachs and exposed thighs that would be considered as "fat" by today's standards. In his "The Garden of Love," the artist himself appears with his young second wife. In this tribute to the joy of love, he again uses figures that are short in stature and wide of girth. The bosoms are mildly large and the flesh overflowing rather than taut. Today soft, fleshy, and plump women are still referred to as Rubenesque.[4]

Later, an emotional reaction against the established order began in all respects, including people's views of their own body. In this period labeled the Romantic Movement, the wild and the strange, nature and freedom were idolized by artists who felt synchronized with them. Benjamin West of Pennsylvania specialized in depicting pictures of brave, noble characters as in his "Death of General Wolfe at Quebec." The prominent figure of an unidentified Indian brave is a lesson in physical perfection for males of the time. Robust, lean, and very muscular limbs assist in projecting the strength of the character. His body frame lends itself to the marvel of the human body in perfectly balanced dimensions.[4]

Later in the Romantic period, Eugene Delacroix helped redefine the female figure. In Delacroix's "Greece Expiring on the Ruins of Misslonghi," as well as Jean-Auguste Dominique Ingres' "Odalisque," a new view of women is seen. The models have elongated proportions, small rounded breasts, small waist, and more apparent firmness to the overall body. This change in the "waistline of women" coincides with the period in history when radicalism and freedom were becoming pronounced to women. Women were gaining freedom and losing weight. With more political liberties and domestic issues such as birth control arising, women were not content to be seen as passive vessels.[7]

Toward the later half of the nineteenth century, this trend continued as depicted in Guillaume-Adolphe Bouguereau's "The Birth of Venus" and Thomas Conture's "Romans of the Decadence." Women are portrayed as more lifelike; darker-haired females are more present in the arts; and the ideal human form is now thinner and more agile. The skin remains alabaster but the torsos are not weighted by mounds of flesh or huge tree trunklike thighs.[4]

Toward the last years of the nineteenth century a more systematic examination of the properties of three-dimensional space, expressive qualities of line, pattern, and color, and of the symbolic character of subject matter was undertaken by the great Postimpressionist artists. In Edgar Degas' "Cafe Concert at Les Ambassadeurs" and George Seurat's "A Sunday Afternoon on the Grande Jatte," the women are portrayed with tiny waistlines and "bubble" type buttocks. By this time, fashion was restricting the woman's waistline and projecting a higher, less flat derriere. It should be noted that especially in Seurat's "Sunday Afternoon" the women do appear taller and less squat than previously portrayed.[4]

Moving into the early 1900s suffragist striving to end male dominance was beginning to materialize. In 1911 there were about 1,000,000 women in private domestic service. During World War I, 400,000 of these women left to do other work. Between 1914 and 1918 a total of 792,000 women entered industry.[12] As seen through the eyes of Pablo Picasso and Henri Matisse, the female torso was being transformed into the more elongated and graceful form that is more common today.

During postwar time, with such phenomena as "the flapper," a unique trend developed: women were "permitted" to be shaped in a way that was not totally unobtainable. Flappers were thin but not anorectic looking, with medium-sized legs, flat chests, and small buttocks. Again, a thin silhouette was associated with an expansion of female liberties.

Through the 1900s, art has continued to depict and influence the "shaping of women" with the communications media unconsciously conveying a rapidly evolving concept of beauty to women. Nowhere in history do we see such profound changes in women's ideal body move so quickly as now. The 1950s and early 1960s returned to the ideal voluptuous prototype of women's body forms but without the mounded flesh on the abdomen. Hips, breast, and buttocks were larger but waistlines were delicate. This coincided with the return of the relatively independent "Rosie the Riveter" to a passive female role. Through the volatile 1960s and 1970s, a thinner woman emerged with a more elongated body. Thinness had again regained its power, replaced with longer legs and smaller hips.[4]

In the 1980s and early 1990s, thinness has again become a symbol of success for high-achieving young women. Even classically beautiful women may see themselves as fatter than they really are and push to be "stringbean" thin.[11] Thinness has thus come to symbolize independence as well as attractiveness.

Primarily the media focused on beautiful women as thin but unusually tall. The early 1990s appear to show slightly bigger breasted women, and "more ample bosoms" with larger shoulders have become the rage. The focus has been on a lithe, powerful frame reflecting the increased status of women.[13]

References

1. Huyghe R. L'art et l'homme. Auge, Gillon et cie. Paris, France, 1957.
2. Brink PJ (exec ed). The fattening room in Nigeria. *Western Journal of Nursing Research* 1989; Vol. 11.

3. Durant W. The Life of Greece. New York, Simon and Schuster, 1939.
4. Delacroix H, Tansey RG, Garner H. Art Through the Ages (fifth edition). New York Chicago San Francisco Atlanta, Harcourt, Brace and World Inc, 1970.
5. Taylor R. Party Politics in the Age of Caesar. Los Angeles, University of California Press, 1949.
6. Lewis N, Meyer R. The Republic—Roman Civilization, Source Book I. New York, Harper Torch Books, 1951.
7. Janson HW, Caumon S. History of Art. New York, Harry N. Abrams Inc, 1971.
8. Durant W. The Reformation—The Story of Civilization VI. New York, Simon and Schuster, 1957.
9. Erikson C. Mistress Ann—The Exceptional Life of Ann Boleyn. New York, Summit Books, Simon & Schuster, 1984.
10. Coister S, Gibson R, Rogers M, Simon J. The National Portrait Galley. London, National Portrait Galleries Publications, 1988.
11. Ives E. Ann Boleyn. Great Britain, T.J. Press, 1986.
12. Roubotham S. Hidden from History. New York, Pantheon Books (Division of Random House), 1974.
13. Wooly S, Wooley W. Thinness Mania—Why are Successful Women Starving Themselves? American Health Magazine.

4
The Presentation of Obesity

JAMES R. HODGE and ERWIN A. MASEELALL

By today's standards the Venus de Milo was fat . . . or at least "pleasingly plump." The subjects of the great painter Rubens were definitely overweight. It is an art historian's bromide that "No artist ever immortalized a skinny woman until Modigliani came along in the 19th century." The history of art shows us that thin has become beautiful during periods of upheaval, periods of transition, periods or war, and when new knowledge becomes important. Plumpness is seen as more attractive during periods of stability. During the Renaissance, a period of great change and upheaval, thinness was accepted as more attractive. Following that was the period of mercantilism, a period of relative stability, when plumpness was more attractive. More recently, the world has been involved with the industrial revolution during which men and women tended to be thinner. As the industrial revolution became stabilized, plumpness became more frequent. In the twentieth century, thinness and hemlines seemed to have correlated with wars and periods of rapid change while in the interval periods weight tended to increase while hemlines would fall. At this time we are moving from the industrial revolution to the stage of information gathering and processing, and thinness and higher hemlines are the vogue.

One speculation about the relationship between thinness and social turmoil is that during periods of social turmoil women have left their homes, have become more involved with the work force and less involved with rearing a family, have become more concerned with appearance for members of the opposite sex which has been less available in those times, have been more concerned with the freedom of movement of their bodies as they have been more active; and often food has been less available. In the more stable historical periods women have become more interested in and involved with the accumulation of material goods, with having children and developing a stable home, with displaying wealth, and with having a less active lifestyle. Food is also more available as is time to prepare and use it.

It is interesting to review the development of the concept of the physical attractiveness of women in America. No colonial American man would have wanted to marry today's beauty ideal. She would have been too skinny, unable to prepare the hearty meals desired or to do the physical work necessary at that time or even able to keep her man warm. The Miss America of today is far different from the Miss America of fifty years ago. This is not just due to the style of the bathing suits. Today's beauty is taller, slimmer, and lighter. The fabled Gibson Girls, the Billy Rose Follies girls, Jenny Lind, and Lillie Langtree were examples of beauty in their times. Though they were thinner than most of their contemporaries, today they would be considered a little corpulent. They are a far cry from today's Cher. In the same sense, Army inductees in the 1950s were significantly heavier than those in 1918 during World War I,[1] and Japanese of both sexes were taller and heavier in the 1980s than they were before World War II. This may be related to the general health of the entire world population.

Generally speaking, people in Third World countries tend to be poor, thin, and physically active; obesity is a sign of success, financial security, and prestige. Contrast this with America. The lower socioeconomic classes, who can least afford it, tend to eat and "store fat" almost as if preparing for leaner days to come; and this is often seen as desirable. On the other hand, the women in the higher socioeconomic classes tend to adopt thinness as beauty and work hard at being thin. More able to afford food, they seem to be displaying evidence of their higher socioeconomic class by working hard at being thin. It is also in this "upper" class that most cases of anorexia nervosa develop.

Who sets the standards of weight and beauty? Is it the American male? The American female? Judges of beauty contests? Today it may be argued that the Metropolitan Life Insurance Company has set the standards for weight, height, and health by periodically putting out tables of "ideal weight, Table 4-1. And how is the "ideal established? The ideal is set by correlation of height and weight with the lowest mortality among those who buy life insurance. Factually, these "ideal weights" have little to do with attractiveness or general health yet everyone who sees the tables tends to interpret them in this way.

However, these tables have become obsolete and have been replaced by 1990 guidelines set by the United States Department of Agriculture and the Department of Health and Human Services, Table 4-2. These tables are for both sexes, but higher weights generally apply to men, who tend to have more muscle and bone; the lower weights apply more often to women. Persons over the age of 35 are allowed to weigh more because recent research suggests that people can be a little heavier as they grow older without added risk to health. The new tables are based not only on height and weight, but on body mass index, fat distribution, and the presence or absence of good health.[2] Essentially, the Dietary Guidelines suggest that if the person's weight is within the range in the table and the waist-to-hip ratio (WHR) discussed later in this chapter does not indicate

TABLE 4-1. 1983 Metropolitan height and weight tables.*

Men

Height		Weight, lb		
Ft	In	Small Frame	Medium Frame	Large Frame
5	2	128–134	131–141	138–150
5	3	130–136	133–143	140–153
5	4	132–138	135–145	142–156
5	5	134–140	137–148	144–160
5	6	136–142	139–151	146–164
5	7	138–145	142–154	149–168
5	8	140–148	145–157	152–172
5	9	142–151	148–160	155–176
5	10	144–154	151–163	158–180
5	11	146–157	154–166	161–184
6	0	149–160	157–170	164–188
6	1	152–164	160–174	168–192
6	2	155–168	164–178	172–197
6	3	158–172	167–182	176–202
6	4	162–176	171–187	181–207

Women

4	10	102–111	109–121	118–131
4	11	103–113	111–123	120–134
5	0	104–115	113–126	122–137
5	1	106–118	115–129	125–140
5	2	108–121	118–132	128–143
5	3	111–124	121–135	131–147
5	4	114–127	124–138	134–151
5	5	117–130	127–141	137–155
5	6	120–133	130–144	140–159
5	7	123–136	133–147	143–163
5	8	126–139	136–150	146–167
5	9	129–142	139–153	149–170
5	10	132–145	142–156	152–173
5	11	135–148	145–159	155–176
6	0	138–151	148–162	158–179

* Source of basic data: 1979 Build Study, Society of Actuaries and Association of Life Insurance Medical Directors of America, 1980. Courtesy of "Statistical Bulletin," Metropolitan Life Insurance Company.

a risk, and if there is no medical problem that indicates a change in weight, there is probably no health advantage to changing the weight.

If the standards of weight and beauty keep changing, and the importance of "ideal weight" has not really been established medically or objectively, how do we judge "how fat is fat?" There is one easy way: the eyeball test;[3] if he (or she) looks fat, he (or she) is fat. Shakespeare said it in a more poetic way: "Beauty is in the eyes of the beholder."

TABLE 4-2. Suggested weights for adults.

Height without shoes	Ages 19 to 34	Ages 35 and over
	(Weight in pounds without clothes)	
5′0″	97–128	108–138
5′1″	101–132	111–143
5′2″	104–137	115–148
5′3″	107–141	119–152
5′4″	111–146	122–157
5′5″	114–150	126–162
5′6″	118–155	130–167
5′7″	121–160	134–172
5′8″	125–164	138–178
5′9″	129–169	142–183
5′10″	132–174	146–188
5′11″	136–179	151–194
6′0″	140–184	155–199
6′1″	144–189	159–205
6′2″	148–195	164–210

USDA and USDHHS, 1990[2]
Source: Derived from National Research Council, 1989.

What is Obesity?

In its simplest terms, obesity can be defined as an excess accumulation of body fat[3] occurring when caloric intake exceeds caloric output. Gray[1] defines obesity as a body fat greater than 25 percent of total body weight for men and 30 percent for woemn. Thus, obesity is an index of fatness. While the terms "obesity" and "overweight" are generally used synonymously in this chapter, the two are really different. "Overweight" refers to the actual amount of body mass and to the recommended weight ranges of the height and weight tables. "Obesity" refers more to appearance, circumferential measurements of the body and its parts, and to skinfold tests. An example of this distinction would be the weight of a professional football player, who is typically heavier than the height and weight tables would indicate to be healthy but who has a higher body mass with a lower amount of body fat than the typical American male. Generally, however, obese persons are overweight and overweight persons are obese.

The above are formal and somewhat simplistic definitions. Obesity is much more than these definitions indicate. For example obesity is a common condition. In 1985 approximately 12 million Americans were considered to be obese.[4] The prevalence is estimated at about 35 percent of men and 40 percent of women. Based on ideal weight, being simply overweight is estimated at 23 percent of men and 30 percent of women; moderate obesity, based on skinfold tests, is 19 percent of men and 28 percent of women. The prevalence of severe obesity, however, is no more than 0.5 percent of the total obese population.[3] Further, obesity tends to run in families. Approximately 80 percent of children with two obese parents are obese whereas 40 percent of children of one obese parent are obese and only 10 percent of children of lean parents are obese.[3] Is this a matter of genetics, of training, and/or of role modeling? Most childhood obesity is related to hyperplasia (increase in number) of fat cells, and the number of fat cells does not change after adolescence. This can be an indicator of a genetic aspect of obesity. However, people receive their genes from the same people with whom they live and who serve as role models and who teach them eating patterns. This "nature-nurture problem" of etiology has yet to be resolved. Certainly, childhood obesity is a risk factor for later obesity, whether by nature or by nurture, but most adult obese people have the onset of obesity after childhood.

There are three demographic factors closely associated with obesity that may help to determine it.[3] These are gender (obesity is far more common among women than among men), age (there is a steady increase in obesity up to the age of 50 with a twofold to threefold increase between the ages of 20 and 64), and social factors. Goldblatt et al.[5] showed that in modern America obesity is six times more prevalent among lower class women than among upper class women. It is also more common in lower class children. He demonstrated that the socioeconomic status of the obese person was closely related to the socioeconomic class of origin. Although socioeconomic class may influence obesity and obesity may influence the socioeconomic class, this can hardly have influenced the social class of one's parents. According to Goldblatt the social class must have influenced the obesity.

Obesity in adolescents is generally of the hyperplastic (excessive number of fat cells) as well as the hypertrophic (excessive size of fat cells) type. It is one of the most common presenting complaints in adolescent clinics in the United States. Primary endocrine or metabolic disorders are uncommon in spite of the wishes of the (generally obese) parents and adolescents themselves. Often the adolescents will present with the same secondary medical problems seen in overweight adults such as low back pain and knee pain or with the wish to lose weight for appearance and social approval. Interestingly, according to Dietz[6] although obese children do not necessarily become obese adults, about 80 percent of obese adolescents do. In another study he[6] found that the time a child spent watching television between the ages of 6 and 11 was the most powerful predictor of obesity in adolescence.

Obesity is a Spectrum Disorder

Obesity exists on the far end of a continuum beginning on one end with cachexia, followed by leanness, then normal, followed by mild obesity or simply "overweight" (20–40 percent above the ideal weight), moderate obesity or "obese" (41–100 percent over ideal weight), and severe obesity or "morbidly obese" (more than 100 percent above the ideal weight). These conventions are arbitrary approximations but more precision is not necessary from a clinical point of view though there may be some treatment implications within these parameters.

Obesity is an Excessive Accumulation of Body Fat

Weight consists of fat and nonfat components of the body. Most obesity is caused by an increase in the body fat components. Body fat is measured by laboratory and by clinical methods. The laboratory techniques at present are basically for research, are generally quite expensive, and have little clinical utility. Among the clinical methods of measuring obesity are:[1]

a. Correlations of height and weight. The Metropolitan Tables are currently the most common methods used in clinical practice and depend on the concept of "ideal weight." Standard weights do not exist, but the new government tables will be increasingly used as standard weights. These are based on the concept of the body mass index (BMI) which is defined as the weight in kilograms divided by the height in meters raised by the power of 2 (W/H^2). This is also known as the Quetelet Index. It has been shown that minimum mortality is associated with a BMI of about 22 kilograms per meter^2 in both sexes, Figure 4-1.
b. Skinfolds. Skinfold-thickness measurement with calipers measures the skinfolds in the areas of the biceps, triceps, subscapular, and suprailiac areas. It has been shown that trunk adiposity compared with thigh adiposity was greater in subjects who developed coronary artery disease; a high subscapular-to-triceps skinfold ratio (an indicator of truncal versus peripheral fat distribution) was associated with a high rate of diabetes mellitus, low density lipoprotein-cholesterol levels, and high triglyceride levels; and also that patients with a higher subscapular skinfold thickness have a higher risk of developing coronary disease. These studies suggest that central body or truncal distribution of body fat may be a more important risk factor than is total body fat. (See Figure 4-1.)
c. Circumferences. "Don't worry about pounds, lose inches" is a statement often used in health spas and weight reduction clinics. Circumferences estimate body fat distribution. In both men and women, a high ratio of waist-to-hip circumferences (WHR) is correlated with the same risks as are the truncal versus peripheral fat distribution levels of the skinfold tests. The WHR is calculated by dividing the waist circumference by the hip circumference. A ratio above 0.85 is a danger signal for women, and a ratio above 0.95 is a danger signal for men. Another

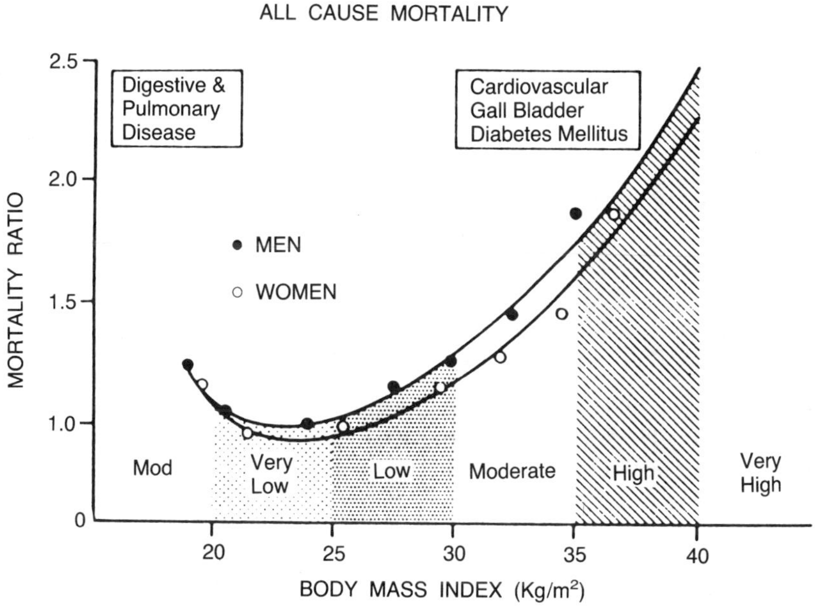

FIGURE 4-1. Mortality ratios are shown for men and women at different levels of body mass index. From Gray DS. Diagnosis and prevalence of obesity. *Medical Clinics of North America*. 1989; 73:1–13, 5. (Data from Lew EA, Garfinkel L. Variations in mortality by weight among 750,000 men and women. *J Chronic Dis* 1979; 32:563–576.) (Reproduced with permission of W.B. Saunders Company.)

ratio is the abdominal-gluteal ratio (AGR) which is also called the android-gynoid ratio. Patients with an elevated AGR (greater than 0.9 for men and 0.8 for women) are said to have abdominal, android, or male pattern obesity while patients with a low AGR are said to have gluteal, gynoid, or female pattern obesity. The "eyeball test" can be of value here, too. If a person looks more like an apple than a pear, he (she) is more likely to be safe.

Obesity is a Metabolic Disorder

Although obesity is occasionally related to a glandular dysfunction that may cause a relatively recognizable fat distribution pattern, these cases are so rare that they hardly need to be considered. There are two important metabolic aspects to regulation of body weight: (a) caloric intake greater than caloric output, and (b) the concept of the "set point".[3] The human body has a tendency to adopt a set point for weight regulation that is relatively constant but that may change with a regular pattern of overeating or undereating. The body tends to regulate weight at around this set point. Because of sociological pressures, obese people attempt to reduce their weight below the set point that is biologically normal for them so that they become biologically underweight (and feel starved) while remaining statistically overweight.[7] One reason for the elevated set point in obese persons can be the elevated number of fat cells (hyperplasia) that they may have; however, almost all obesity is primarily related to hypertrophy of the fat cells regardless of their numbers. The set point can only be changed after several months of changed eating patterns, but it can be reset.

Obesity is Evidence of Overeating in the Past or Present

We typically think of the obese person as either overeating or under-exercising at the present time. In fact, this person may be merely maintaining his or her weight around the biological set point that was established by overeating during some previous period in the person's life.

Obesity is a Highly Individualized Problem with Psychological Aspects

Obesity can be said to be the final common path of an intake versus output problem. What applies statistically to the general population may or may not apply to the individual person. We should always keep in mind that it is not the disorder "obesity" that we are treating, but it is the person who is obese that we are treating. For example, Roden et al.[8] describe how the obese and those at risk for obesity appear to have a lower threshold for physiological arousal than other people do, especially to the presence of food. People who are easily arousable are also more subject to arousal by the symbolic as well as the factual appearance of food, much as were Pavlov's dogs. However it should be kept in mind that highly arousable individuals exist in all weight categories and not all of them become obese.

Locus of Control (LOC)

Locus of control is a psychological term defining the source of factors influencing a person's life. A person with an internal locus of control feels that he is capable and competent and is "master of his own fate," and that external impediments are only to be overcome. The person with an external locus of control feels that he is the helpless victim of external events and circumstances, and that it does not matter what he does because external forces are more powerful. It is easy to hypothesize that persons with an external LOC will attribute their obesity to events that are beyond their control, for example glands, hormones, illness, genetics, constitution, allergies, socioeconomic status, etc. Such patients are commonly seen clinically and they often take the position that, "I might as well eat because I can't do anything about my obesity anyway." This can be emphasized because they have unsuccessfully tried. A high internal LOC can be a good predictor of success in weight control programs, though surprisingly a high external LOC is not a good predictor.[9]

Obesity is a Value Judgment

Is it always "bad"? Certain individuals and population subgroups find that severe obesity is not only desirable but is sensually stimulating. There are many obese men who will marry only an obese woman, and vice versa. There are a number of extremely obese strip teasers and belly dancers who show off their obesity to admiring audiences. Beauty is truly in the eyes of the beholder. Certainly many of our parents have looked upon us as children and even as adults as being "healthy" only if overweight. The more frequent value, however, is that obesity is undesirable. In an unpublished study Hodge and Maseelall[10] made of obese medical patients, almost all of them felt that obesity is undesirable, and there were only three frequently mentioned factors involved: appearance, health, and social acceptance.

Obesity is a Risk Factor for Morbidity and Mortality

Though current statistics[1,3] indicate that there may be no significant adverse mortality and morbidity in patients with mild obesity, the risk factors are certainly increased especially with moderate and severe obesity. The mortality and morbidity even from accidents and from surgery are higher in these groups. The earlier section on skinfold measures and circumferences detailed the associations of fat distribution with various illnesses. The three most potent factors for coronary heart disease (hypertension, diabetes, and hyperlipidemia) are far more prevalent among obese patients. Skin disorders[11] are frequent among the obese due to impaired heat loss and an increase in sweating, especially after meals. Disorders of the feet, knees, hips, and low back are frequent; and obesity is the most frequent aggravator of osteoarthritis (degenerative joint disease). Emotional factors should not be ignored; anxiety, depression, social isolation, and disparagement of the body image are common, creating a poor self-concept with low self-esteem. In extreme cases a Pickwickian syndrome may occur as may obstructive sleep apnea.[12] Obesity, then, is also a risk factor for premature death.

Obesity is a Result of Eating Habits

It is a common assumption that most obese persons can be observed to eat much more than do normal-weight subjects. Roden[9] summarizes studies from the general population, showing that statistically there is no real difference between the eating patterns of the obese and the nonobese in terms of quantity and of speed. She points out that it is not always possible to define an eating style from the behavior with one meal. Some obese patients will deny overeating at all; some of these can actually be observed to be overeating. They are denying what other people can see.

There are two special types of eating patterns that contribute to obesity in some people.[12] The first is bulimia,[12] which refers to repetitive episodes of sudden, compulsive ingestion of large amounts of food, usually accompanied by anxiety and agitation and frequently preceded by stress and followed by self-condemnation and frequently by vomiting. Bulimia is a clinical condition and is to be distinguished from "binge eating" which is something that nonobese persons frequently do but allow the natural body regulatory systems to prevail. Bulimia also occurs frequently along with anorexia nervosa. Some people mistakenly use the term "bulimia" to include anorexia nervosa, but this should not be done. Sometimes it is appropriate to use the term "bulimorexia" when these two occur together. Most obese bulimics do not vomit after binging;[3] many thin bulimics do vomit after binging. About five percent of obese persons may be bulimic.[3] The complications of binging and vomiting include enlarged parotid glands, esophageal inflammation, dental problems such as caries and pyorrhea and erosion, fluid and electrolyte imbalances especially with low potassium mostly due to vomiting, and pneumonitis. Laxatives lead to damages in the colon, impaired intestinal activity, metabolic acidosis, and sometimes to chemical dependency upon laxatives. Not only do bulimics binge, they also diet; and the psychological factors of dieting are an additional complication. Most dieters are depressed about having to diet, feel deprived, and feel depressed and anxious about their lack of success. Not only do dieters feel deprived, they feel starved, and they may actually be starving according to their regulatory set points. Bulimics are especially prone to self-mutilation and suicide attempts, and there may be a history of a major affective disorder in the patient or in the relatives. Up to 15 percent have been victims of incest and sexual abuse. The other particular eating pattern often resulting in obesity is the "night-eating syndrome" consisting of morning anorexia, evening hyperphagia, and insomnia. This syndrome occurs primarily in women, appears to be precipitated by stressful life circumstances, and may represent a form of depression. It may also become a habit. Stunkard[12] adds that weight reduction as the primary treatment in these two eating problems is usually ineffective.

Obesity is a Psychiatric Dilemma

Does psychopathology cause obesity or does obesity cause psychopathology? Obesity is associated with endomorphism, but is endomorphism present before and/or after obesity? In the heyday of the psychoanalytic movement, obesity was considered to be a clear-cut psychosomatic condition representing a partial fixation at the oral stage of development between the ages of 0 and 2. Food was a pacifier and parents solved problems. This led to the development of a passive, dependent, helpless, clinging person who had a tendency to depression, anxiety, and problems with separation reactions. The goal of treatment according to Stunkard[3] was to "cure" obesity forever. However, psychoanalysis did and does focus on the underlying personality problem rather than on the specific symptom, and the symptom was often relieved almost incidentally. Stunkard[3] states that today the search for psychopathology as the cause of obesity has been largely abandoned and that psychopathology is the result of obesity, yet he also states that psychoanalysis is one of the most effective treatments for obesity.[13] Roden[14] summarizes general population studies showing that obese people in general do not differ significantly from the nonobese in psychopathology or other psychological characteristics. Persons who do not feel good about themselves may become obese, but not all depressed people will overeat, nor are all obese persons depressed.

The fact is that both obese and nonobese people can have psychopathology and psychopathology may precede, accompany, or follow the problem of obesity. There is no typical or necessary personality type preceding obesity. Individual patients are not always well described by statistics. Actually it appears that depressed patients who are obese, or patients who are depressed about being obese, are those who are more likely to present for treatment. Two case examples illustrate these points.

1. Miss AB came to therapy because of depression and was noted to be approximately 50 percent over the maximum for the height and weight tables. As is typical in such cases, by the time she came to me she had been through many weight reduction programs but always gained her weight back and she probably knew more about diets, calories, exercise, etc. than most physicians do. When asked how things are different when she is thin she replied that she is more assertive, expects more of herself especially socially, and is afraid of becoming a sex object. Her weight gain began just after puberty when she became the "mother" of the household which included many nonobese children and nonobese parents. She recalls staying indoors doing household chores while the other children were out playing, and she would bake cookies to entice the others to come in for a while with her. She also ate the cookies. Later she left home at a relatively young age "to get away from that," and within a year she had lost a significant amount of weight, but she gained it back. Her only significant relationship with a man was brief and occurred when she was at her thinnest.
2. An obese schizophrenic patient who had been gaining weight declared that, "Eating is the last coping mechanism I have. It's the only gratification I can get."

Obesity can be defense against sexuality and a defense against control by others. It can also be a "way out" of ongoing problems such as marriage or social life. It can be a classical passive aggressive mechanism of expressing hostility while helplessly communicating, "I can't help it." It can also be a method of punishing oneself for past behavior and preventing oneself from engaging in it again. Obese patients, as do anorexic patients, may have a pathological disturbance of their body image; but this occurs in only a minority of obese persons, most of whom have some other psychopathology, have been obese since childhood, and who have low self-esteem.

At the Fourth International Symposium on Eating Disorders, Fornari[15] described how nearly 70 percent of patients treated for eating disorders met the lifetime criteria for at least one other form of major psychopathology. Bulimia seemed to be more closely associated with lifetime psychiatric disorder than did anorexia. He reported that in another study patients who had anorexia nervosa, bulimia nervosa, or a combination of the two showed 45 percent of anorexics having anxiety disorders, 60 percent of bulimics, and 68 percent of patients with both. At the same conference Marcus pointed out the similarities between the behaviors associated with substance abuse and eating disorders. Both types of patients present "repetitive compulsive self-destructive behaviors, which are extremely resistant to change." The behavior of binge eaters is often similar to that of binge alcoholics in the sense that they may be able to refrain from eating (at times other than meal times) for long periods of time so long as they do not take one bite. However, like the alcoholic, one bite is too much and a thousand bites are not enough. This is particularly characteristic of patients with the night-eating syndrome.

Summary: How the Patient Presents

Typically, the patient presents herself to the physician with symptoms and/or signs of physical problems, emotional problems, patterns of overeating, complications of dieting, and disparagement of the body image. She may also present with the primary desire to lose weight in order to look better, feel better, or be more socially acceptable.

Physical Problems

Frequently the patient does not present with a desire to lose weight. She may come in with a physical problem such as low back pain or may on routine examination be found to have a physical problem such as hypertension and may then be unhappy to learn that one of the most important aspects of the treatment for that problem is to lose weight.

Emotional Problems

Obese patients who are physically well and happy with themselves do not present for treatment. Those who do wish to lose weight are generally unhappy, depressed, or anxious, though this may not be of sufficient degree to catch the attention of the physician. Many of the other psychosocial factors mentioned earlier may be present but not mentioned. Rarely is a patient told that she should lose weight to help with her anxiety or depression. Patients do not complain of a disturbed body image because they do not believe that it is disturbed. Patients presenting to a weight loss center, typically women, were noted to be generally depressed and to feel that they had been "picked on" by others. They resented other people who had never had a weight problem, and they were critical and hostile to other people. They complained both that their social lives interfered with their weight loss and that their excessive weight interfered with their social lives. There is almost always some biopsychosocial problem that precipitates the decision to get help.

Patterns of Overeating

The two most typical pathological forms of overeating are bulimia and the night-eating syndrome. Other patterns of overeating include "picking" without realizing it and night eating on the basis of a habit that was developed earlier in life. The patient describes her eating habits as: (a) "I eat like a bird but I can't lose weight," but upon further inquiries states that she used to eat a great deal; (b) "I can't help overeating. I eat between meals and I eat a lot at meals and I just can't resist it"; (c) "I have periods of binge eating, mostly at night, that I can't control. I only eat a regular diet during the day and I try not to binge but sometimes when I'm bored or lonely or just get hungry I may take a piece of candy and then I'm off on a binge. If I don't take that first bite I can avoid binging. If I drank, I'd be an alcoholic"; (d) "A couple of hours after supper I start to eat and I just can't stop. I'm not hungry in the morning, but that may have something to do with not sleeping well after eating so much the night before."

Family History

The family history typically reveals that the mother and father are both obese or that major affective disorder or alcoholism occurred in one or more primary relatives. Siblings tend to be obese but this is not necessarily so. Typically the parents are from a low socioeconomic class whose parents were of a low socioeconomic class in the country of origin. The mother always imparted the attitude that, "You should clean your plate," and "Eat! You are too thin and your mother knows best."

Developmental History

The developmental history may indicate that the patient is one of several children and has been obese since childhood, puberty, or adolescence. The patient was teased unmercifully by children at school, was unable to fight back, and withdrew. She was always sensitive to her obesity, and she rarely had dates. Mostly she sufffered in silence about this, and put on a happy face when in fact she was mildly depressed, lonely, and almost came to hate her body. She really tended to lose weight after high school when she left home, but again the weight returned within five years of marriage or after the birth of a child. This has led to conflicts with her husband and to an interference with their sex life. Unless specifically asked, and perhaps not even then, she will not reveal that she was sexually molested as a child. The patient has made several attempts at losing weight through crash diets which sometimes have produced a moderate weight loss that has been unable to be maintained; and/or the patient has attended TOPS, Overeaters Anonymous, or commercial weight loss programs and has either dropped out after no results or after an unsatisfactory weight loss. The patient is thoroughly familiar with counting calories and with the nutritional aspects of food. The patient has "tried everything, but nothing works." She states that she has been mildly depressed and anxious for as long as she has been obese, but she recalls little about what she was like before then since it was so long ago. If her obesity started in adulthood she gives a history of being "happy" or "normal" until she became obese, but depression or social conflicts may have immediately preceded her obesity and her presentation for weight loss. She looks upon her body as unattractive, perhaps even loathsome. She is frustrated with herself for not being able to lose weight or maintain her weight loss. She cannot get her mind off food and diets. She leads a sedentary existence, though episodically she will involve herself in some mild exercise though it is clear that this is not enough to use up the calories that she ingests.

References

1. Gray DS. Diagnosis and prevalence of obesity. *Med Clin NA* 1989; 73:1–13, 8.
2. U.S. Department of Agriculture and U.S. Department of Health and Human Services. Dietary guidelines for Americans (third edition). U.S. Government Printing Office. Home and Garden Bulletin No. 232. November, 1990.
3. Stunkard AJ. Obesity. In Hales RE, Francis AI (eds): *American Psychiatric Association Annual Review—Vol. 4.* Washington, DC, American Psychiatric Press, Inc; 1985; 419–437. (42).
4. Raymond CA. Biology, culture, and dietary changes conspire to increase incidence of obesity. *JAMA* 1986; 256:2157–2158.

5. Goldblatt PB, Moore ME, Stunkard AJ. Social factors in obesity. *JAMA* 1965; 192:1039–1044.
6. Dietz JW Jr. Cited by: Raymond CA. Biology, culture, dietary changes conspire to increase incidence of obesity. *JAMA* 1986; 256:2157–2158.
7. Nisbett R. Hunger, obesity, and the ventromedial hypothalamus. *Psychol Rev* 1972; 79:433–453.
8. Roden J, Elman D, Schachter S. Emotionality and obesity. In Schacter S, Roden J (eds): Obese Humans and Rats. Washington, DC, Erlbaum/Wiley, 1974.
9. Roden J, Schrank D, Striegel-Moore R. Psychological features of obesity. *Med Clin NA* 1989; 73:47–66.
10. Hodge JR, Maseelall E. Unpublished study.
11. Stunkard AJ. Obesity. In Berkow R (ed): The Merck Manual of Diagnosis and Therapy (fifteenth edition). Rahway, NJ, Merck Sharp & Dohme Research Laboratories, 1987; 950–955.
12. Stunkard AJ. *Merck Manual*, 1987; 951–952.
13. Rand SW, Stunkard AJ. Cited by: Stunkard AJ. *Annual Review* 1985; 422.
14. Roden J, Schrank D, Striegel-Moore R. *Med Clin of NA* 1985; 49.
15. Fornari V. Cited by: Unnamed reporter. Co-morbid psychopathologies often accompany eating disorders: Panel. Obesity '90 Update. September/October 1990; 7.

5
The Biological Basis of Bulimia

PETER M. BOLO

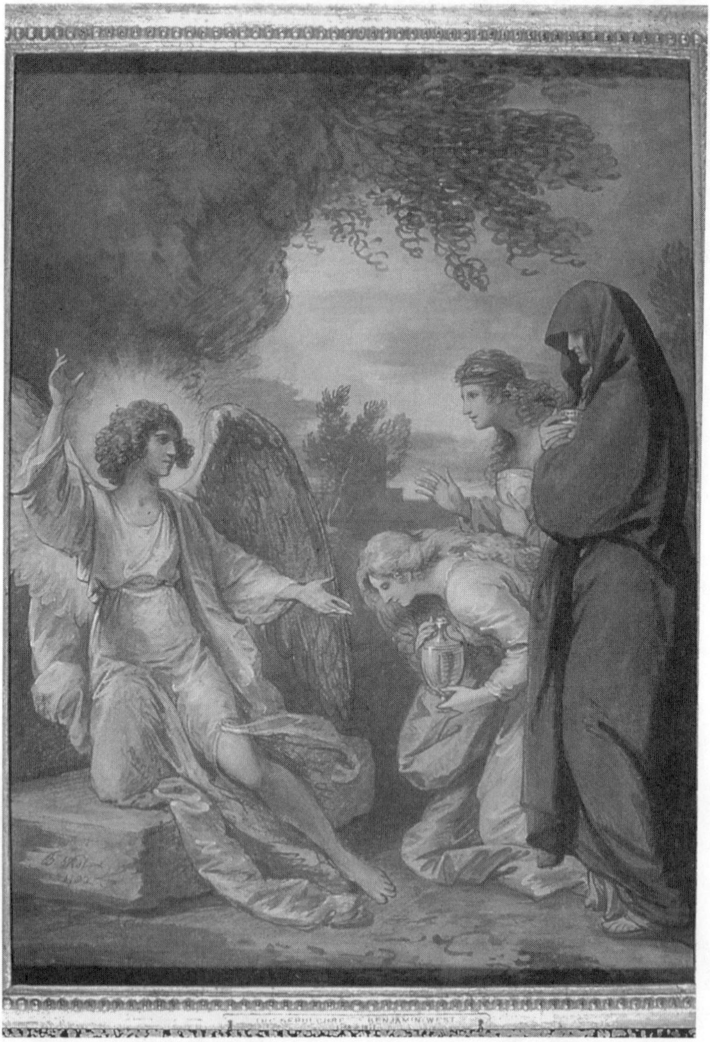

West, Benjamin—*The Sepulchre*—(Butler Institute of American Art, Youngstown, Ohio)

Introduction

It is widely held that the etiology of bulimia nervosa involves a complex interplay of biological, psychological, and sociological factors. This is reflected in the wide range of treatment strategies now employed for this illness. Bulimia fits a biopsychosocial model of psychiatric illness well.

Biological theories concerning bulimia derive in large part from two sources. The first of these is animal research—predominantly in rats—as to the brain's control of appetite and eating behavior. The second source is medication trials in human beings, usually suggested by relating bulimia to other psychiatric or neurologic disorders. Little is definitively understood in this area. Theorizing in humans based upon beneficial response of bulimic symptoms in drug trials is troublesome for several reasons: response to treatment does not necessarily define illness etiology; the list of drugs purported to be beneficial is long and varied; and the drugs in question each possess multiple physiological effects that might contribute to treatment response.

Despite these limitations, it is important to explore what is known to date about the biological basis of bulimia. We begin by summarizing our understanding of the brain's regulation of appetite and feeding. Next, we explore the relationship between bulimia and affective disorders, which led to multiple drug trials in humans. We then explore the early conceptualization of bulimia as a form of seizure disorder, and associated medication trials. Finally, we discuss more recent drug trials conceived to modulate specific neurotransmitter systems believed to play a role in the control of appetite and feeding.

Brain Regulation of Appetite and Feeding

The central control of appetite and feeding is complex and incompletely elucidated. An exhaustive description is beyond the scope of this chapter; we summarize in large part from the excellent works of Leibowitz[1] and of Morley.[2]

The hypothalamus plays a pivotal role by acting as a transducer of many sensory and metabolic inputs and coordinating the response of the animal in feeding behavior. The hypothalamus provides an interface between the brain and the periphery. Mapping studies performed on the rat brain reveal specific sites most sensitive to injected neurotransmitters or drugs that release neurotransmitters, suggesting their involvement in feeding behavior.

Within the ventral hypothalamus, two important regions have been defined; a satiety center in the ventromedial hypothalamus and a feeding center in the lateral hypothalamus. Electrical stimulation of the satiety center (ventromedial hypothalamus) inhibits eating, and destructive lesions here result in hyperphagia and obesity. The opposite effects are seen in the feeding center (lateral hypothalamus). Here, electrical stimulation increases eating, even in sated animals, and destructive lesions result in the inhibition of eating. The satiety center is thought to coordinate the "stop feeding" response; the feeding center integrates the "start feeding" signal.

A long list of brain neurotransmitters have been implicated in the regulation of food intake: the monoamines (norepinephrine, serotonin, dopamine), opioid peptides, gamma-aminobutyric acid (GABA), hormone-releasing factors, pancreatic polypeptides, and gut-brain peptides. We focus on the monoamines and opioid peptides here, as they pertain to bulimia studies in humans.

Norepinephrine, serotonin, and dopamine pathways run through the hypothalamus. The serotonergic pathway, originating in the raphe nuclei of the pontine-midbrain area, courses through the ventromedial (satiety center) hypothalamus. Adrenergic pathways run through the perifornical area adjacent to the ventromedial hypothalamus and give projections to the lateral (feeding center) hypothalamus. The nigrostriatal tract, a dopaminergic pathway, is also associated with the lateral hypothalamus. Opiate receptors for endogenous opioid peptides exist on dopaminergic neurons in the nigrostriatal tract.

In the lateral (feeding center) hypothalamus, release of norepinephrine inhibits feeding. The other monoamines are likewise inhibitory here. In the ventromedial (satiety center) hypothalamus, serotonin input predominates and is stimulatory; that is, release of serotonin produces satiety and decreased eating. Depletion of serotonin here results in hyperphagia and obesity. On the other hand, norepinephrine inhibits the satiety center, leading to increased eating. Note that norepinephrine produces opposite effects upon eating in the two centers, increasing eating at the ventromedial hypothalamus via alpha$_2$-noradrenergic receptors, and decreasing eating at the lateral hypothalamus via beta-noradrenergic receptors.

Endogenous opioid peptides in the hypothalamus are believed to produce an overall drive to feed. This is supported by studies in which naloxone—a specific opiate antagonist—reduces feeding centrally under a variety of circumstances, including in obese human beings. Opiate receptors are found on dopaminergic neurons in the nigrostriatal tract that are stimulatory to feeding behavior. Of the three known opiate receptors in the brain—mu, delta, and kappa—the kappa receptor is believed to be the most important in the regulation of feeding.

Bulimia and Affective Disorders

In the early 1980s, much effort was focused on defining the relationship between bulimia and affective disorders. This topic is expanded upon in

Chapter 17, however we summarize here as this relationship led to much theorizing on the biological basis of bulimia.

Evidence linking the two disorders was found in the high rates of depression in bulimic individuals and their family members, as well as in the positive response of bulimic symptoms to antidepressant medications. Finally, similar neuroendocrinologic and polysomnographic abnormalities were noted in both disorders. Levy et al.[3] recently reviewed this area and summarized arguments against this hypothesized relationship between bulimia and affective disorders.

A number of authors noted a significant prevalence of major depression among bulimic patients. Hudson et al.[4] found that 59 percent of the normal weight bulimics they studied met DSM-III criteria for major depression some time during their lives, with 40 percent of these individuals reporting episodes of depression prior to the onset of bulimic behaviors. Walsh et al.[5] reported a 71 percent lifetime prevalence of major depression among a population of 50 bulimics, with 30 percent having a concurrent diagnosis of RDC major depression.

Levy et al.[3] counter such reports by suggesting that depression may result from the negative psychosocial consequences of deranged feeding behavior or may result from malnutrition itself, even in normal weight bulimics. Additionally, they point out that there have been no large studies comparing rates of depression in bulimics versus controls with interviewers blind to diagnosis; this type of study would minimize interviewer bias which might lead to overestimates of depression in bulimic patients. They also note that the DSM-III defines bulimia with a depressive criteria—"depressed mood and self-deprecating thoughts"—that likely encouraged excessive estimates of depression in bulimics. Finally, they remark that research samples of bulimics are typically obtained from individuals seeking treatment, which may skew toward a population with more depression hoping for symptomatic relief.

A number of early family studies reported a high incidence of affective disorders in the first degree relatives of bulimic individuals. These included, by self-report, 16 of the 34 bulimics studied by Pyle et al.[6] and 33 among 56 bulimics studied by Lee et al.[7] However, neither of these studies compared a control sample. In a population of 20 bulimics and 20 normal controls, Musisi and Garfinkel[8] noted no increased incidence of depression in the families of bulimics. Stern et al.[9] estimated the prevalence of affective disorders in first and second degree relatives of bulimics to be 9 percent, and that of controls to be 10 percent. These better controlled studies suggest that bulimics do not have a higher family incidence of affective disorders.

Initial reports of sleep abnormalities in bulimics suggested they had shortened REM latency, as is characteristic of patients with major depression. Katz et al.[10] studied 17 bulimics and noted shortened REM latencies compared to controls. However, some of their bulimic subjects clearly had concomitant severe major depression. Others have not corroborated this finding, including Levy et al.[11] who found no polysomnographic differences between 9 bulimics and 10 healthy controls; none of these bulimic subjects had concomitant major depression. It appears that, in the absence of concomitant major depression, bulimics do not have shortened REM latency.

Abnormal dexamethasone suppression tests (DST) have been reported in both major depression and bulimia and are another purported link between the two illnesses. However, the specificity of the DST is low; it is abnormal in many other conditions as well. The significance of this and other such neuroendocrine tests is unclear at this juncture, and certainly does not provide strong evidence to support a relationship between bulimia and affective disorders.

Drug Trials I—Suggested by Theorized Relationship of Bulimia to Affective Disorders

Tricyclic Antidepressants

There have been five double-blind placebo-controlled trials using tricyclic antidepressants in bulimics: two each with imipramine and desipramine, and one with amitriptyline. All demonstrated benefit in decreasing bulimic behaviors, except the amitriptyline study.

Pope et al.[12] studied 22 chronic bulimics, giving half imipramine 200 mg daily and the others placebo for six weeks. They reported a 70 percent decline in binge frequency in the imipramine group, including 35 percent becoming abstinent from binging altogether, compared to no change in the placebo group. They also found that imipramine was associated with decreased intensity of binges, decreased preoccupation with food, greater subjective global improvement, and significantly reduced Hamilton rating scale scores of depression. Pope et al. argue that imipramine's benefit was due to its antidepressant action rather than some other separate antibulimic property because decrease in Hamilton rating scale scores correlated significantly with reduction in binge eating. Further support for this postulate was found in a two-year follow-up study of the patients enrolled in their imipramine study.[13] At follow-up, 19 of the 20 subjects reported at least a partial improvement in bulimic symptoms, with 50 percent experiencing complete remission. However, many had responded to antidepressants other than imipramine, such as desipramine, trazodone, or phenelzine; changes in antidepressant choice were typically prompted by lack of benefit or adverse effects. Agras et al.[14] also performed a double-blind placebo-controlled study using imipramine in dosages up to 300 mg daily among 22 bulimics; their trail extended to 16 weeks. They corroborated the benefit noted by Pope et al.,[12] but found a slower rate of response. At six weeks, Agras et al. reported imipramine reduced binge frequency by 39 percent, in contrast to 70 percent reported by Pope et al. However, binge frequency reduction improved further to 72 percent by the end of 16 weeks in the Agras et al. study. They also found 30 percent to be abstinent from binging altogether at 16 weeks. In contrast to Pope et al., Agras et al. found no correlation between improvement in depression and improvement in bulimia. In fact, a number of subjects improved markedly with imipramine who had no evidence of depression at any time. Agras et al. suggest that any correlation between decreased binging and improvement in mood could mean that depression lifts in response to normalization of eating behavior. They see evidence for an antibulimic property of imipramine aside from its antidepressant effect.

In contrast to the positive results with imipramine noted previously, a study of 32 bulimics conducted by Mitchell and Groat[15] failed to demonstrate a significant difference in outcome between those receiving placebo and those receiving 150 mg daily of amitriptyline for eight weeks. The most striking finding was the marked improvement in bulimic symptoms in both the placebo and amitriptyline groups, though there was a non-statistically significant trend toward better response with active drug. There was a 72.1 percent reduction in binges per week with amitriptyline, compared to a 51.8 percent reduction with placebo. Mitchell and Groat divided their subjects into depressed and nondepressed groups; they noted less bulimic symptom improvement in the depressed group whether treated with placebo or amitriptyline. Amitriptyline did, however, have significant antidepressant effect among the depressed bulimic subjects. Although the depressed bulimics experienced less improvement in bulimic behaviors as a group, there was a positive correlation in individual responses; that is, depressed subjects whose depression improved fared better in improvement of bulimic symptoms than those whose depression did not lift. Mitchell and Groat suggested that the presence of depression is a negative prognostic indicator, but that improvement in depression allows for improvement in bulimic behaviors. The significant positive response to both placebo and amitriptyline was attributed to the minimal behavioral treatment that was provided to each subject in this study and/or to the high level of subject motivation. Subjects in this study were gathered from individuals presenting for treatment, whereas in the Pope et al.[12] imipramine study where placebo response was minimal, subjects were recruited through advertisements. Finally, multiple authors attribute the lack of greater-than-placebo response in this study to inadequate dose of amitriptyline. Mitchell and Groat themselves note that, based on some serum levels obtained, as many as half of the subjects may have received inadequate doses of the drug.

Hughes et al.[16] published the first double-blind placebo-controlled crossover study demonstrating desipramine beneficial in a population of 22 bulimics that excluded subjects with significant depression. Using desipramine 200 mg daily for six weeks, there was a 91 percent decrease in binge frequency, with 68 percent of subjects attaining complete remission of binge and purge behaviors. Serum desipramine levels were found to vary widely, measured at week five of the study, with half of the subjects being subtherapeutic. When dosage was adjusted to obtain therapeutic levels is those still partially symptomatic, there was an additional 51 percent decrease in binge frequency in these subjects. Hughes et al. believe that, because they excluded depressed individuals from their study, they demonstrated an antibulimic effect of desipramine separate from its antidepressant property. Barlow et al.[17] performed a second double-blind placebo-controlled crossover study among 24 bulimics using desipramine 150 mg daily for six weeks, with a sample containing both depressed and nondepressed individuals. Desipramine effectively reduced both binging and vomiting compared to placebo; however, they rated the clinical effects as modest. They noted significant improvement on desipramine beginning at one week, with maximal decrease in binge/purge frequency at the end of the sixth week. Serum desipramine levels revealed three-quarters of the subjects tested to have levels below the range generally accepted for treatment of depression. Of note, desipramine treatment did not result in any significant improvement in depressive symptoms. Barlow et al. conclude that desipramine has an antibulimic effect independent of its antidepressant property based on its rapid benefit (improvement within one week for bulimia as opposed to the several week lag for antidepressant action) and effectiveness at subtherapeutic serum levels. They postulate[18] that its antibulimic effect is likely mediated through increased norepinephrine activity, given that desipramine is a relatively specific norepinephrine reuptake inhibitor. Recall that norepinephrine is inhibitory in the feeding center of the lateral hypothalamus, thus reducing hunger.

Mianserin

Sabine et al.[19] reported an early double-blind placebo-controlled trial of mianserin, a tetracyclic piperazino-azepine antidepressant used for many years in England. Mianserin 60 mg daily was compared to placebo for eight weeks in 36 bulimic patients without severe depression. They noted some overall improvement in abnormal eating behaviors, attitudes, anxiety, and depression, but noted no significant benefit of mianserin compared to placebo. They attributed the improvement noted to regular contact with a psychiatrist interested in their condition and progress, as well as to high subject motivation for treatment response. These are similar arguments to those used by Mitchell and Groat[15] to account for the equivalent positive response they noted with placebo and amitriptyline in their study. Pope et al.[20] offer a different explanation for the lack of superiority of mianserin over placebo: the dosage of 60 mg daily was inadequate, especially given that McGrath et al.[21] reported that dosages up to 150 mg daily were necessary to treat depression. There have been no further important studies of mianserin in bulimia, and this medication has not been made available for use in the United States.

MAO Inhibitors

There have been two double-blind placebo-controlled studies of MAO inhibitors in bulimia—one each examining phenelzine and isocarboxazid—both demonstrating significant benefit. Clinical drawbacks to these agents include difficult-to-tolerate side effects, clinician and patient concern about possible dietary indiscretion causing hypertensive crisis, and patient reluctance to accept a tyramine-free diet.

Walsh et al.[22] studied 50 bulimics, administering either eight weeks of phenelzine in a dosage between 60 mg and 90 mg daily or placebo. Phenelzine was significantly superior to placebo in reducing binge frequency: 64 percent with phenelzine versus 5 percent with placebo. By the end of the phenelzine trial, 35 percent ceased binging altogether. The benefit of phenelzine was not limited to a depressed subgroup, speaking against phenelzine treating bulimic symptoms through stabilization of a mood disorder. Walsh et al. hypothesized that phenelzine works by relieving prebinge anxiety; however, there was no significant improvement in anxiety noted in the one anxiety scale they used. They also postulated a possible direct effect of phenelzine on neurobiological systems that regulate feeding. They were unable to elaborate on this further, citing the wide range of effects MAO inhibitors have on the central nervous system, including the elevation of postsynaptic concentrations of all monoamines. Unfortunately, about half the subjects who responded to phenelzine were unable to remain on the drug after the study due to side effects, the most common being orthostatic hypotension and sedation. No hypertensive crises occurred, although patients were carefully screened and educated to maximize tyramine-free diet compliance.

Kennedy et al.[23] reported isocarboxazid beneficial in a double-blind placebo-controlled crossover study among 24 bulimics in a six-week trial at a dosage of 60 mg daily. Of subjects given active drug initially, all experienced a more than 50 percent decrease in vomiting and most noted a more than 50 percent reduction in binging; 33 percent abstained entirely from binging and 39 percent abstained from vomiting. Platelet MAO inhibition on average was documented to be greater than 85 percent, suggesting adequate dosage and compliance. Of note there was no correlation between improvement in bulimic and depressive symptoms, supporting an antibulimic effect independent of the antidepressant effect of isocarboxazid. Kennedy et al., like Walsh et al.,[22] discussed the possibility that central MAO inhibition alters noradrenergic and serotonergic activity in the hypothalamic centers regulating feeding behavior, accounting for its antibulimic property.

Trazodone

Pope et al.[24] have published the only double-blind placebo-controlled study of the effect of trazodone on bulimic behavior. They gave 42 bulimic patients trazodone in a dosage between 200 mg and 400 mg daily—dependent upon side effects—or placebo for six weeks. They found trazodone significantly superior to placebo: binge frequency was halved in 41 percent of those taking trazodone, although only 12 percent experienced complete remission. They noted mininal adverse effects; only one patient dropped out due to side effects (headaches). Though they cite the serotonergic agonist property of trazodone, they hesitate to suggest this as its mode of antibulimic action since desipramine is equally beneficial and has virtually no serotonergic effect.

Lithium

Hsu[25] initially reported lithium to be beneficial in controlling bulimic symptoms. In an open-label, four-week trial of lithium maintained at serum levels between 0.6 and 1.0 mEq/l, 12 of 14 bulimic subjects experienced a 75 to 100 percent decline in binging. Of note, eight patients received behavioral therapy simultaneously. Lithium's benefit was not supported by a later double-blind placebo-controlled study by Hsu et al.[26] They reported preliminary findings on the first 13 bulimics in the study: on average, the frequency of binge and purge episodes diminished by 70 percent after eight weeks on either lithium or placebo. Hsu suggested that the patients responded to simple cognitive techniques provided to them at their eating disorders clinic, including dietary instruction and self-monitoring of bulimic behaviors, rather than medication. They cite a similar finding in the amitriptyline study of Mitchell and Groat.[15]

Nomifensine

Nomifensine is a novel antidepressant that was briefly approved for use in the United States but was withdrawn subsequently due to associated reports of hemolytic anemia and hypersensitivity reactions. Prior to its removal from the market, Pope et al.[27] conducted an open-label trial of nomifensine among 12 bulimics who took from 200 mg to 400 mg daily for two to six months. Two subjects dropped out early because of febrile reactions. Of the remaining ten, nine subjects showed moderate or more reduction in binge frequency, with minimal side effects.

Bupropion

Bupropion, another novel antidepressant with fewer anticholinergic, sedative, and hypotensive side effects compared to the standard tricyclic agents, was examined in a double-blind placebo-controlled study by Horne et al.[28] For eight weeks, 81 nondepressed bulimics took either placebo or bupropion in a dosage between 225 mg and 450 mg daily. The drug was significantly superior to placebo in diminishing the frequency of binge and purge behaviors. Side effects were minimal, with the important exception of grand mal seizures in four of those receiving bupropion. This finding prompted termination of this study and led the manufacturer to warn against administration of bupropion to patients with bulimia. The seizure complication is not clearly understood. Horne et al. did cite earlier studies that conceived of bulimia as a form of seizure disorder.

Drug Trials II—Suggested by Theorized Relationship of Bulimia to Seizure Disorder

Phenytoin

In 1974, Green and Rau[29] published an open-label trial of ten patients with compulsive eating disorders—roughly equivalent to bulimia by today's nomenclature—treated with phenytoin 400 mg daily. Their subjects included several who were underweight, normal weight, and overweight. They reported that nine out of ten responded with normalization of eating, though they hastened to caution that a double-blind placebo-controlled trial was needed to confirm this. They undertook this study based on a belief that episodic dyscontrol of eating—a binge—represents an epileptic equivalent.[30] They described one patient: "The salient characteristics, then, of Laura's syndrome consisted of an episodic, ego-dystonic, non-predictable, irregular 'seizure' involving compulsive eating preceded by an apparent aura and followed by a probable postictal phase involving loss of consciousness, amnesia, and confusion." Knowing that lesions in the ventromedial hypothalamus produce hyperphagic rats and lesions in the lateral hypothalamus produce anorectic rats, Green and Ray hypothesized that subcortical electrical dysfunction involving the hypothalamus could result in abnormal eating behavior in humans. In fact, they reported EEG abnormalities in nine of their ten subjects. Six showed 14- and 6-per-second positive spiking in the temporal and occipital areas which they believe consistent with underlying subcortical dysfunction. Four patients showed spiking in the temporal and occipital areas consistent with cortical dysfunction, but possibly associated with subcortical abnormalities as well.

Wermuth et al.[31] subsequently reported a double-blind placebo-controlled crossover study of phenytoin in a dosage of 300 mg daily for six weeks among 19 bulimics of varying weight. The response to phenytoin, though statistically significant, was much more modest than that noted by Green and Rau.[29] Curiously, in the group of patients who took phenytoin followed by placebo, the benefit from phenytoin carried over through the entire placebo period. This is particularly remarkable given that the anticonvulsant action of phenytoin terminates quickly upon discontinuation of the drug. Also in contrast to the Green and Rau study, EEG abnormalities were not correlated with treatment response. In fact, definite EEG abnormalities were found in only three patients, with four showing 14- and 6-per-second positive spikes. Wermuth et al. conclude that bulimia does not fit a seizure disorder model, even though clinically the episodic, uncontrollable nature of binges and occasional favorable response to phenytoin noted suggests a variant of psychomotor epilepsy. They point out that Green and Rau implicated hypothalamic involvement based upon observing 14- and 6-per-second positive spikes, which most encephalographers consider a nonpathological, normal variant. The anticonvulsant property of phenytoin does not appear important here as diminished binging was reported in some bulimics with subtherapeutic phenytoin serum levels. Also, there was no correlation between EEG abnormality and treatment outcome. Wermuth et al. did admit that phenytoin is felt to have actions beyond its anticonvulsant property that might impart some antibulimic effect.

The abnormal EEG patterns referred to previously are controversial.[32] Rau and Green[33] reported 38 of 59 patients with "binge-eating syndrome" to have EEG abnormalities, the most common being the 14- and 6-per-second positive spiking pattern. However, this EEG finding is also common among an asymptomatic control population, especially in adolescents: Wegner and Struve[34] reported the incidence among adolescents to be anywhere from 25 to 58 percent. In the literature, it is generally felt that such positive spikes are infrequent in the very young, peak in frequency during adolescence, and become rare by adulthood. It also bears mentioning that the phenytoin studies reported previously did not use modern diagnostic criteria for bulimia and that samples included both obese and anorexic individuals; these factors limit their current applicability.

Carbamazepine

Kaplan et al.[35] undertook a double-blind placebo-controlled crossover study of carbamazepine—a tricyclic similar in structure to imipramine—in normal weight bulimics. Their rationale: carbamazepine treatment is effective in partial complex epilepsy and bipolar disorder, both conditions believed to be related etiologically to subcortical dysregulation. Dosage of carbamazepine was titrated to maintain high-therapeutic serum levels, and subjects were treated for six to ten weeks. Of 16 patients, one experienced complete remission of bulimic symptoms, another showed marked improvement, and three others demonstrated partial response though this was continued after crossover to placebo.[32] Kaplan et al. concluded that carbamazepine was ineffective for the majority of bulimics, but that there may be a small minority who do respond dramatically. They liken this to phenytoin. Of interest, the one patient who experienced complete remission of bulimic symptoms with carbamazepine treatment had a history suggestive of bipolar disorder.

Sodium Valproate

Like carbamazepine, sodium valproate is an anticonvulsant known to be efficacious in some cases of bipolar disorder. Though no double-blind placebo-controlled trial has been performed in bulimics, Herridge and Pope[36] reported on one woman with bulimia and rapid-cycling bipolar disorder who experienced complete remission of her symptoms while being treated with sodium valproate in therapeutic serum levels. This case is reminiscent of the patient reported to experience remission of bulimic symptoms on carbamazepine.[32]

Drug Trials III—Suggested by Theorized Neurotransmitter Control of Appetite

Opiate Antagonists: Naloxone and Naltrexone

Considerable data collected in animal studies points to an important role for endogenous opioid peptides in the activation of feeding behavior through their actions in the hypothalamus. Of the various opiate receptors, the kappa receptor plays a pivotal role in the initiation of feeding.[37] Mitchell and Morley[38] summarized the animal data which demonstrates that opiate antagonists inhibit feeding, including in stress-induced feeding models. This led to trials in humans with eating disorders of both naloxone—a short-acting, parenterally administered opiate antagonist—and naltrexone, which is a long-acting, orally administered opiate antagonist used commonly in the medical management of opiate addiction.

Mitchell et al.[39] reported a double-blind placebo-controlled trial of naloxone among five normal-weight, hospitalized bulimics. Naloxone was administered intravenously just prior to a daily scheduled binge. They found the number of kilocalories consumed per binge was significantly reduced by naloxone as compared to placebo. They note that naloxone is a relatively weak antagonist to the kappa receptor, and suggest that an opiate antagonist with greater specificity for the kappa receptor might attenuate binge eating behavior more effectively.

The impact of naltrexone treatment on bulimic behavior was explored by Jonas and Gold[40] in an open-label trial of 20 bulimics who had each failed a prior antidepressant trial. Thirteen subjects took naltrexone in a dosage from 200 mg to 300 mg daily for six weeks; seven others took naltrexone in addition to continuing on an antidepressant that had resolved a recent episode of major depression but had not impacted upon bulimic symptoms. The authors selected this antidepressant nonresponder population in hopes of identifying a subgroup of bulimics in whom opioid systems play a more pivotal role than monoamine systems in the regulation of feeding behavior. Among the 13 patients taking naltrexone alone, six demonstrated complete remission of binging and purging; four experienced a 75 percent reduction; and three did not respond. In follow-up that occurred between two and eleven months later, most maintained their level of clinical improvement. Similar benefit was also noted among the seven subjects taking naltrexone in combination with an antidepressant. Jonas and Gold speculate that endogenous opioids are involved in the pathogenesis of eating disorders since naltrexone is a nearly pure opiate antagonist. However, they caution that naltrexone's effect could relate to its altering of other neurotransmitter systems, such as the monoamines, by blockade of opiate receptors. Jonas and Gold further suggest that involvement of opioid systems could account for the compulsive and irresistible urge to binge and purge, which has been likened in quality to the urges of substance abuse (e.g., heroin addiction). Although only one patient experienced mildly elevated liver function tests which corrected with lowering of naltrexone dose, they warn that several studies using similar high dosages of naltrexone in obese subjects were associated with significant incidence of hepatotoxicity.

In a further open-label trial, Jonas and Gold[41] examined the effect of six weeks of low dose (50 mg to 100 mg daily) versus high dose (200 mg to 300 mg daily) naltrexone among 16 bulimics who, too, had failed a prior antidepressant trial. Jonas and Gold found that only those receiving high dose naltrexone benefitted significantly. Several subjects who did not respond initially to low dose subsequently improved when dosage was increased into the 200 mg to 300 mg range. Jonas and Gold note that low dose naltrexone is effective in the medical management of opiate dependence. They explain this by citing a much greater naltrexone affinity for the mu receptor—important in mediating opioid dependency—than the kappa receptor, which is thought to be key in the regulation of feeding behavior; high dose naltrexone may be required to impact the kappa receptor.

Mitchell et al.[42] performed a double-blind placebo-controlled crossover study of low dose (50 mg daily) naltrexone for three weeks among 16 normal weight bulimics. Confirming the preceding negative report of low dose naltrexone, Mitchell et al. found no significant benefit of naltrexone compared to placebo.

Serotonin Agonists: Fenfluramine and Fluoxetine

Serotonin is known to play an important role in the ventromedial hypothalamus in producing satiety. Goldbloom has summarized[43] a number of studies in the rat that show that intraventricular injection of serotonin decreases feeding, as do a variety of peripheral interventions which increase serotonin centrally. These included the administration of the serotonin agonists fluoxetine and fenfluramine.

Over the past several years, attention has been focused on the theory that bulimic behavior results from a hyposerotonergic state; that is, a state of decreased satiety. In humans, direct evidence for this is limited and difficult to obtain. However, one study by Kaye et al.[44] of weight-restored bulimic and nonbulimic anorectics suggests lowered serotonin function in bulimics. They measured cerebrospinal fluid (CSF) 5-hydroxyindolacetic acid (5-HIAA) levels in 16 anorectic patients. CSF 5-HIAA concentration is thought to reflect the level of serotonin activity/metabolism in the central nervous system since 5-HIAA is the principal metabolite of serotonin. Five of the 16 anorectics had lost weight by restricting food intake only (nonbulimic anorectics) and 11 had also engaged in binge-purge behaviors (bulimic anorectics). There was no significant difference in CSF 5-HIAA levels between the two groups prior to restoration of normal weight. However, following weight restoration, the bulimic patients had lower CSF 5-HIAA levels than the nonbulimic group, consistent with lower serotonin activity among the bulimics. It was less clear whether there was a significant difference in CSF 5-HIAA levels between weight-restored bulimic anorectics and the normal control group. The failure of CSF 5-HIAA—and therefore serotonin activity—to return to normal levels in bulimic anorectics after weight recovery suggests that a hyposerotonergic state may perpetuate binging in even normal-weight bulimics.[43]

Dextrofenfluramine, a known appetite suppressant, increases presynaptic serotonin release and inhibits it reuptake. Robinson et al.[45] chose to investigate its effect on binge behavior after noting that methylamphetamine, another appetite suppressant, improved bulimic symptoms when administered intravenously.[46] They wished to clarify that it was the appetite suppressant effect, rather than the euphoriant or stimulant properties, of methylamphetamine that was antibulimic; fenfluramine, being a pure appetite suppressant, would clarify this point if beneficial for bulimic symptoms. They administered 60 mg of fenfluramine orally under double-blind placebo-controlled conditions to 15 hospitalized bulimics. Two hours later, food for binging was provided. The amount consumed was significantly less following fenfluramine, and was correlated with fenfluramine serum levels. Blouin et al.[47] point out that the rapid onset of diminished binging in this study suggests that fenfluramine acts by producing satiety. They performed another double-blind placebo-controlled crossover study of fenfluramine among 22 bulimics. For six weeks each, subjects received either fenfluramine 60 mg daily or desipramine 150 mg daily. Fenfluramine significantly reduced vomiting beginning the day after first administration, and this was maintained throughout the trial. They also found desipramine beneficial and within the first week of treatment, suggesting an antibulimic effect separate from its antidepressant property (see earlier discussion). Blouin et al. note that fenfluramine was tolerated well by their patients.

Russell et al.[48] performed a double-blind placebo-controlled trial of fenfluramine among 42 bulimics at a dosage of 30 mg daily for 12 weeks. Unfortunately, 17 subjects withdrew midway through the study. Fenfluramine was not significantly superior to placebo among those who completed the trial. Curiously, when the patients who withdrew prematurely were assessed, they showed significant improvement in bulimic symptoms while taking fenfluramine. The authors suggest that persistence of depression or other features of the eating disorder led to the high drop-out rate, rather than serious side effects of the medication.

Fluoxetine, a popular novel antidepressant agent, is a potent serotonin reuptake inhibitor that does not significantly impact upon the catecholamine system. Fuller et al.[49] demonstrated that fluoxetine selectively increases serotonin levels in the rat hypothalamus. This led to investigation of its role in promoting satiety; in nondepressed obese females, fluoxetine does have an anorexic effect.[50]

Several double-blind placebo-controlled trials of fluoxetine in bulimics demonstrate a clear beneficial response. Enas et al.[51] performed a double-blind placebo-controlled trial of fluoxetine in 382 outpatient bulimics, comparing eight weeks of fluoxetine in a dosage of 60 mg daily or 20 mg daily to placebo. At 60 mg daily, fluoxetine was significantly superior to placebo in decreasing the frequency of binging and vomiting; at 20 mg daily, fluoxetine was intermediate in benefit. Fluoxetine was well tolerated, as evidenced by a low drop-out rate that was consistent across the placebo and active drug groups. Depressive symptoms, pathological eating attitudes and behaviors, and carbohydrate craving also improved with fluoxetine treatment.

Foss et al.[52] reported on 40 bulimic outpatients given either fluoxetine 60 mg daily or placebo for between 6 and 24 weeks. Fluoxetine had a highly significant effect on bulimic symptoms as compared to placebo. In another double-blind placebo-controlled study, Freeman et al.[53] also demonstrated fluoxetine to be of benefit in bulimia.

Conclusion

Animal studies demonstrate the important role of the hypothalamus in regulating appetite and feeding behavior, including deranged feeding behavior. Multiple medication trials among human bulimics suggest that manipulation of various neurotransmitter systems impacts beneficially upon binge and purge behaviors. These medications include a range of noradrenergic and serotonergic antidepressants, as well as opiate antagonists. These presumably alter the noradrenergic, serotonergic, and endogenous opioid systems within the hypothalamus. It is likely that antidepressants work through an antibulimic property separate from their mood-stabilizing effect. Anticonvulsants and lithium have been shown largely ineffective. Understanding biological issues in bulimia is only one piece of the puzzle; prudent use of medication demonstrated effective in controlling binge/purge symptoms is an important part of the comprehensive treatment of a bulimic individual.

References

1. Leibowitz SF. Brain neurotransmitters and drug effects on food intake and appetite: Implications for eating disorders. In Walsh BT (ed): Eating Behavior in Eating Disorders. Washington, DC, American Psychiatric Press, 1988; 21–35.
2. Morley JE, Levine AS. The central control of appetite. *Lancet* 1983; 1:398–401.
3. Levy AB, Dixon KN, Stern SL. How are depression and bulimia related? *Am J Psychiatry* 1989; 146:162–169.
4. Hudson JI, Pope HG, Jonas JM. Phenomenologic relationship of eating disorders to major affective disorder. *Psychiatry Res* 1983; 9:345–354.
5. Walsh BT, Roose SP, Glassman AH. Bulimia and depression. *Psychosom Med* 1985; 47:123–131.
6. Pyle RL, Mitchell JE, Eckert ED. Bulimia: A report of 34 cases. *J Clin Psychiatry* 1981; 42:60–64.
7. Lee NF, Rush AJ, Mitchell JE. Bulimia and depression. *J Affective Disord* 1985; 9:231–238.
8. Musisi S, Garfinkel P. Comparative dexamethasone suppression test measurements in bulimia, depression and normal controls. *Can J Psychiatry* 1985; 30:190–194.
9. Stern SL, Dixon KN, Nemzer E. Affective disorder in the families of women with normal weight bulimia. *Am J Psychiatry* 1984; 141:1224–1227.
10. Katz JL, Kuperberg A, Pollock CP. Is there a relationship between eating disorder and affective disorder? New evidence from sleep recordings. *Am J Psychiatry* 1984; 141:753–759.
11. Levy AB, Dixon KN, Schmidt H. Sleep architecture in anorexia nervosa and bulimia. *Biol Psychiatry* 1988; 23:99–101.
12. Pope HG, Hudson JI, Jonas JM, Yurgelon-Todd D. Bulimia treated with imipramine: A placebo-controlled double-blind study. *Am J Psychiatry* 1983; 140:554–558.
13. Pope HG, Hudson JI, Jonas JM, Yurgelon-Todd D. Antidepressant treatment of bulimia: A two-year follow-up study. *J Clin Psychopharmacol* 1985; 5: 320–327.
14. Agras WS, Dorian B, Kirkley BG, Arnow B, Bachman J. Imipramine in the treatment of bulimia: A double-blind controlled study. *Int J Eating Disord* 1987; 6:29–38.

15. Mitchell JE, Groat R. A placebo-controlled, double-blind trial of amitriptyline in bulimia. *J Clin Psychopharmacol* 1984; 4:186–193.
16. Hughes PL, Wells LA, Cunningham CJ, Ilstrup DM. Treating bulimia with desipramine: A double-blind, placebo-controlled study. *Arch Gen Psychiatry* 1986; 43:182–186.
17. Barlow J, Blouin J, Blouin A, Perez E. Treatment of bulimia with desipramine: A double-blind crossover study. *Can J Psychiatry* 1988; 33:129–133.
18. Blouin J, Blouin A, Perez E, Barlow J. Bulimia: Independence of antibulimic and antidepressant properties of desipramine. *Can J Psychiatry* 1989; 34:24–39.
19. Sabine EJ, Yonace A, Farrington AJ, Barratt KH, Wakeling A. Bulimia nervosa: A placebo-controlled double-blind therapeutic trial of mianserin. *Br J Clin Pharmacol* 1983; 15:195S–202S.
20. Pope HG, Hudson JI. Antidepressant drug therapy for bulimia: Current status. *J Clin Psychiatry* 1986; 47:339–345.
21. McGrath PJ, Quitkin FM, Stewart JW. An open trial of mianserin. *Am J Psychiatry* 1981; 138:530–532.
22. Walsh BT, Gladis M, Roose SP, Stewart JW, Stetner F, Glassman A. Phenelzine vs placebo in 50 patients with bulimia. *Arch Gen Psychiatry* 1988; 45:471–475.
23. Kennedy SH, Piran N, Warsh JJ, Prendergast P, Mainprize E, Whynot C, Garfinkel PE. A trial of isocarboxazid in the treatment of bulimia nervosa. *J Clin Psychopharmacol* 1988; 8:391–396.
24. Pope HG, Keck PE, McElroy SL, Hudson JI. A placebo-controlled study of trazodone in bulimia nervosa. *J Clin Psychopharmacol* 1989; 9:254–259.
25. Hsu LKG. Treatment of bulimia with lithium. *Am J Psychiatry* 1984; 141: 1260–1262.
26. Hsu LKG, Clement L, Santhouse R. Treatment of bulimia with lithium: A preliminary study. *Psychopharmacol Bull* 1987; 23:45–48.
27. Pope HG, Herridge PL, Hudson JI, Fontaine R, Yurgelon-Todd D. Treatment of bulimia with nomifensine. *Am J Psychiatry* 1986; 143:371–373.
28. Horne RL, Ferguson JM, Pope HG, Hudson JI, Lineberry CG, Ascher J, Cato A. Treatment of bulimia with bupropion: A multicenter controlled trial. *J Clin Psychiatry* 1988; 49:262–266.
29. Green RS, Rau JH. Treatment of compulsive eating disturbances with anticonvulsant medication. *Am J Psychiatry* 1974; 131:428–432.
30. Rau JH, Green RS. Compulsive eating: A neuropsychologic approach to certain eating disorders. *Comp Psychiatry* 1975; 16:223–231.
31. Wermuth BM, Davis KL, Hollister LE, Stunkard AJ. Phenytoin treatment of the binge-eating syndrome. *Am J Psychiatry* 1977; 134:1249–1253.
32. Kaplan AS. Anticonvulsant treatment of eating disorders. In Garfinkel PE, Garner DM (eds): The Role of Drug Treatments for Eating Disorders. New York, Brunner/Mazel, 1987; 96–123.
33. Rau JH, Green RS. Binge-purge syndrome. Neurological factors affecting binge eating: Body over mind. In Hawkins RG, Fremouw WJ, Clement PF (eds): Diagnosis, Treatment and Research. New York, Springer, 1984; 123–143.
34. Wegner JR, Struve FA. Incidence of the 14- and 6-per-second positive spike pattern in an adult clinical population: An empirical note. *J Nerv Ment Dis* 1977; 164:340–345.

35. Kaplan AS, Garfinkel PE, Darby PL, Garner DM. Carbamazepine in the treatment of bulimia. *Am J Psychiatry* 1983; 140:1225–1226.
36. Herridge PL, Pope HG. Treatment of bulimia and rapid-cycling bipolar disorder with sodium valproate: A case report. *J Clin Psychopharmacol* 1985; 5:229–230.
37. Morley JE, Levine AS, Grace M. An investigation of the role of kappa opiate receptor agonists in the initiation of feeding. *Life Sci* 1982; 31:2617–2626.
38. Mitchell JE, Morley JE. Endogenous opioid peptides and feeding. In Hudson JI, Pope HG (eds): The Psychobiology of Bulimia. Washington, DC, American Psychiatric Press, 1987; 101–113.
39. Mitchell JE, Laine DE, Morley JE, Levine AS. Naloxone but not CCK-8 may attenuate binge-eating behavior in patients in with the bulimia syndrome. *Biol Psychiatry* 1987, 21:1399–1406.
40. Jonas JM, Gold MS. Opiate antagonists as clinical probes in bulimia. In Hudson JI, Pope HG (eds): The Psychobiology of Bulimia. Washington, DC, American Psychiatric Press, 1987; 117–127.
41. Jonas JM, Gold MS. The use of opiate antagonists in treating bulimia: A study of low-dose versus high-dose naltrexone. *Psychiatry Res* 1988; 24: 195–199.
42. Mitchell JE, Christenson G, Jennings J, Huber M, Thomas B, Pomeroy C, Morley J. A placebo-controlled, double-blind crossover study of naltrexone hydrochloride in outpatients with normal weight bulimia. *J Clin Psychopharmacol* 1989; 9:94–97.
43. Goldbloom DS. Serotonin in eating disorders: Theory and therapy. In Garfinkel PE, Garner DM (eds): The Role of Drug Treatments for Eating Disorders. New York, Brunner/Mazel, 1987; 124–149.
44. Kaye WH, Ebert MH, Gwirtsman HE, Weiss SR. Differences in brain serotonergic metabolism between nonbulimic and bulimic patients with anorexia nervosa. *Am J Psychiatry* 1984; 141:1159–1161.
45. Robinson PH, Checkley SA, Russell GFM. Suppression of eating by fenfluramine in patients with bulimia nervosa. *Br J Psychiatry* 1985; 146:169–176.
46. Ong YL, Checkley SA, Russell GFM. Suppression of bulimic symptoms with methylamphetamine. *Br J Psychiatry* 1983; 1143:288–293.
47. Blouin AG, Blouin JH, Perez EL, Bushnik T, Zuro C, Mulder E. Treatment of bulimia with fenfluramine and desipramine. *J Clin Psychopharmacol* 1988; 8261–8269.
48. Russell GFM, Checkley SA, Feldman J, Eisler I. A controlled trial of d-fenfluramine in bulimia nervosa. *Clin Neuropharmacol* 1988; 11:S149–S159.
49. Fuller RW, Perry KW, Molloy BB. Effect of an uptake inhibitor of serotonin metabolism in rat brain. *Life Sci* 1974; 15:1161–1171.
50. Ferguson JM. Fluoxetine-induced weight loss in overweight, non-depressed subjects. *Am J Psychiatry* 1986; 143:1496.
51. Enas GG, Pope HG, Vevine LR. Fluoxetine in bulimia nervosa: A double-blind study [abstr]. Presented at the American Psychiatric Association. San Francisco, May 11, 1989.
52. Foss I, Trygstad O, Jettestad S. Double-blind study of fluoxetine and placebo in treatment of bulimia nervosa [abstr]. Presented at the Fourth International Conference on Eating Disorders. New York, April 28, 1990.

53. Freeman CP, Morris JE, Cheshire KE. A double-blind controlled trial of fluoxetine versus placebo for bulimia nervosa [abstr]. Presented at the Second International Conference On Eating Disorders. New York, April 22–24, 1988.

6
Biological Factors in Obesity

William S. Rea and Irl L. Extein

Overview

Obesity is an extremely common disorder in many societies—both industrial and preindustrial. Like many other pathological conditions, obesity results from a combination of biological, psychological/behavioral, behavioral, and social factors. It is at times very difficult to separate physical findings that are a complication of obesity, rather than a biological factor underlying it. In this chapter, we deal only with biological factors that may contribute to obesity, leaving the issue of complications to others.

If we view obesity as an interaction between host and environmental factors, it seems natural to look at the host factors most likely to lead to increase in weight. Among these areas, much research has been done in the fields of genetics, in the essential biochemistry and neuroanatomy of feeding and satiety, in the early life growth of adipose tissue, and in endocrine interactions with weight and appetite regulation. We shall examine each of these areas in turn.

Genetics

The genetic contribution to human obesity is a complex one. Studies can be divided into animal studies, studies of families with members affected by idiopathic obesity, and studies of families with members affected by unusual genetic illnesses with associated obesity (e.g., Prader-Willi syndrome).

Animal Studies

Few animals are naturally obese. In the search for an animal model of this disorder, Ingalls et al. bred a strain of mice in which weight was connected to a single-locus gene. In this strain, a mouse that was homozygous for the recessive gene was severely obese.[1] Other strains have since been isolated, including the Żucker-fatty rat, which also inherits obesity as an autosomal Mendelian recessive trait.[2] These rats are obese, hyperphagic, and hyperinsulinemic, but their blood glucose remains at normal levels. Their adipocytes are increased in both size and number. This strain of rat also shows increased excretion of corticosteroids and diminished pituitary responsiveness to corticotropin-releasing factor.[3]

Overall, these strains of genetically obese animals show some alterations in cell sensitivity to corticosteroids, insulin, and glucagon, probably connected with the single gene locus. These strains have been useful in clarifying the interrelationships of hormonal and cellular responsiveness to feeding, and to examining some hypotheses regarding the human obese. However, there is no indication that most idiopathic human obesity has a single gene locus, and in fact some evidence that it is multigenic in transmission, with partial penetrance. However, human studies have shown a genetic parent-child linkage in obesity.

Obesity genes in the mouse have been mapped to chromosome 4 (the db gene) and 6 (the ob gene). Genetic mapping has also been done for genes regulating the production of adipsin, calcitonin, cholecystokinin, Gi alpha and Gs subunits of G proteins, insulin, and lipoprotein lipase. None of these sites are syngenic with the obesity genes. It seems unlikely that any of the other transmitters currently under investigation will map specifically to the obesity gene. In mice, it seems likely that posttranscriptional and/or posttranslational factors are involved in effecting the specific changes seen in the obese animals.[4]

Animal models of obesity other than the genetic have included dietary ones and hypothalamic ones, examined below.

Human Studies

Epidemiologic

Mayer looked at the weight of offspring of obese and nonobese parents. If both parents were obese, about 80 percent of the offspring also were. If only one parent was obese, about 50 percent of the offspring were obese. If neither parent was obese, only 10 percent of the offspring were obese.[5] This study demonstrated a clear connection between parent and child weight. An important question is whether this is truly a genetic transmission, or possibly a product of home environment or early feeding practices. The question becomes one of "nature versus nurture" and is at least partly answered by adoption studies. Studies of identical twins have examined how efficient the body is in converting excess dietary energy to fat. The results show that this property is, to a large extent, inherited.[6] Individuals seem to inherit a predetermined disposition to store fat efficiently (and thus to be at risk for obesity) or not (and thus to be thin).

Epidemiologic data regarding childhood obesity,[7] like that noted for animal studies, argues against a single genetic site for inheritance, and for a complex interaction of host and environmental factors. Like many other human disorders, environmental effects may contribute as much, if not more, to the expression of the syndrome than genetic factors.

Bouchard[8] studied 1698 individuals from 409 families in French Quebec, and found that the heritability of amount of subcutaneous fat was almost zero, while the additive genetic effect was about 25 percent of the variation. This epidemiologic data also argues against a single-gene mode of transmission of the disorder.

Racial/Ethnic Variations

Looking at racial or ethnic groups that have been relatively isolated genetically, and that have a high incidence of obesity, can also yield interesting insights. One such group is the Pima Indian tribe of the southwestern United States, with about eight thousand members. The data about climate during the past several hundred years in the area in which the Pima Indians live suggests there was inadequate rainfall at least every other year, and severe drought (lasting at least two years) every 25 years.[9] These climatic conditions could be expected to lead to frequent periods of severe famine.

The prevalence of type II diabetes in this population exceeds 45 percent and more than 75 percent of the Pimas are obese. Longitudinal studies of metabolic measurements have been conducted in 200 nondiabetic members of this tribe. In comparing members of this study population, there is quite a large variability in the resting metabolic rate at any given body weight and body composition. It did seem that metabolic rate after adjustment for body composition and body weight is a familial trait. The researchers found that a low metabolic rate is a risk factor for body weight gain and that, in response to body weight gain, there is a "normalization" of the resting metabolic rate. These researchers suggest that these individuals are predisposed to the development of obesity because of an inherited tendency for a "thrifty" metabolic rate, or in other words an efficient mechanism for converting excess dietary energy into fat.[10] Such a mechanism would have favored survival of affected individuals during times of famine, as they would have increased adipose energy stores to draw upon.

In this tribe the prevalence of diabetes is increasing. A likely link between obesity and diabetes is tissue insulin resistance. There is some evidence to suggest that a useful correlation of metabolic rate in these people is the fat-free mass, and that insulin resistance in this tribe is not secondary to inhibition of glucose metabolism by free fatty acids. Rather, obesity among the Pima is associated with an increase in fat-free mass as well as in fat mass, with a hypothesized increase in tissue insulin resistance as a consequence.[11]

Adoption Studies

Stunkard[12] reviewed genetic contributions to human obesity. In Denmark, where comprehensive data is kept on adopted children and where there is a centralized health care system, adoption studies showed a high correlation of body mass index of adopted children with their biological parents and no correlation with their adopted parents. The body mass of the adoptees was also highly correlated with that of their biological siblings. Bivariate analysis of identical twins however showed high intrapair correlations among normal weight twins and low correlations among the obese twins distributions, suggesting a strong environmental influence.

Data on identical twins reared apart nonetheless shows evidence of high levels of heritability.

Summary of the adoption studies shows a clear hereditary component in the illness, with some evident additional environmental contribution.

Rare Genetic Studies

There are interestingly a few severe genetic disorders in which obesity plays a compelling role, including Laurence-Moon-Biedl syndrome,[13] and the Prader-Willi syndrome.[14] One case diagnosed clinically as Prader-Willi syndrome was shown by Giemsa banding to have 15/15 chromosome translocation.[15] The significance of this finding is unknown.

A case was also described of a young woman with syndromic obesity and her normal mother, who both have an abnormal chromosome 15. The patient had marked obesity, acanthosis nigricans, short fingers, and severe cone degeneration of the retina. She had high plasma insulin levels, hypothyroidism, and an empty sella on CT scan. High-resolution chromosome banding demonstrated an increase in band 15q12. Further analysis showed the same abnormal 15 in her normal mother but not in her normal sister. This case and recent reports in the literature indicate that duplication of chromosome 15q in the PWS region may be associated with a syndrome of obesity, acanthosis nigricans, empty sella, and rodcore dystrophy as well as with a normal phenotype.[16]

Another rare genetic disorder is the Cohen syndrome, consisting of mental retardation, obesity, hypotonia, and a characteristic craniofacial appearance. Since its original description, 18 patients have been reported. This disorder is most probably transmitted as an autosomal recessive trait, and may involve a basic defect in connective tissue.[17]

Perinatal Factors

Adipose Cell Hypothesis

Hirsch formulated the adipose cell hypothesis of obesity.[18] His basic tenet was that obese individuals had not only increased size of their adipose cells, but also increased numbers. He also postulated that the increase in numbers of adipose cells was determined early in life due to genetic and perinatal feeding factors.

Knittle and Hirsch examined nonobese children, and showed two periods in their lives in which fat cells (adipocytes) markedly proliferated. These periods generally coincided with ages birth to two years, and with the years just prior to puberty.[19] Although these perinatal factors are important in the development of obesity (especially the childhood variant), they are clearly not the primary biological determinants of development of the syndrome.

Neuroanatomy and Neurochemistry of Eating

It has been known since the 1940s that lesions made in the ventromedial hypothalamic region (VMH) can lead to enormous hyperphagia and consequent obesity.[20,21] Stimulation of this area in normal animals would lead to cessation of eating, so that the VMH became known as the "satiety center" of the brain. Nobrega and Coscina found that dopamine and norepinephrine interactions partially mediated the development of hyperphagia and obesity following VMH lesions in animals.[22] Bray reviewed the literature and reported on eight human patients who suffered from severe obesity following lesions of the ventromedial hypothalamus.[23] Christiansen et al. reported a case of a 19 year old woman who developed severe hyperphagia and who doubled her body weight within four months after a probable pituitary cerebrovascular accident.[24] It should be noted that hypothalamic damage as an etiology for obesity is likely to be quite rare.

In the 1950s, a separate area in the lateral hypothalamus was labeled as the "feeding center," after ablation studies showed that destruction of it led to cessation of feeding, weight loss, and eventual death of the animal.[25] Unfortunately, subsequent studies have revealed that the separation of "satiety" and "feeding" centers is an oversimplification, as many areas quite near each other anatomically seem to have diametrically opposed functions.[26]

There are a plethora of neurotransmitters involved in regulation of eating, many of them operating via hypothalamic mechanisms. An excellent recent review by Leibowitz[27] separates them broadly into those that stimulate eating and those that inhibit it.

Amines

Catecholamines

Administration of catecholamines into the medial hypothalamus causes a short-term increase in overall food intake.[28,29] Chronic infusion of norepinephrine into the hypothalamic paraventricular nucleur also lead to increased eating and increased weight.[30] Vagotomy below the diaphragm reverses this syndrome,[31] suggesting a strong autonomic component in its full expression. Injection of amphetamine (which acts via release of catecholamones) into the lateral hypothalamus causes a marked suppression of initiation of eating. Injection of amphetamine, dopamine, or epinephrine led to a strong inhibition of protein consumption, with no effect on carbohydrates and little on fats.[32]

Another factor that may mediate some of the suppression of eating on administration of amphetamine is the heat production from this compound,[33] as increased thermogenesis from brown adipose tissue may also function as a signal to stop eating.[34] Cocaine, which facilitates dopaminergic neurotransmission in the brain, suppresses appetite. Part of the cocaine withdrawal syndrome, hypothesized to be related to dopamine depletion, includes rebound increase in appetite.[35]

Serotonin

The involvement of serotonin in the regulation of appetite has been quite complex. Recent receptor research has helped clarify the situation, as it develops that two different serotonin receptors are involved in feeding regulation, the 5-HT-1A and 5-HT-1B receptors.[36] The 1A receptor seems to stop feeding, while the 1B receptor augments it.

Serotonin has been implicated in carbohydrate craving.[37,38] There appears to be a subgroup of obese people who have excessive snacking on carbohydrates. These individuals show in preliminary studies some positive response to serotonin-reuptake blockers. They also show increased incidence of depression.[39] Fenfluramine, a serotonergic agonist, causes rats to eat less carbohydrates[40] and causes similar effects in human beings.[41] Preliminary data from studies of the use of the serotonin-reuptake inhibitor antidepressant fluoxetine suggest an associated loss of weight.[42] Whether fluoxetine may have actual clinical utility as a diet aid awaits more definitive studies.[43]

Dopamine

As noted previously, infusion of dopamine into the lateral hypothalamus leads to diminished protein consumption. In addition, the dopaminergic compound bromocriptine stimulates eating.[44] However, unlike norepinephrine and serotonin, there does not seem to be increased brain levels of dopamine in genetically obese mice.[45] One study reports an increased number of dopamine receptors in the brains of these animals.[46] The role of dopamine in the development or maintenance of obesity is at this time still ambiguous.

Neuropeptides

Opioids

In the early 1960s it was demonstrated that use of exogenous opiates in rats could stimulate eating.[47] Conversely, opiate antagonists including naloxone[48] and naltrexone[49] had some appetite-suppressing properties. In fact, Mitchell and Morley[50] reviewed five studies systematically looking at the use of opiate antagonists in obesity, with little indication that naltrexone aids weight loss in human beings.

It should be noted that animal studies have shown that the kappa opiate receptor is the one primarily involved in regulation of appetite.[51] Morley and Levine[52] have identified dynorphin (an endogenous opioid peptide that preferentially binds to this receptor), and Schultz et al. alpha-neo-endorphin[53] as primary opioids involved in the regulation of eating. Beta endorphin is increased in the pituitaries of obese rodents.[54]

The use of opioid antagonists in genetically obese mice has shown the rodents to be extremely sensitive to minute doses of naloxone and naltrexone, which suppress their eating at doses of an order of magnitude lower than control animals.[55]

Facchinetti et al. looked at hypothalamic regulation of many chemicals in obese individuals as compared with normal-weight controls. In a study of eight obese patients, beta-endorphin, cortisol, ACTH, and beta-lipotropin were measured at baseline periods and sequentially after administration of 1 milligram (mg) of dexamethasone orally (the dexamethasone suppression test). In comparison with the normal controls, the beta-endorphin levels in the obese patients were three times as high, and failed to suppress with the administration of the synthetic corticosteroid. In addition, three of the eight obese patients showed an elevation of cortisol sampled 17 hours after administration of the dexamethasone (a so-called "late-escape pattern"). This correlated highly with the presence of depression in these patients as shown by concurrent psychological testing (as it does in depressed, normal weight individuals). These data are overall consistent with a hypothesis of beta-endorphinemia in these obese individuals.[56]

In addition, a significant subgroup may suffer from biological depression. Other studies have found a blunted response to corticotropin-releasing hormone of cortisol in obese adults[57] and beta-endorphin in obese children.[58]

In a comprehensive review of the role of opioid receptors and energy balance, Margules[59] notes that kappa and delta receptors in the central nervous system allow the body to expend energy, while epsilon receptors in the periphery promote energy conservation.

Polypeptides

Neuropeptide Y is a 36 amino acid peptide that occurs both in the central and peripheral nervous systems, with a concentration of receptors in the paraventricular nucleus of the hypothalamus, as well as in the olfactory bulb, superficial layers of the cortex, ventral hippocampus, lateral septum, and area postrema.[60] Injections of neuropeptide Y into the hypothalamus produce a marked increase in ingestion of carbohydrates, with little or no alteration in fat or protein intake. As a result, chronic injection of this peptide leads to obesity.[61] This peptide not only increases the rate of eating, but also its duration. This chemical triggers eating even in satiated rats, and is much longer in action than the catecholamines.[62]

Human studies of peptides have looked at a related polypeptide, PYY, in anorectic and bulimic patients. Cerebrospinal fluid levels of PYY were found to be markedly increased in bulimic women who had abstained from binging for 30 days, as compared to both normal controls and to their own values during times when they were binging. No change was found in PYY levels in anorectics. It is quite possible that binges may be triggered in the bulimic group as a response to elevated PPY levels.[63] The functioning of PYY in obesity bears further investigation.

Cholecystokinin[64] and bombesin, peptides present in the gut, may convey satiety signals to receptors in the hypothalamus.[65]

Nutritional Factors

Cultural Variations in Diet and Ideals

It should be noted that obesity has not always been seen as a disorder, and in fact there are cultures today in which obesity is viewed as a sexually desirable trait. In these cultures, obesity may be genetically selected for as a result.

Availability of Food (Poverty or Feast-or-Famine)

Brown and Konner have advanced an anthropological theory of the evolutionary benefit from obesity, centering on the frequency of "feast-or-famine" conditions throughout much of prehistory, and among many nonindustrialized contemporary societies.[66] Whiting[67] surveyed 115 pre-industrial societies and found that many societies had frequent severe food shortages (at least annually in 47 percent of these societies). Brown and Konner hypothesize that in these conditions evolution favored individuals who could store metabolic energy in the form of adiposity during feasts for use during famines. This hypothesis would fit well with the data regarding the Pima Indians noted previously.

Metabolic Factors

Endocrine

The common myth attributes obesity to a glandular problem. Surprisingly few severely obese people are found to suffer from endocrine disturbance, however. Some disorders that can lead to mild-to-moderate obesity are hypothyroidism, adrenal hyperplasia, and hypogonadism.

Biological Models of Obesity

Most models of obesity recognize that it is a problem of storage of excess dietary energy. Early models of obesity were similar to a bank account model. In these, weight (or the balance in the bank account) was seen as calorie equivalents. Eating more (or making deposits) would increase the balance and increased activity (withdrawals) would decrease it. There are several problems with this model, including wide individual variation in metabolic rates, and the fact that hyperphagia in most people produces only limited obesity.[68] Fuller and Yen[69] pointed out that an increased efficiency in converting dietary energy into fat is usually necessary to produce obesity. Much current research is focused on clarifying the factors that might lead to such an increase. One possibility is in the field of heat production: some genetically obese rodents show signs of altered thermogenesis preceding development of obesity.[70] There is still some controversy regarding the relative importance of thermogenesis as a contributing factor for the development of obesity in humans,[71] but it is a promising area for further study.

Whether or not thermogenesis is a core defect in the development of obesity, it seems quite clear that the development of this disorder involves a complicated interaction of host and environmental factors. Further exciting research into neurotransmitter regulation of both eating behavior and other vegetative functions may lead to *effective pharmacologic* interventions.

References

1. Ingalls AM, Dickie NM, Snell GD. Obese, new mutation in the mouse. *J Heredity* 1950; 41:317–318.
2. Bray GA. The Zucker-fatty rat: A review. *Fed Proc* 1977; 36:148–153.
3. Cunningham JJ, Calleses J, Garrido F, Carr DB, Bode HH. Hypercorticosteronuria and diminished pituitary-responsiveness to corticotropin-releasing factor in obese zucker rats. *Endocrinology* 1986; 118:98–101.
4. Johnson PR, Greenwood MR, Horwitz BA, Stern JS. Animal models of obesity: Genetic aspects. *Ann Rev Nutr* 1991; 11:325–353.
5. Mayer J. Genetic factors in human obesity. *Ann NY Acad Sci* 1965; 131:142.

6. Van Itallie TB. Obesity, genetics, and ponderal set point. *Clin Neuropharmacol* 1988; 11 Suppl 1:S1–7.
7. Dietz WH, Bandini LG, Gortmaker S. Epidemiologic and metabolic risk factors for childhood obesity. *Klin Pediatr* 1990; 202:69–72.
8. Bouchard C. Genetique et obesite chez l'homme. *Diabete Metab* 1988; 14: 407–413.
9. Minnis PE. Social Adaptation to Food Stress: A Prehistoric Southwestern Example. Chicago, University of Chicago Press, 1985.
10. Ravussin E, Bogardus C. Energy expenditure in the obese: Is there a thrift gene? *Infusionstherapie* 1990; 17:108–112.
11. Lillioja S, Bogardus C. Obesity and insulin resistance: Lessons learned from the Pima Indians. *Diabetes Metab Rev* 1988; 4:517–540.
12. Stunkard AJ. Genetic contributions to human obesity. *Res Publ Assoc Nerv Ment Dis* 1991; 69:205–218.
13. Laurence HE. Obesity, mental retardation, polydactylis, retinal pigmentation, and hypogenitalism (Laurence-Moon-Biedl Syndrome). Case report. *Bull N Engl J Med* 1944; 6:285–290.
14. Hofnagel R. The Prader-Willi syndrome. *J Ment Defic* 1967; 2:1–10.
15. Hawkey CJ, Smithies A. The Prader-Willi syndrome with a 15/15 translocation. Case report and review of the literature. *J Med Genet* 1976; 13: 152–157.
16. Shohat M, Shohat T, Rimoin DL, Mohandas T, Heckenlively J, Magenis RE, Davidson MB, Korenberg JR. Rearrangement of chromosome 15 in the region q11.2—q12 in an individual with obesity syndrome and her normal mother. *Am J Med Genet* 1990; 37:173–177.
17. Friedman E, Sack J. The Cohen syndrome: Report of five new cases and a review of the literature. *J Craniofac Genet Dev Biol* 1982; 2:193–200.
18. Hirsch J. The adipose cell hypothesis. *N Engl J Med* 1976; 295:389.
19. Knittle JL, Hirsh J. Effect of early nutrition on the development of fat epididymal fat pods: Cellulosity and metabolism. *J Clin Invest* 1968; 47: 2091.
20. Heatherington AW, Ranson SW. Hypothalamic lesions and adiposity in the rat. *Anatomical Records* 1940; 78:149–172.
21. Heatherington AW, Ranson SW. The spontaneous activity and food intake of rats with hypothalamic lesions. *Am J Physiol* 1942; 136:609–617.
22. Nobrega JN, Coscina DV. Dopamine-norepinephrine interactions in the development of hyperphagia and obesity following medial hypothalamic lesions. *Pharmacology, Biochemistry and Behavior* 1986; 25:401–409.
23. Bray GA, Gallagher TF. Manifestations of hypothalamic obesity in man: A comprehensive investigation of eight patients and a review of the literature. *Medicine* 1975; 54:301–330.
24. Christiansen KH, Petersen P, Lindholm J. Rapid development of a Pickwickian syndrome after pituitary apoplexy. *Int J Eating Disord* 1988; 7:701–704.
25. Anand BK, Brobeck JR. Hypothalamic control of food intake in rats and cats. *Yale J Biol Med* 1952; 24:123–140.
24. Morley JE, Levine AS, Krahn DD. Neurotransmitter regulation of appetite and eating. In: Blinder BJ, Chaitlin BF, Goldstein RS (eds): The Eating Disorders: Medical and Psychological Bases of Diagnosis and Treatment. New York, PMA Publishing, 1988; 11–19.

27. Leibowitz SF. Hypothalamic neutrotransmitters in relation to normal and disturbed eating patterns. *Ann NY Acad Sci* 1987; 499:137–143.
28. Grossman SP. Direct adrenergic and cholinergic stimulation of hypothalamic mechanisms. *Am J Physiology* 1962; 303:872–882.
29. Leibowitz SF. Neurochemical systems of the hypothalamus in control of feeding and drinking behavior and water-electrolyte excretion. In Morgane PJ, Panksepp J (eds): Handbook of the Hypothalamus. New York, Marcel Dekker, 1980; 3A:299–437.
30. Lichtenstein SS, Marinescu C, Leibowitz SF. Chronic infusion of norepinephrine and clonidine into the hypothalamic paraventricular nucleus. *Brain Res Bull* 1984; 13:591–595.
31. Bray GA. Hypothalamic and genetic obesity: An appraisal of the autonomic hypothesis and the endocrine hypothesis. *Int J Obesity* 1984; 8(Suppl 1): 119–137.
32. Leibowitz SF, Shor-Posner G, MacLow C, Grinker JA. Amphetamine: Effects on meal patterns and macronutrient selection. *Brain Res Bull* 1986; 17: 681–689.
33. Wellman PJ. Influence of amphetamine on brown adipose tissue thermogenesis. *Res Commun Chem Pathol Pharmacol* 1983; 41:173–176.
34. Glick ZV. Inverse relationship between brown fat thermogenesis and meal size: The thermostatic control of food intake revisited. *Physiol Behav* 1982; 29:1137–1140.
35. Jaffe JH. Drug addiction and drug abuse. In Gilman AG, Rall TW, Nies AS, Taylor P (eds): The Pharmacological Basis of Therapeutics. New York, Pergamon Press, 1990; 522–573.
36. Dourish CT, Huston PH, Kennett GA, Curzon A. 8-OH-DPAT-induced hyperphagia: Its' neural basis and possible therapeutic relevance. *Appetite* 1986; 7(Suppl):127–145.
37. Li ETS, Anderson GH. 5-Hydroxytryptamine: A modulator of food composition but not quantity? *Life Sci* 1984; 34:2453–2460.
38. Caballero B. Brain-serotonin and carbohydrate craving in obesity. *Int J Obesity* 1987; 11:179–183.
39. Wurtman JJ. Disorders of food intake: Excessive carbohydrate snack intake among a class of obese people. *Ann NY Acad Sci* 1987; 499:197–202.
40. Wurtman JJ, Wurtman RJ. Fenfluramine and other serotonergic drugs depress food intake and carbohydrate consumption while sparing protein consumption. *Curr Med Res Opin* 1979; 6(Suppl 1):28–33.
41. Wurtman JJ, Wurtman RJ. d-Fenfluramine selectively decreases carbohydrate but not protein intake in obese subjects. *Int J Obesity* 1985; 8:79–84.
42. Feighner JP. A comparative trial of fluoxetine and amitriptyline in patients with major depressive disorder. *J Clin Psychiatry* 1985; 46:369–372.
43. Ferguson JM. Fluoxetine-induced weight loss in overweight, nondepressed subjects. *Am J Psychiatry* 1986; 143:1496.
44. Morley JE, Levine AS, Grace M, Kneip J. Dynorphin (1–13), dopamine and feeding in rats. *Pharmacol Biochem Behav* 1982; 16:701–705.
45. Lorden JF, Oltmans GA. Hypothalamic and pituitary catecholamine levels in genetically obese mice (ob/ob). *Brain Res* 1977; 131:162–166.
46. El-Refai MF, Chan TM. Possible involvement of a hypothalamic dopaminergic receptor in development of genetic obesity in mice. *Biochim Biophys Acta* 1986; 880:16–25.

47. Martin WR, Wikler A, Eades CG, et al. Tolerance to and physical dependence on morphine in rats. *Psychopharmacology* 1963; 4:247–260.
48. Holtzman SG. Behavioral effects of separate and combined administration of naloxone and d-amphetamine. *J Pharm Exp Ther* 1974; 189:51–60.
49. Atkinson RL, Berke LK, Drake CR, Bibbs ML, Williams FL, Kaiser DL. Effects of long-term therapy with naltrexone on body weight in obesity. *Clin Pharmacol Ther* 1985; 38:419–422.
50. Mitchell JE, Morley JE. Endogenous opioid peptides and feeding. In Hudson JI, Pope HG (eds): The Psychobiology of Bulimia. Washington, DC, APA Press, 1987; 99–114.
51. Morley JE, Levine AS, Grace M, Kniep J. An investigation of the role of kappa opiate receptor agonists in the initiation of feeding. *Life Sci* 1982; 31:2617–2626.
52. Morley JE, Levine AS. Dynorphin (1–13) induces spontaneous feeding in rats. *Life Sci* 1981; 29:1901–1903.
53. Schulz R, Wilhelm A, Dirlich G. Intracerebral injection of different antibodies against endogenous opioids suggests alpha-neoendorphin participation in control of feeding behavior. *Naunyn Schmiedebergs Arch Pharmacol* 1984; 326:222–226.
54. Margules DL, Moisset B, Lewis MJ. Beta-endorphin is associated with overeating in genetically obese mice (ob/ob) and fats (fa/fa). *Science* 1978; 202: 988–991.
55. Ferguson-Segall M, Flynn JJ, Walker J, Margules DL. Increased immunoreactive dynorphin and leu-enkephalin in posterior pituitary of obese mice (ob/ob) and supersensitivity to drugs that act at kappa receptors. *Life Sci* 1982; 31:2233–2238.
56. Facchinetti F, Giovannini C, Barletta C, Petraglia F, Buzzetti R, Burla F, Lazzari R, Genazzani AR, Scavo D. Hyperendorphinemia in obesity and relationships to affective state. *Physiology and Behavior* 1986; 36:937–940.
57. Kopelman PG, Grossman A, Rees LH, Lavender P, Coy D, Besser GM. The cortisol response to corticotrophin-releasing factor is blunted in obesity. *Clin Endocrinology* 1988; 28:15–18.
58. Bernasco S, Petragli F, Iughetti L, Marcelli C, Lamborgh A, Facchine F, Genazzan AR. Impaired beta-endorphin response to human corticotropin-releasing hormone in obese children. *Acta Endocrinologica* 1988; 119:7–10.
59. Margules DL. Energy balance and opioid receptors: Epsilons in the periphery promote conservation; kappa and delta in the CNS permit expenditures. In Blinder BJ, Chaitlin BF, Goldstein RS (eds): The Eating Disorders: Medical and Psychological Bases of Diagnosis and Treatment. New York, PMA Publishing, 1988; 21–27.
60. Martel JC, St. Pierre S, Quirion R. Neuropeptide Y receptors in rat brain: Autoradiographic localization. *Peptides* 1986; 7:55–60.
61. Morley JE, Levine AS, Gomell BA, Kneip J, Grace M. Studies on the effect of neuropeptide Y on ingestive behaviors in the rat. *Am J Physiology* 1987; 252:599–609.
62. Stanley BF, Leibowitz SF. Neuropeptide Y: Stimulation of feeding and drinking by injection into the paraventricular nucleus. *Life Sci* 1984; 35: 2635–2642.

63. Berrettini WH, Kaye WH, Gwirtsman H, Albright A. Cerebrospinal fluid peptide YY immunoreactivity in eating disorders. *Neuropsychobiology* 1988; 19:121–124.
64. McHugh RP, Moran TH. The stomach, cholecystokin, and satiety. *Fed Proc Fed Am Soc Exp Biol* 1986; 45:1384–1390.
65. Gibbs J, Smith GP. Satiety: The roles of peptides from the stomach and the intestine. *Fed Proc Fed Am Soc Exp Biol* 1986; 45:1391–1395.
66. Brown PJ, Konner M. An anthropological perspective on obesity. *Ann NY Acad Sci* 1987; 499:29–46.
67. Whiting MG. A Cross-Cultural Nutrition Survey. Doctoral Thesis. Cambridge, MA, Harvard School of Public Health, 1958.
68. Sims EAH, Danforth E, Horton ES, Bray GA, Glennon JA, Salans LB. Endocrine and metabolic effects of experimental obesity in man. *Recent Prog Horm Res* 1973; 29:457–496.
69. Fuller RW, Yen TT. The place of animal models and animal experimentation in the study of food intake regulation and obesity in humans. *Ann NY Acad Sci* 1987; 499:167–178.
70. Trayhurn P, Thurlby PL, James WPT. Thermogenic defect in preobese ob/ob mice. *Nature* 1977; 266:60–63.
71. Himms-Hagen J. Brown adipose tissue thermogenesis as an energy buffer. Implications for obesity. *N Engl J Med* 1984; 311:1549–1558.

7
Clinical Laboratory Aspects of Eating Disorders

DAVID M. MARTIN, CARLTON E. TURNER and BRIAN K. LONG

Introduction

Clinical laboratory studies have only recently been applied to the diagnosis and treatment of eating disorders. The most remarkable laboratory investigations in this area have been in etiology and sequelae of anorexia nervosa and bulimia nervosa. Although distinct medical illnesses, both anorexia and bulimia have a spectrum of clinically overlapping symptoms that also may exist with other disorders such as depression, substance abuse, and endocrinopathies. The accurate diagnosis of the specific underlying or coexisting disorders associated with the clinical presentations of anorexia or bulimia is essential for the development of an effective treatment strategy. Clinical laboratory studies routinely provide physicians with a means of objectively assessing the medical status of patients and can also provide invaluable information on the course and medical condition of anorectic and/or bulimic patients. The following provides an overview of the clinical utility and cost effectiveness of a variety of laboratory studies in the diagnosis and management of the anorectic and/or bulimic patient.

General Laboratory and Medical Considerations

The spectrum of eating disorders commonly referred to as anorexia and bulimia carry with them grave medical consequences that can ultimately result in death.[1,2,3] Accurate and rapid diagnosis of the general medical condition of anorectic and bulimic patients is key to the development of an effective and often lifesaving treatment plan. Comprehensive medical laboratory evaluations can aid and augment the clinician's treatment program for individual patients independent of their current weight status, reported medical history, or cursory clinical observations. Although there are few obvious physical abnormalities in bulimic patients there are subtle and serious physical changes that range from dental erosion and parotid enlargement to significant serum electrolyte and metabolic derangements.[3,4,5] These electrolyte losses are derived from the individual or additive effects of vomiting, and laxative and/or diuretic use leading to serum potassium depletion. Eventually this lowered serum potassium will compromise myocardial contractility and may result in a fatal arrhythmia.[6]

In anorectic patients weight loss often draws attention first as they outwardly "wear their symptoms." However, the medical complications are more diverse and catastrophic than simple weight loss. There is extensive involvement of all major body systems especially with regard to endocrine and metabolic abnormalities including hypothalamic and pituitary brain tumors, thyroid disease, diabetes mellitus, Addison's disease, gastrointestinal disorders, peptic ulcers, and inflammatory bowel diseases to mention but a few. Virtually every endocrine and metabolic system is affected in anorexia correlating with some of the effects expected in starvation but may be confused with other endocrinopathies such as hypopituitarism and hyperthyroidism.

The diagnosis and treatment of anorexia nervosa is further complicated by the distinct differences in patients who accomplish weight loss by simply restricting the amount of food they eat (restricters) and those who have bulimic behaviors such as the binge/purge cycle and abuse of diuretics and laxatives (bulimics). Patients who have both anorectic and bulimic profiles will have the medical consequences of both disorders, for example, electrolyte imbalance, substance abuse, and starvation effects while restricters primarily display the effects of starvation. The differential diagnosis of restricter versus bulimic anorexia is vital to effective treatment planning and can be helped by comprehensive laboratory workups.

Laboratory evaluations, although in their infancy in these disorders, can objectively provide clinicians with independent verification of the patient's medical status. A comprehensive general medical laboratory evaluation should be done on all eating disorder patients to ascertain hematologic, electrolyte, liver, cardiac, thyroid, renal, and overall nutritional status of the individual. This evaluation should be viewed as an enhancement but not as a replacement of medical observation and clinical judgment. As each patient presents a unique constellation of medical, psychological and psychiatric events no single approach or diagnostic panel fits all situations.

Basal Luteinizing, Follicle Stimulating Hormone, and Gonadotropin Releasing Factor (GnRF) Challenge Studies

The gonadotropins, luteinizing hormone (LH) and follicle stimulating hormone (FSH), are the pituitary hormones that initiate ovulation and the menses cycle in females by stimulating the secretion of progesterone and estrogenic hormones. Disruption of this cycle is characteristic of anorectic patients with greater than 80 percent reporting amenorrhea well before noting significant weight loss or anorectic behaviors. A number of studies have reported subnormal basal LH and FSH levels in anorectic patients as well as bulimic patients. A suppressed response to gonadotropin releasing hormone (GnRH, also known as LHRH) and an immature 24 hour LH secretory profile are found in anorectic patients as well as normal weight and underweight bulimic patients.[7,8,9] This offers an interesting theory that the hypothalamic-pituitary-gonadal dysfunction is common to both disorders and may be antecedents rather than sequelaes of the illnesses.[10] Consequently, LH and FSH testing should be considered in this patient group as a means of identifying an ongoing or concurrent endocrine abnormality, categorizing endocrine maturity and documenting normal ovulatory endocrine profiles.

LH more so than other hormones is highly variable in the plasma compartment and a single blood level may produce misleading results. LH levels have a distinct 24 hour circadian rhythm that changes with the various stages of maturity.[8,11] The LH pulses or releases increase in amplitude during the sleep cycle with the larger pulse in the early morning. An immature LH secretory profile would be that of pubescence

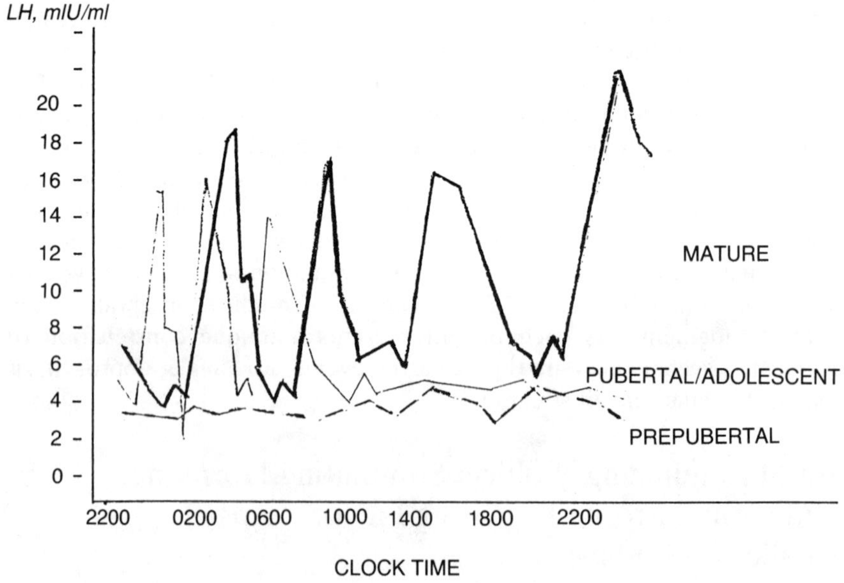

FIGURE 7-1. Example maturation stages of the 24 hour LH secretory profile.

where there is little variation during the day with a notable increase during the sleep cycle. As the rhythm matures past puberty, LH pulses are apparent in the daytime with higher concentrations observed during sleep. Adult LH 24 hour patterns have both day and night LH pulse of somewhat equal magnitude, Figure 7-1.

This variation of LH levels found in a 24 hour cycle and at various stages of maturation leads to difficulty in the interpretation of a single plasma level of LH. A number of alternatives have been offered to compensate for this variation; plasma levels drawn at the same time for three consecutive days, 24 hour plasma monitoring for maturity classification or average (calculated mean) concentration, 24 hour urine collections, and challenge tests with GnRH.

For practical and economic considerations 24 hour plasma monitoring is not a realistic clinical approach to assessment of this system. The same holds true for challenge studies but they should not be discounted entirely in the comprehensive endocrine workup of specific patients. Although not standardized, a GnRH challenge study requires the placement of an indwelling intravenous catheter, the draw of baseline LH and FSH sample, intravenous infusion of 0.18 μg/kg GnRH, and subsequent LH and FSH sampling every 20 minutes for two hours. Anorectic patients have characteristically lower LH responses to GnRH than do patients with bulimia as compared to normals.[12,13] Anorectic and bulimic patients tend to display higher FSH responses to GnRH than normals but the maximum response does not significantly differ between these groups. These GnRH response profiles can help to independently differentiate anorectic patients with and without bulimic characteristics and to corroborate patient history and clinical observations. The complexity of the procedure however limits its routine clinical application.

Recent advances in monoclonal antibody technology has made LH tests more specific and readily available even for at home use to detect ovulation at home in urine.[14] Urine offers an advantage in that it will normalize the LH pulses over a 24 hour period and more accurately reflect average LH concentration. Although comprehensive studies are not yet available on 24 hour urine studies in anorexia amd bulimia nervosa using the newer monoclonal antibody techniques, they promise to offer a cost effective and uncomplicated approach to the assessment of the maturity and function of the LH system.

FSH is less pulsatile in nature and as such less problematic to measure. However, the clinical information the test yields in anorectic and bulimic patients is less significant than that of LH. FSH measurements are indicated in the comprehensive workup of the amenorrheic anorectic and bulimic patient in order to fully ascertain the fertility and hormonal status independent of the eating disorder.

Basal Thyroid, Prolactin, Growth Hormone, and TRH Challenge Testing

Starvation and stress have been associated with alterations in the endocrine status of a number of patient populations including anorectic and bulimic patients.[15,16] Most susceptible to these factors is the balance of the hypothalamic-pituitary-thyroid (HPT) as well as the hypothalamic-pituitary-adrenal (HPA) axis. The pituitary hormones prolactin, growth hormone (GH), and thyroid stimulating hormone (TSH) could be measured basally, or a dynamic evaluation of the entire system can be obtained by a challenge test using the hypothalamic tripeptide thyrotropin releasing hormone (TRH).

Basal thyroid hormones thyroxin (T4) and triiodothyronine (T3) levels in anorexia are generally low whereas TSH is normal to slightly decreased.[11] This helps differentiate euthyroid anorexics from patients with hypothyroidism where T4 and T3 are low and TSH is high. Low weight anorectic patients exhibit thyroid profiles consistent with starvation or euthyroid sick states. In healthy individuals T4 is converted into the more potent T3 producing approximately 90 percent of circulating T3. In euthyroid medically ill patients, starvation and anorexics, this conversion is slowed down yielding decreased serum T3 level. T4 levels are also slightly lower to normal in anorectics which is probably the reflection of reduced carbohydrate, protein, and calorie intake. This is similar to conditions found in medically ill patients. Upon weight gain, peripheral thyroid hormones return to normal and can be used as an indicator of patient compliance. Basal thyroid levels in patients with exclusively bulimic presentations are unremarkable and routinely fall into the normal range.

Basal GH levels are abnormally high in both anorexia and starvation reflecting this hormone's sensitivity to caloric intake and the shared endocrine signature of these disorders. These levels fall rapidly when normal caloric intake is achieved but not always upon regaining appropriate weight. This suggests that other mechanisms may be affecting the GH system in anorectics other than a normal weight set point. Elevated basal GH levels in bulimia have been reported as high as 30 percent in bulimic populations. The etiology of this finding is unclear at the present time. GH is sensitive to excessive stress, and physiological trauma of repeated binge/purge cycles may be the cause of its elevation.

Basal prolactin levels in uncomplicated anorexia and bulimia are unremarkable and often in the normal range. Elevated prolactin levels are useful in teasing out microadenomas of the pituitary which would also cause menstrual irregularities such as amenorrhea, a common occurrence in both the anorectic and bulimic patient.

Prolactin, like GH, is also very sensitive to stress and may be elevated as a consequence of the stress induced in the binge/purge cycle. Because of the variability of both prolactin and growth hormone, basal levels should be drawn similar to LH on three consecutive days at the same time to normalize any pulses and to verify abnormalities.

TRH challenge studies in both anorexia and bulimia have provided a number of interesting clues into the origins of these disorders. The TRH challenge test has been routinely used in the diagnosis of thyroid disease for about 30 years. The procedure used in identification of thyroid disease requires the placement of an indwelling venous catheter, baseline samples for TSH, intravenous bolus of 500 μg of TRH, and sequential sampling for TSH at 15, 30, 45, and 90 minutes post infusion. TSH values normally rise to a peak value at the 30 minute sampling and the delta value (peak TSH minus baseline TSH) in normals ranges from 7 to 20 units. Hypothyroid patients will exhibit an extraordinary delta in excess of 35 units while hyperthyroid patients are unresponsive with deltas that are less than 1 unit.[17]

TRH is a hypothalamic tripeptide that not only stimulates the release of both TSH and prolactin from the pituitary gland but in some pathological cases GH as well. Greater than 80 percent of euthyroid anorectics and approximately 20 percent of bulimics have been reported to have delayed peak (greater than 30 minutes) TSH responses post TRH infusion.[17] Any GH response post TRH infusion is considered pathological yet the same study reported that up to 50 percent of the bulimic anorectic and 13 percent of bulimic patients have an abnormal GH response (delta GH greater than 5) with no association of weight, psychiatric status, or binge/purge cycle.

Prolactin levels normally rise post TRH infusion and conflicting reports[18,19] suggest both a normal and elevated response making these prolactin levels post TRH difficult to apply clinically. In bulimics equally inconclusive reports of normal to elevated responses in some patients suggest that further study is required in order to apply this response in eating disorders. As such, the measurement of prolactin and growth hormone is not a cost effective and clinically significant aspect of the TRH test.

Delta TSH values have been reported as blunted (less than 7) in both anorexia and bulimia in up to 50 percent of the patients. However, this is not a consistent marker and is highly variable within this patient population. Blunted delta TSH levels have also been reported in a number of psychiatric disorders especially major depression.[17,20,21] This finding can serve to aid the clinician in the differential diagnosis between major depression and hypothyroidism, two conditions sometimes found to be associated with eating disorders. Patients who are hypothyroid will exhibit exaggerated delta scores of 35 or greater while some patients with major depression and eating disorders have blunted responses of less than 7. These findings suggest that HPT axis abnormalities cannot be attributed solely to starvation or from binging and purging.

		Anorexia	Bulimia
Baseline	TSH	Decreased-Normal	Normal
	PRL	Elevated	
	GH	Elevated	Normal-Elevated
Peak	TSH	Delayed	Normal-Delayed
	PRL	Normal	Normal
	GH	Elevated	Normal-Elevated
Delta	TSH	Blunted-Normal	Blunted-Normal
	PRL	Blunted	Elevated
	GH	Elevated	Normal-Elevated

FIGURE 7-2. Summary of TRH test results in eating disorders.

Although these studies are sometimes conflicting, Figure 7-2, this may be due to the nonuniformity of analytical methods, control groups, and experimental design. The TRH challenge, as it dynamically tests the hypothalamic-pituitary-thyroid axis, offers valuable information over basal studies. With further standardization of technology and streamlining of procedures, such as only sampling for TSH at baseline and at 45 minutes, it promises to be a routine and cost effective laboratory procedure in the diagnosis and treatment of eating disorders.

Dexamethasone Suppression Testing

Hypothalamic-pituitary-adrenal (HPA) axis disturbances have been studied over the years by a number of laboratory testing strategies. Cortisol, the adrenal hormone regulated by the pituitary secretion of adrenocorticotropic hormone (ACTH), is routinely measured in clinical laboratories in the serum, urine and, most recently, the saliva compartments.[22,23] The case and availability of cortisol measurements have produced a wealth of literature on basal HPA hormone testing using serum or urine cortisol and dynamic testing of this axis using the dexamethasone suppression test (DST).

The DST was initially used as a diagnostic tool in patients with Addison's or Cushing's disease but has received widespread comment over the past decade as a marker for endogenous depression.[24,25] The test is administered by sequential sampling of cortisol after the patient is given 1.0 mg of dexamethasone orally at 12 midnight. There have emerged a number of suggested sampling points post dexamethasone and method-dependent criteria for a positive test but nonsuppression of cortisol values greater than 5.0 μg/dl of serum cortisol is generally considered non-suppression or a positive result.

Anorectic patients almost uniformly demonstrate a positive DST and, unlike patients with malnutrition or starvation, have an increased production of cortisol rather than a decrease typically associated with starvation states.[10,26] Although endogenous depression does not exist in all patients with anorexia nervosa, their HPA axis profile is similar to that found in depression. In addition to a positive DST some depressed patients also exhibit a lack of diurnal circadian rhythm of cortisol. Cortisol production in normals follows a distinct circadian cycle with the lowest point being at 12 midnight and the highest occurring in the early morning hours.

Some anorectic patients demonstrate a loss of cortisol diurnality in addition to their overproduction of cortisol and DST nonsuppression. These are endocrine findings that are shared with depression. As the anorectic patient attains normal weight, cortisol production drops, diurnality reestablishes, and DST nonsuppression normalizes. It is unclear whether these events are independent of endogenous depression or a sign of a similar but unrelated endocrine dysfunction. It is clear that starvation alone would not produce these results and the clinical assessment of the HPA axis in anorexia is indicated. This should be combined with a comprehensive psychiatric evaluation in patients with DST nonsuppression.

HPA axis profiles in bulimic patients parallel those found in anocretic patients with DST nonsuppression noted in 50 percent of patients. Bulimics like anorectic and depressives have increased basal cortisol production.[27] These elevated levels may be a function of stress induced by the binge-purge cycle but the DST nonsuppression suggests that other factors are involved. Several studies report DST nonsuppression in bulimics independent of depressive symptomatology. Unfortunately, there are fewer studies on the utility of the DST in bulimia than there are in anorexia making clinical application problematic. DST nonsuppression in bulimic patients has been suggested in one study to be a function of lower plasma levels of dexamethasone.[28] This finding requires further study but suggests there may be altered metabolism of dexamethasone in bulimic patients as has been noted in other patient populations.

Anorexics who have attained normal weight as well as bulimics who are not actively binging and purging show a decline in basal cortisol levels into the normal range. In addition to this finding, DST nonsuppression has been noted to normalize. These findings suggest that the DST may have some limited clinical value in certain patients. Neuroendocrine testing along the HPA axis may prove to be a sensitive indicator to bulimics in the binge-purge cycle and monitoring subtle endocrine shifts in the active anorectic patient.

Drugs of Abuse, Diuretics, and Laxative Testing

Probably the most important and overlooked area of laboratory investigation in bulimic patients is the determination of a psychoactive substance use disorder. The most frequently encountered drugs of abuse are amphetamines, cocaine, sedatives, or alcohol.[2,29] The treatment for substance abuse or dependence would be necessary as part of the overall treatment plan of the individual. Even though alcohol abuse has been identified as the most common form of drug abuse associated with bulimic patients,[30] few programs have been established to address this complicated syndrome. Bulimic patients also abuse stimulants to curb their appetite and to produce rapid and consistent weight loss. In addition, they are also frequent abusers of diuretics and laxatives to achieve their goals of weight gain prevention. As bulimic patients are often overly concerned about their weight, they regularly engage in strict dieting, fasting, or vigorous exercise to prevent weight gain. They also make repeated attempts to control their weight by self-induced vomiting often with the use of cathartic agents, the most frequent being ipecac. The use of laxatives or diuretics is also quite common for the same end in these patients and only recently has adequate attention been focused on these compulsive behaviors.

The purging behavior of bulimic and bulimic anorectic patients is often induced by the self-administration of cathartic agents such as ipecac to induce vomiting. A frequent medical complication associated with this behavior in bulimic patients is ipecac (emetine) intoxication. This intoxication results in cardiomyopathy which leads to cardiac failure. Some of the clinical findings associated with this life-threatening situation are precordial pain, dyspnea, muscle weakness, hypotension, and tachycarida. EKG abnormalities which include fatal arrhythmias and certain laboratory findings are also evident in acute ipecac intoxication. These laboratory findings can include elevated liver enzymes (alkaline phosphatase, ALT, AST, GGT) and increased sedimentation rate (ESR).[30] Testing for ipecac is usually unremarkable. Due to the rapid clearance and low dosages associated with ipecac metabolism it is rarely detected.[31]

Unlike the bulimics where impulsivity and drug abuse are associated features, anorectic patients are more conservative and restrained. They have a decreased interest in sex and compulsive behavior and as such are less likely to become involved with drug abuse in general. However, the bulimic form of anorexia previously described is vulnerable to impulsive behaviors such as suicide attempts, self-mutilation, stealing, and substance abuse as well.[30]

Clearly both the anorectic and bulimic patient populations are at risk of substance abuse, and appropriate drug testing strategies should be developed according to the individual patient's clinical presentation.

Although a tremendous amount of attention has been paid to drug testing both in the media and legislative bodies with the advent of mandatory drug testing, there still exists a wide variation of quality among laboratories.[31,32] Simply ordering a "drug screen" without specifying the components and sensitivities or cutoffs to be tested is a dangerous practice as the results can be misleading. A negative drug screen does not mean the patient has not taken drugs; it simply means that for a particular patient's sample no drugs were found using a specific test. As such, a familiarity with drug testing is key to its accurate interpretation.

Although extensive reports have emerged on the technology and design of drug testing procedures little attention has been given to the specific requirements of drug screens applied to eating disorders. Drug testing in the bulimic patient and those anorectics with bulimic characteristics should be viewed in three distinct categories: general drug screening, diuretic screening, and laxative screening.

General screening for drugs of abuse in both the anorectic and bulimic patients should be done as early in the assessment as possible. It is preferable to obtain the first morning void as it is most concentrated and yields the higher rate of positive findings. It is important to only order drug screens that employ antibody-based technology such as enzyme immunoassay (EIA) or radioimmunoassay (RIA) systems and not to order tests using thin layer chromatography (TLC) as the latter is not sensitive enough to detect low level substance abuse often seen in these patients.[32]

Although there is a wide range of compounds that can be screened, only a very few can be readily detected on a consistent and cost effective basis. The compounds of most interest in anorectic and bulimic patients are listed in Figure 7-3 indicating the initial screening sensitivity or cutoff and the confirmation level by an alternative method if needed. In routine clinical situations confirmation may not be required if abuse is readily admitted by the patient. If the patient denies the finding, the sample can always be confirmed at a later point. This strategy allows for more frequent testing as a deterrent to continued abuse in a very cost effective manner.

Diuretic screening is not widely available on a clinical basis. The widespread attention being paid to abuse of diuretics in athletics as a means of negating drug tests has increased the demand for diuretic

Class	General screen ng/ml	Positive conf. ng/ml	Detection time days
Marijuana	50	10	3–30
Amphetamines	300	100	1–2
Cocaine	300	50	2–4
Opiates	300	100	1–2
PCP	25	25	2–8
Barbiturates	300	100	10–14
Benzodiazepines	300	100	10–14
Methaqualone	300	25	10–14
Optional: Methadone, Propoxyphene, Alcohol			

FIGURE 7-3. Eating disorders drug abuse screening guidelines.

Acetazolamide
Amiloride
Bendroflumethiazide
Benzthiazide
Bumetanide
Canrenone
Chlormerodrine
Chlorthalidone
Diclofenamide
Ethacrynic Acid
Furosemide
Hydrochlorothiazide
Mersalyl
Spironolactone
Triamterene

Note: Specific gravity may also be used to indicate the need for the diuretic screen if below 1.010

FIGURE 7-4. Eating disorders diuretic screen.

analysis.[33,34] Anorectic and bulimic patients also use diuretics as a means of weight reduction often obtaining the medications illegally and using them without any medical supervision. Diuretic self-induced weight loss of greater than 3 percent can induce leg and stomach cramps, basal temperature dysregulation, altered electrolyte balance, exhaustion, arrhythmia, coma, and eventually death. The recent speculation of a high occurrence of anorexia and bulimia in female athletes raises the need for diuretic testing to become available to clinicians on a routine level.

The standard panel of diuretics screened for in athletics is readily applicable to the anorectic and bulimic patient. Figure 7-4 lists the most commonly abused diuretics. Unfortunately the "diuretic screen" is not as well defined as the general "drug screen" as diuretic screening has not received the attention and scrutiny that drug abuse screening has received in the last few years. As such, there are no standards of methodology or recommended cutoffs in diuretic testing as there are in drugs of abuse testing. Clinicians should ask if the laboratory provides diuretic testing to professional sports organizations and ask where their diuretic testing is performed. As with any laboratory test the more familiar the clinician is with the analysis the better an interpretation can be made upon receiving the results. As testing in this area varies greatly with individual laboratories, the clinician would be well advised to develop a comfortable understanding and association with the provider of this service.

Diuretics cause rapid weight loss by the elimination of water stored in tissues. This excess water is filtered through the glomerular system and eliminated via the urine compartment. As this process is chemically induced by diuretics, the specific gravity of the patient's urine is greatly diluted. This dilution of urinary specific gravity is readily apparent if measured on the urine specimen either at the point of collection or upon analysis in the laboratory. Normal specific gravity varies upon the methodology used, however for simple gravimetric analysis by refractometry a reference range of 1.010 to 1.030 is commonly reported. As the diuretic analysis is nonroutine, it can be costly. An alternative strategy would be only to run a diuretic screen if the specific gravity is below 1.010. This again would provide a cost effective way to insure the patient is abstinent by increased frequency of testing as a relapse deterrent.

Although 20 to 40 percent of bulimic and bulimic anorectic patients abuse laxatives at least once a week to control weight, laxative screening, Figure 7-5, is rarely requested by clinicians. There are few clinical situations where such testing would be helpful and as such the technology to measure these agents is not fully developed. Panels for the analysis of specific laxatives have been developed[35] but the cost is so prohibitive at times that laxative screens should only be considered if the patient denies abuse and if medical judgment suggest otherwise. Like the diuretic technology, laxative analysis is not widespread and the clinician ordering the test should request a technical and clinical briefing on the procedure.

A comprehensive toxicology evaluation would not be complete if the patient is on medication and therapeutic monitoring is not done. Individual patient metabolism and medical condition can effect the plasma concentration and clearance of medications up to fiftyfold.

This enormous interindividual variation can not be clinically predicted nor readily apparent upon the initiation of the medication regime. A careful medication history supported by therapeutic monitoring of the patient's blood levels will insure that an adequate amount of medication is administered and that unnecessary accumulations in the patient are avoided.

Anthraquinones
cascara
danthron
senna
Bisacodyl
Caster oil
Mineral oil
Magnesium
Oxphenisatin
Phenolphthalen
Phosphate

FIGURE 7-5. Eating disorders laxative screen.

Additional Considerations

Although out of the realm of clinical laboratory testing, research on the biological basis of eating disorders suggests several novel areas that may lead to a better understanding of the mechanisms involved and more productive testing strategies for these patients in the near future. The endogenous opiate hypothesis suggests the bulimic has a chronic deficit of endorphins initiating feeding to stimulate this down regulated system; alternately, the anorexic has an excess of endorphins, shutting down the feeding system and inhibiting LH release thus initiating amenorrhea.[36] The key role serotonin plays in the down regulation of the natural feeding cycle is reflected in decreases in urinary and spinal fluid 5-hydroxyindoleacetic acid (5-HIAA), plasma tryptophan, and platelet serotonin binding sites in anorectic patients.[37] Serotonin has been associated with the central regulation of the production of cortisol, gonadotropins, prolactin, and thyroid hormones[38,39] potentially explaining alterations in these systems in eating disorders. Bulimics who spontaneously halted the binge-purge cycle had an increased ratio of plasma tryptophan to other competing amino acids whereas those who continued this behavior had lower ratios suggesting serotonergic involvement in this disorder.[40] Cholecystokinin, a brain-gut peptide associated with satiety, has recently been shown to be serotonin dependent for its anorexic effects.[41] To make this system even more challenging, serotonin has a circadian and seasonal rhythm.[39]

Endorphin, platelet serotonin binding, amino acid ratios, and cholecystokinin testing suggest exciting possibilities for the future direction of laboratory evaluations in eating disorders. They also offer a fascinating approach to explaining the role of the central nervous system on the regulation of normal eating behaviors. Due to the complexity of analysis and the studies that must be conducted to account for circadian and seasonal variation of neurotransmitters, near term clinical application is confined to research settings.

Conclusion

Clinical and laboratory testing has emerged as a useful adjunct in the diagnosis, management, and research evaluation of eating disorders. Along with the standard routine screening, additional tests should be considered (see Figure 7-6) to evaluate suspected conditions often associated with eating disorders such as drug abuse and depressive disorders. Complicating physical conditions such as electrolyte imbalances, anemias, cardiac irregularities, and renal and endocrine abnormalities can also be clarified with selected testing. For example, drug screens for the common drugs of abuse with the addition of screens for laxative, diuretic,

[ ] Complete blood count (CBC)
[ ] Chemistry profile:
  electrolytes
  liver function
  cardiac enzymes
  renal function
[ ] Urinalysis
[ ] Thyroid Panel:
  T4
  T3 uptake
  TSH
[ ] B12 Folate
[ ] Zinc
[ ] Thyrotropin releasing hormone (TRH Challenge)
[ ] Dexamethasone suppression test (DST)
[ ] LH
[ ] FSH
[ ] Prolactin
[ ] Growth Hormone
[ ] Drug of abuse, Diuretics, and Laxatives
[ ] Therapeutic Drug Monitoring

Note: Checklist only suggests possible testing options; appropriate application must be determined for each patient must be evaluated individually

FIGURE 7-6. Eating disorders lab checklist.

and cathartic agents is indicated in known or suspected bulimics and bulimic anorexics. Finally, though, many questions still need to be answered; neuroendocrine testing suggests tremendous potential in providing clues to the etiology, pathophysiology, treatment, and eventually prediction of these serious and sometimes fatal medical disorders.

References

1. Morley JE, Silver AJ. Anorexia in the elderly. Neurobiology of Aging. *Pergamon Journal Ltd* 1988; Vol. 9:9–16.
2. Pope Jr HG, Hudson JI. Eating disorders. In Kaplan HI, Sadock BJ (eds): Comprehensive Textbook of Psychiatry (fifth edition). New York 1989; Vol. 2:1854–1864.
3. Spack NP. Medical complications of anorexia nervosa and bulimia, Chapter 1. In Emmet SW (ed): Theory and Treatment of Anorexia Nervosa and Bulimia. New York 1985; 5–19.
4. Fenley J, Powers PS, Miller J, Rowland M. Untreated anorexia nervosa: A case study of the medical consequences. *General Hospital Psychiatry* 1990; 12:264–270.
5. Hall RCW, Beresford TP. Medical complications of anorexia and bulimia. *Psychiatric Medicine* 1989; 7(4):165–192.

6. Pope H, Hudson J. Biological treatments of eating disorders. In Emmet SW (ed): Theory and Treatment of Anorexia Nervosa and Bulimia. New York 1985; 72–92.
7. Apter D, Cacciatore B, Alfthan H, Stenman UH. Serum luteinizing hormone concentrations increase 100-fold in females from 7 years of age to adulthood as measured by time-resolved immunofluorometric assay. *J Clin Endocrinol Metab* 1989; 68:53–57.
8. Devlin MJ, Walsh BT, Katz JL, et al. Hypothalamic-pituitary-gonadal function in anorexia nervosa and bulimia. *Psychiatry Research* 1982; 28:11–24.
9. Kulin HE, Bell PM, Santen RJ, Ferber AF. Integration of pulsatile gonadotropin secretion by timed urinary measurements: An accurate and sensitive 3-hour test. *J Clin Endocrinol Metab* 1975; 40:783–789.
10. Doerr P, Ficher M, Pirke KM, Lund R. Relationship between weight gain and hypothalamic pituitary adrenal function in patients with anorexia nervosa. *J Steroid Biochem* 1980; 13:529–537.
11. Newman MM, Halmi KA. The endocrinology of anorexia and bulimia nervosa in endocrinology of neuropsychiatric disorders. *Endocrinology Clinics of North America* 1988; 6:195.
12. Gwirtsman ME, Roy-Byrne P, Yager J, Gerner RH. Neuroendocrine abnormalities in bulimia. *Am J Psychiatry* 1983; 140:559–563.
13. Pettersson KSI, Soderholm JR-M. Individual differences in lutropin immunoreactivity revealed by monoclonal antibodies. *Clin Chem* 1991; 37:333–40.
14. Vermes I, Bonte HA, Veer GvdS, Schoemaker J. Interpretations of five monoclonal immunoassays of lutropin and follitropin: Effects of normalization with WHO standard. *Clin Chem* 1991; 37:3, 415–421.
15. Portnay GI, O'Brian JT, et al. The effect of starvation of the concentration and binding of thyroxin and triiodothyronine in serum and on the response TRH. *J Clin Endocrinol Metab* 1974; 39:191–194.
16. Vigersky RA, Anderson AE, Thompson RH, Loriaux DL. Hypothalamic dysfunction in secondary anorexia associated with simple weight loss. *N Engl J Med* 1977; 297:1141–1145.
17. Loosen PT, Prangue AJ. Serum thyrotropin response to thyrotropin-releasing hormone in psychiatric patients: A review. *Am J Psychiatry* 1982; 139:4: 405–416.
18. Levy AB. Neuroendocrine profile in bulimia nervosa. *Biol Psychiatry* 1989; 25:98.
19. Levy AB, Malarkey WB. Growth hormone and somatomedin-C in bulimia. *Psychoneuroendocrinology* 1988; 12:126–139.
20. Gold MS, Pottash ALC, Extein I, et al. The TRH test in the diagnosis of major and minor depression. *Psychoneuroendocrinology* 1981; 6:159–169.
21. Roy A, Karoum F, Linnoila M, Pickar D. TRH test in unipolar depressed patients and controls: Relationship to clinical and biological variables. *Acta Psychiatr Scand* 1988; 77:151–159.
22. Martin DM, Santana R, Zani J. Salivary cortisol analysis continued evidence as to its clinical utility in the dexamethasone suppression test. Society of Biologocial Psychiatry 1989 Convention & Scientific Program, Abstract #79, 1989.
23. Morse DR, Furst ML, Schacterle GR. Saliva: The misunderstood and underrated fluid. *Stress Med* 1986; 2:13–25.

24. Carroll BJ, Feinberg M, Greden JF, et al. A specific laboratory test for the diagnosis of melancholia. *Arch Gen Psychiatry* 1981; 38:15–22.
25. Extein I, Pottash ALC, Gold MS. Relationship of TRH test and dexamethasone suppression test abnormalities in unipolar depression. *Psychiatry Research* 1981; 4:49–53.
26. Copeland PM. Neuroendocrine aspects of eating disorders, Chapter 3. In Aimed SW (ed): Theory and Treatment of Anorexia Nervosa and Bulimia. 1985; 51–71.
27. Kiriike N, Nishawaki S, Izumiya Y, et al. Dexamethasone suppression test in bulimia. *Biol Psy* 1987; 21:325–328.
28. Levy AB, Dixon KN. DST in bulimia without endogenous depression. *Biol Psychiatry* 1987; 22:783–786.
29. American Psychiatric Association: Diagnostic and Statistical Manual of Mental Disorders (third edition). Washington, DC, APA, 1987.
30. Halmi KA. Eating disorders. In Talbott JA, Hales RE, Yudofsky SC (ed): The American Psychiatric Press Textbook of Psychiatry. 1988; 753–766.
31. Executive Order Number 12564 for a Drug-Free Federal Workplace Federal Register, September 15, V. 51 N. 32:899, 1986.
32. Miller NS, Giannini AJ, Gold MS, Philomena JA. Drug testing: Medical, legal and ethical issues. *J Subst Abuse Treatment* 1990; 7:239–245.
33. Tisdall PA, et al. Liquid-chromatographic determination of thiazide diuretics in urine. *Clin Chem* 1980; 26/6:702–706.
34. Voy R. Drugs, Sport, and Politics. Champaign, IL, Leisure Press, 1991.
35. DeWolff FA, et al. A screening method for establishing laxative abuse. *Clin Chem* 1981; 27(6):914–917.
36. Gillman MA, Lichtigfeld FJ. The opioids, dopamine, cholecystokinin and eating disorders. *Clin Neuropharmacology* 1986; Vol. 9, No. 1, 91–97.
37. Blundell JE. Serotonin and appetite. *Neuropharmacology* 1984; 23:1537–1551.
38. Brewerton TD, Mueller EA, Brandt HA. Evidence for serotonin dysregulation in anorexia. New Research Abstracts of the 140th Annual Meeting of the American Psychiatric Association. Chicago, 1987; 123.
39. Leibowitz SF. The role of serotonin in eating disorders. *Drugs* 1990; 39(Suppl 3):33–48.
40. Kaye WH, Gwirtsman HE, Brewerton TD, et al. Bingeing behavior and plasma amino acids: A possible involvement of brain serotonin in bulimia nervosa. *Psychiatry Research* 1988; 23:31–43.
41. Geracioti TD, Kling MA, et al. Meal-related cholecystokinin secretion in eating and affective disorders. *Psychopharmacology Bulletin* 1989; Vol. 25, No. 3, 444–449.

Bibliography

Crouch DJ, et al. Quantitative analysis of emetine and cephaeline by reverse-phase high performance liquid chromatography with fluometric detection. *J Analytical Tox* 1984; 8:63–65.

Garattini S, Bizzi A, et al. Progress in assessing the role of serotonin in the control of food intake. *Clinical Neuropharmacology* 1988; 11(Suppl 1):S8–S32.

Garfinkel PE, Brown GM, Stancer HC, Moldofsky H. Hypothalamic pituitary function in anorexia nervosa. *Arch Gen Psychiatry* 1975; 32:739–744.

Garfinkel PE, Kaplan AS. Psychoneuroendocrine profiles of disorders of eating behavior. In Ferrari FR, Brambilla GL (eds): Disorders of Eating Behavior. A psychoneuroendocrine approach. Oxford, Pergamon Press, 1986; 1–8.

Gerner RH, Gwirtsman HE. Abnormalities of dexamethasone suppression test and urinary MHPG in anorexia nervosa. *Am J Psychiatry* 1981; 138:650–653.

Gold P, Goodwin F, Wehr T, Rebar R. Pituitary thyrotropin response to thyrotropin-releasing hormone in affective illness: Relationship to spinal fluid amine metabolites. *Am J Psychiatry* 1977; 134:1028–1031.

Hales RE, Frances AJ. American Psychiatric Association Annual Review-Vol. 4. 1985; Section 4, Eating Disorders, pp. 399–524.

Kiriike N, Nishiwaki S, Izumiya Y, et al. Thyrotropin, prolactin and growth hormone response to thyrotropin-releasing hormone in anorexia and bulimia. *Biol Psychiatry* 1986; 22:167.

Martin DM, Weinstein ME, Dozoretz RI. Clinical implications of federal regulations on laboratory testing for alcohol and drugs of abuse/addiction. In Miller N (ed): The Comprehensive Handbook of Drug and Alcohol Addiction. 1991; 825–841.

Mitchell JE, Bantle JP. Metabolic and endocrine investigations in women of normal weight with the bulimic syndrome. *Biol Psychiatry* 1983; 18:355–365.

Moffat AC. The measurement of diuretics in urine. In Clarke's Isolation and Identification of Drugs (second edition). London, The Pharmaceutical Press, 1986.

Muhlbauer HD, Ziolko HV. Abnormalities of anterior pituitary responsiveness to hypothalamic hormones in bulimia. *Pharmacopsychiatry* 1986; 19:241–242.

Stallone D, Nicolaidis S, Gibbs J. Cholecystokinin-induced anorexia depends on serotonergic function. *American Journal of Physiology* 1989; 256:1138–1141.

Weiner H. Psychoendocrinology of anorexia nervosa. Women's Disorders, *Psychiatric Clinics of North America* Vol. 12, No. 1, March 1989.

8
Neuropsychiatric Approach to the Eating Disorder Patient

David A. Gross

Introduction

The neuropsychiatric examination of the patient with an eating disorder poses a distinct challenge to the psychiatrist. Not only do we have to consider the metabolic secondary pathophysiologic effects of disturbances of input and output but we must be attentive to clues that might implicate a central nervous system (CNS) cause.

As mentioned in the DSM III R,[1] the eating disorders are phenomena in search of etiological clarification. A plethora of theories abound suggesting a spectrum of causality including biologic,[2] psychologic, and societal. Has the increased prevalence of these disorders reflected a troubling shift in the psychopathology of modern industrial technosocieties or have we become more sensitive diagnosticians? We certainly could blame these disorders on the greenhouse effect but should we ignore environmental influences? Diet, toxin/pollutants, etc., come to mind. Does the prevalence of perfectionistic competitiveness and slimness in our societal families have an impact on the child's developing brain? After all, posttraumatic stress disorder has been hypothesized to be a psychological syndrome reflecting pathological brain mechanisms arising out of traumatic life experience(s).[3] The animal[4] and human[5] kindling models represent a possible analogous paradigm.

As psychiatrists rediscover their medical roots, it becomes increasingly apparent that many if not most of the major psychiatric syndromes have a biologic central nervous system dysfunction. This biological core contributes to the clinical presentation. Because of the familial prevalence of many of these psychiatric syndromes, the genetic influences have added to, and in some cases supplanted, the traditional psychodynamic theories of origin.

In summary, the spectrum of eating disorders forces the clinician to consider the biopsychosocial medical model. At first glance, the signs and symptoms described in this text suggest primary or secondary CNS dysfunction. However, one cannot help but be impressed with the individual and familial psychodynamic difficulties these patients share. It is equally intriguing to consider the sociologic explanations for the individuals presenting with eating disorders in the past two decades. Are these the result of societal ills impacting upon familial and individual dynamics with resultant biological dysfunction or are there other commutations that arise through systems? The answer is not yet in but we can still ensure that a careful systematic diagnostic and treatment approach is pursued.

Medical Mimics

It is by no means a coincidence that extra-CNS organ system dysfunction is frequently associated with changes in mental state. Also, not surprisingly, has been the relationship between major psychiatric mood disorders and neuroendocrine abnormalities: this has been the case in the relationship among major depression, the dexamethasone suppression test, and thyrotropic releasing hormone test. Appetite satiety and weight change are also commonly seen in both psychiatric and nonpsychiatric medical illness. The common underpinning linking these seemingly disparate states and pathological processes is the temporal lobe-limbic-hypothalamus axis. This collection of nuclei and tracts serves to sample and process exteroceptive (external world) and interoceptive (internal bodily milieu) stimuli. Basic neurovegetative and autonomic nervous function as well as emotional tone are modulated by this axis. It may be that the human concept of the separation of "I" and "them" derives from this primitive set of interactions. Sense of self, body image, and personality may be the result of such influences on association cortex.[6]

The brain is an electrical organ system that relies upon chemical processes for the production and modification of its electronic transmissions. Therefore neuronal function and dysfunction can result from anything that interferes with the normal transmission of data. Disturbances of the brain's chemical milieu can be due to primary processes (e.g., pituitary hypersecretion; central neurotransmitter imbalance in affective illness, and schizophrenia; or the destructive lesions found in tumors, strokes, and demyelinating plaques) as well as secondary processes (e.g., extra-CNS electrolyte, hormonal, or toxic abnormalities) that cross the blood-brain barrier and impact upon synaptic function.

It is no surprise that changed mental states accompany the wide fluctuations of blood sugar in diabetes, the abnormal thyroxine levels that result from hypothyroidism and hyperthyroidism or the effects of low B12 stores in pernicious anemia.[7] Clinical experience and recent literature suggest that change on personality (mental state) may be the sentinel sign of HIV infection and AIDs. Thus, the brain may truly be the "least forgiving organ." Dependence upon a complicated electrochemical homeostasis requires that there be redundancy and flexibility built into CNS processes. We are rarely aware of the neurophysiologic fluctuations that constantly take place.

Therefore, the assessment of a patient with any of the spectrum of eating disorder complaints must begin with a comprehensive medical history, review of systems, and physical examination. Laboratory screening is a must and should include a multipanel SMA (electrolytes, liver functions, renal functions, lipids, glucose), CBC with differential, thyroid functions including TSH (thyroid stimulating hormone), RPR (if not done in past year), sedimentation rate, urinalysis, pregnancy test in females, and in this day and age, a comprehensive urine drug screen for substances.

Neuropsychiatric Investigation

When the possibility of a straightforward neuropsychiatric medical mimic is ruled out, a more focused assessment must investigate the significant variables in the biopsychosocial systems. Although psychodynamic formulations are intellectually quite stimulating, they should not be relied upon as the sole etiology or treatment modality. Psychological underpinnings should be considered within a broad framework of predisposing factors that include biologic and psychosocial variables. The stress-ulcer model[8] can be an illustrative example. It is not the stressful situation alone or the "power" of the personality style that single-handedly leads to peptic ulceration. Rather, it is the biological predisposition (via genetically based hyperacidity or mucosal sensitivity to injury) that permits a confluence of psychosocial factors to result in a pathological end product.

In the patient with an eating disorder, the biologic, psychologic, and social (i.e., current reality life situation issues) components must be isolated and weighed. The psychosocial data base is incorporated into appropriate psychotherapeutic modalities as part of an overall treatment plan. Successful recovery cannot depend solely upon biological somatic intervention. There is growing evidence that psychotherapeutic intervention may result in enduring mental change because of neurobiological alteration.[9] The rational belief that "what is good for the mind is good for the body, and what heals the mind aids the body" may be based on this understanding of the mind-brain-body trichotomy. The comprehensive treatment plan must therefore be a well-balanced mixture of these systems.

What then is the purpose of the neuropsychiatric assessment? What are we seeking to reveal? After all, not every eating disorder patient can be "run through" a PET scanner or be exposed to the risk of depth electrode electroencephalographic recording of the limbic system. Therefore, we must be able to systematically examine the patient to reveal the presence of signs and symptoms that result from neurochemical, electrical, or structural (disturbance of cellular integrity resulting in combined electrical and chemical disruption) CNS pathology. What is responsible for the pathological body image; the excessive, bizarre, or restrictive nutritional intake; the postprandial emesis and the motoric hyperactivity of the eating disorder patient?

Disturbances of affective modulation are commonly seen and may include complaints of frank depression or dysthymia. Hypomanic episodes are not unusual and may coincide with excessive exercising and energy expenditure. Certain cognitive features are commonly noted in anorectic and bulimic patients. Obsessive preoccupation with physical image, food types eaten, calories consumed, and perfectionistic life style complement compulsive rituals involving eating, vomiting, and hoarding behaviors. Body image distortion suggests the existence of delusional processes yet these patients fail to fulfill major criteria for psychotic disorders.

The biological common denominator for such a wide spectrum of pathology probably rests within a system of interconnecting brain regions called the temporal lobe-limbic-hypothalamic axis (TLLHA).[10] Multivariate connections with the association and the executive cortex provide for the production of higher cortical functions that develop over time into the concept of self-identity. The presence of abstract reasoning, attitude, belief systems, and emotional coloring interact with basic neurovegetative drive states (pleasure, hunger, thirst, satiety, sociality, novelty, arousal) and internal milieu (metabolic) homeostasis. We are seldom aware of these automatic interchanges and therefore implicitly believe in our own "reality" as normal. For example, the undiagnosed Hashimoto thyroiditis patient tries to attribute the hyperthyroid-driven anxiety, agitation, and tremulousness to some external factor as marriage or life situation. Similar attribution occurs in the episodic undiagnosed major depressive. Even after diagnosis is made, it is difficult to accept that one's pathological state is due to subcortical neurotransmitter imbalance. For general psychiatrists, the treatment of the major depressive is the most straightforward of tasks, yet patients don't always see it this way. Thus, the anorexia nervosa victim sometimes attribute their myriad signs and symptoms entirely to family dynamics and faulty individuation/differentiation rather than acknowledge a pathological TLLHA? Much depends on the manner in which the patient is approached in the evaluation phase as well as the type of patient education furnished during therapy. If we look for family and individual psychopathology as the sole probable cause, we will then most likely find it to the exclusion of everything else.

The neuropsychiatric evaluation must take into account the nature of brain dysfunction that may be present. "Fixed deficits" indicate persistent abnormality of CNS function. Dyslexia and aphasia are examples. That does not mean to say that the degree of deficit remains fixed over time, because, in actuality, it will fluctuate. However, there will be no period free from some amount of pathology. Metabolically based deficits by nature wax and wane much the same way as noted in the course of delirium. The changeable nature of the symptoms can be most striking.

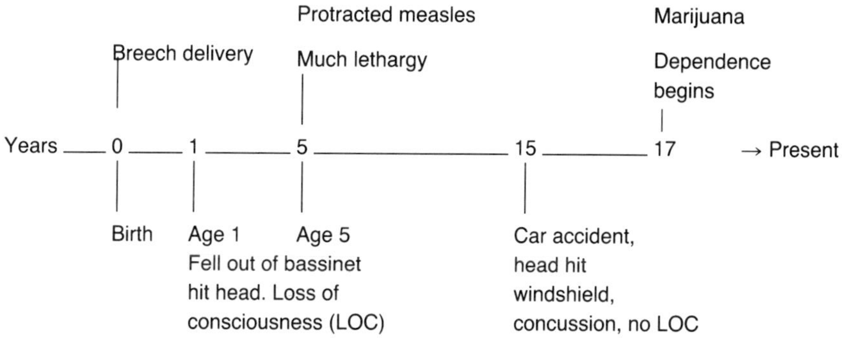

FIGURE 8-1. Example of an event time line for CNS risks.

Such would be the fluctuating mental state of the bulimic patient in electrolyte imbalance. Paroxysomal deficits by definition come and go "spontaneously" and in rapid fashion. Cerebral dysrhythmia, epileptiform states, and true epilepsy comprise the best examples of paroxysmal signs and symptoms.

The neuropsychiatric assessment must include a careful inventory of life events that would suggest CNS pathology, thus the need to ask pointed questions to determine the presence of a past history of CNS risk factors. Draw a life event time line, Figure 8-1, as part of your record.

Table 8-1 provides a list of some of the CNS risk factors to be assessed in the clinical interview. It is necessary to determine the presentation of

TABLE 8-1. CNS Risk factors.

- Parental chromosomal damage risks.
- In utero events—unusual maternal illnesses, drugs, trauma.
- Birth complications—prematurity, delayed birth, breech delivery, placenta previa, complicated forceps delivery, cord around neck, meconium staining, cyanosis, low Apgar Score.
- Unusual childhood illness—especially viral (e.g., measles, subclinical encephalitis), child abuse.
- Head trauma—falls, fights, car accidents, specify degree of LOC, if any, note concussive signs and symptoms, outcome of neurological examinations and testing, presence of neurologic (including mental state change) sequelae.
- Substance abuse—includes primary and secondary CNS effects. Examples of primary effects include toxic damage (LSD, PCP, marijuana, alcohol, amphetamines). Secondary influences include, for example, those seen in cocaine use: vasoconstriction ischemia, contamination and cerebral anoxia, cardiovascular collapse, and postinjection foreign body contamination.
- Heavy metal exposure—being raised in an old mill town, lead based paint in tenement.
- Other toxin exposure—hazardous waste dumps, air pollution.
- HIV risk.

- Construct a circle and place numbers in it so it becomes a clock face. Make the clock read 8:30 (spatial organization, tests perseveration in one continuous pen, eye, hand integrity).

- Copy simple geometric figures and label them with their names.

△	✚	□	
triangle	cross	square	(all of the above plus naming of geometric shapes)

- copy repetitive figures (see greater perseverative and impulsive errors here)

  +OOO++OOO+++OOO

FIGURE 8-2. Nondominant hemisphere bedside neuropsychological screen.

symptoms and signs to see if they are fixed, fluctuant, or paroxysmal. A WAIS-R (Wechsler Adult Intelligence Scale—Revised)[11] can be very helpful for many fixed deficits but unfortunately is not always accessible or affordable. The same is true for neuropsychological batteries as the Halstead-Reitan[12] or Luria-Nebraska.[13] The traditional bedside mental status examination can be most productive, but like most mental state exam models, relies heavily on analytic and logical language use (dominant hemisphere) but essentially ignores visuo-spatial, part-whole, gestalt organized tasks (nondominant hemisphere). This, however, can be remedied by using some simple neuropsychological tests[14] that can be administered at the time of the clinical interview. Figure 8-2 presents some examples.[15]

TABLE 8-2. Additional neuropsychological screens.

- "Please use your right arm to point to the source of illumination in this room and tell me what it is called." (right-left discrimination, body part recognition, verbal command response, comprehension and naming)
- Have patient identify part of a watch, shoe, telephone. (part-whole naming)
- "Cover your right eye with your left hand:" and all other combinations of right and left eye and hand placements. (right-eye and body part recognition, integrity of corpus callosum, ideomotor capability)
- "Make believe that you have a lit candle in your left hand and blow it out." (ideomotor praxis)
- "Please repeat after me, no ifs, and, or buts" (speech fluency, comprehension)
- "If Bob can buy 5 pencils for a dollar, how many pencils can he buy with 60 cents?" (comprehension, multistep problem solving)
- "Please picture this scene in your head. You are walking down the street and see a group of guys and gals milling around a store. They have black leather jackets on, are making quite a racket, and are drinking something out of cans. Next to them on the street can be seen several parked motorcycles. Tell me what you think is happening and what you would do." (visuo-spatial mediated social judgment)

Table 8-2 lists some additional neuropsychological tasks that can detect fixed defects.

Fluctuating deficits require observation from others when the patient is hospitalized. This is a much easier task; nursing staff can look for changes in sensorium, affect, and behavior across shifts. Outpatients require co-operative family members and/or significant others to be briefed on pertinent signs. It is helpful to pick out 3 to 5 target symptoms or signs to focus on and then train the patient or observer to compile an occurrence record. Symptom presentation may be sleep-cycle dependent (e.g., hypnogogic and hypnopompic hallucinosis) cortisol-rhythm dependent (diurnal mood fluctuation), or ambient light-sensitive (as in the "sundowning" phenomena of organic brain syndromes). It is important to note the frequency and duration of symptom presentation and to correlate them with any warning signs or environmental occurrences.

Paroxysmal symptoms and/or signs often point to abnormal electrical discharges in the TLLHA. Table 8-3 presents a helpful checklist that systematically evaluates TLLHA function. Again, duration, frequency, and longitudinal history of positive responses should be noted (see Table 8-3).

The temporal lobe-limbic hypothalamic checklish (TLLHC) illustrates the wide array of psychopathology that can emanate from TLLHA dysrhythmia. This is best exemplified by the clinical correlates displayed by Table 8-4.

Electroencephalographic evaluation is a valuable component of the neuropsychiatric workup because of the clinical importance of the TLLHA. The existence of deep brain subcortical afterdischarge often eludes surface scalp EEG recordings. Depth electrode placement would provide definitive data but other than use in the preoperative neurosurgical seizure patient, this option is ethically unavailable. Therefore, other maneuvers are utilized to maximize the efficacy of surface recording. Sleep deprivation, sleep recording, and careful attention to temporal leads increases the yield as does hyperventilation and photic driving. When a sleep-deprived recording is obtained, the clinician should be aware that the record will not be an accurate awake sample due to the persistent drowsiness after the patient has been up all night. An additional awake tracing may be required. An ambulatory 24-hour EEG gains in sampling duration what it loses in electrode number and montage sophistication. A relatively new technology, computerized EEG (brain electrical activity mapping) has begun to show some promise in the eating disorder patient.[16,17]

Because PET scanning is prohibitively expensive, relatively unavailable in most areas, and still a research tool, an alternative must be found to help elucidate regional cerebral metabolism. The single photon emission computed tomography (SPECT) scans of the brain provide a semiquantitative measure of regional blood flow and, indirectly, metabolism. This technique may reveal pathology when magnetic resonance imaging (MRI) and computerized tomography (CT) fail.[18]

TABLE 8-3. Temporal lobe-limbic-hypothalamic checklist.

RIGHT TEMPORAL LOBE:
— Micropsia
— Macropsia
— Deja Vu
— Jamais Vu
— Visual Distortions (spots, blur, hallucinations)
— Visual Memory Loss
— Spatial Agnosia
— Sense of Unfamiliarity
— Derealization
— Depersonalization

LEFT TEMPORAL LOBE:
— Word finding difficulty
— Difficulty naming familiar objects
— Episodic Memory Loss for
(1) places
(2) events
(3) words
(4) concepts
— Amnesia for symptomatic episodes
— Episodic confusion
— Episodic disorientation

BI-TEMPORAL PHENOMENA:
— Fugue States
— Partial Fugue States
— Stereotypic behavior
— Other episodic dysfunction
— Autoscopy

LIMBIC LOBE DYSFUNCTION:
— Olfactory Hallucinations e.g., foul smells
— Gustatory Hallucinations e.g., bad tastes
— Lip Smacking
— Tongue Movements
— Rage attacks/violence
— Episodic Anxiety
— Episodic intense depression
— Episodic dysphoria
— Episodic euphoria
— Episodic paranoia
— Sense of impending doom
— Sense of impending ecstasy
— Episodic anhedonia (loss of pleasure, acts that usually give pleasure)

HYPOTHALAMIC SEIZURES:
(Mimic autonomic and organ involvement; limbic phenomena)
— Pallor
— Flushing
— Sweating
— Finger or toe paresthesiae
— Episodic faintness
— Episodic dyspnea

THALAMIC:
— Sense of cold or hot
— Unexplainable intense abdominal pain
— Unexplainable focal pain anywhere

OPTIC RADIATION:
— Visual hallucinations
— Illusions
— Scintillations

OTHER SYMPTOMS:
— Loss of consciousness
— Brief episodes of loss of memory
— Vertigo
— Dizziness
— Grand mal seizure

Clinical Example

Case C.F.

An illustrative case example is that of a 27-year-old female college student. She was a theater major who was seen as an outpatient because of depressed mood, alcohol abuse, and hysterical style. This young woman related an 11-year history of bulimia, anorexia, fad dieting (without pathological weight loss), and alternatively automatic or forced emesis. Surprisingly, she did not describe a disturbance of body image. She noted that her present weight was "just about right," which was in fact the case.

TABLE 8-4. Clinical correlates of TLLHC.

DISTURBANCES OF AFFECT
affective hypertrophy
affective lability
manic and/or depressive mood swings
dysphoric states
anxiety-panic attacks
angry outbursts
anhedonia
DISTURBANCES OF THINKING AND REALITY EXPERIENCE
forced obsessive thoughts—sexual, religious, self-negative, referential themes
racing thoughts—flight of ideas
referential (paranoid) thinking—a secondary compensatory phenomenon?
depersonalization
derealization, unfamiliarity
deja vu, jamais vu, deja entendu
confusion, disorientation, fugue states
word finding difficulties
PERCEPTUAL DISTURBANCES
macropsia, micropsia, visual distortion, visual hallucinosis, visual agnosia
olfactory or gustatory hallucinosis
auditory distortion or hallucinosis
vertigo/dizziness
paresthesiae including focal pain
AUTONOMIC DISTURBANCES
vasomotor lability
sweating
palpitations
piloerection
dyspnea
vascular headaches
DYSMNESIA
visual or language memory loss
amnesia for symptomatic episodes
NEUROVEGETATIVE DRIVE DISTURBANCE
hunger—bulimia and anorexia
thirst—compulsive water drinking
sex—hypersexuality
sleep attacks—narcolepsy
anhedonia
AUTOMATISMS
complex motor—compulsive, purposeless
lip smacking, tongue movements

She described an eight-year history of periods of intense depression and dysphoria marked by psychomotor retardation. She also noted binge drinking episodes that correlated with periods of depression. She did not enjoy the taste of alcoholic beverages but felt a compulsion to drink.

Interspersed between her depressions were periods of motoric hyperactivity, elation, insomnia, and hypersexuality. Her premorbid history failed to illicit significant psychopathology except for obsessive-compulsive traits. Her TLLHC, however, was dramatically positive and revealed olfactory hallucinosis, frequent deja vu, fugue states, visual illusions of size and movement, and spontaneous affective disturbance. Her EEG was only mildly abnormal. As a child, she was noted to have had a severe case of measles with probable signs of temporal lobe dysrhythmia (some sharpwaves unilaterally). The neurological examination and CT scan were negative. An empirical phenytoin trial led to cessation of affective and "eating disorder" signs. While on vacation in Europe, the young woman forgot to take her medicine on her trip and noted symptom return. Reinstitution of phenytoin upon returning to the United States led to complete remission. A several year follow-up demonstrated medication compliance and persistent symptom control.

The neuropsychiatric approach to the eating disorders requires patience, curiosity, and a lot of humility; there is much to be learned and plenty to be "unlearned." Diagnosis should not be based on phenomenology, psychodynamics, or exclusion. The biopsychosocial model provides a good foundation to build upon.

References

1. DSM-III-R. American Psychiatric Association: Diagnostic and Statistical Manual of Mental Disorders (third edition revised). Washington, DC, American Psychiatric Association, 1987.
2. Halmi KA. Eating disorders. In Talbot JA, Hales RE, Yudofsky SC (eds). The American Psychiatric Press Textbook of Psychiatry. Washington, DC, American Psychiatric Press, Inc, 1990; 753–766.
3. Giannini AJ, Martin DM, Turner CE. Beta-endorphin decline in late luteal phase dysphoric disorder. *Int J Psychiatry Med* 1990; 20(3):279.
4. Goddard CV, McIntyre DC, Leech CK. A permanent change in brain function resulting from daily electrical stimulation. *Exp Neurol* 1969; 25:295–330.
5. Post RM, Koponda RT. Cocaine kindling and psychosis. *Am J Psychiatry* 1976; 133:627–634.
6. Williams D. Man's temporal lobe. *Brain* 1968; 92:639–654.
7. Gross DA. Medical origins of psychiatric emergencies: The systems approach. *Int J Psychiatry Med* 1981; 11:1–10.
8. Weiner H, Thaler M, Reiser MF, et al. Etiology of duodenal ulcer. *Psychosom Med* 1957; 19:1–10.
9. Kandel ER. Psychotherapy and the single synapse. *N Engl J Med* 1979; 301:1028–1037.
10. Gross DA. The TLLHA in psychiatry: Its use in psychiatry and neurology. Presented at the International Epilepsy Society Symposium. Neurobehavioral Problems in Epilepsy, New Orleans, February 1989.

11. Wechsler D. The Measurement of Adult Intelligience. Baltimore, Williams & Williams, 1958.
12. Reitan R, Davidson L (eds). Clinical Neuropsychology: Current Status & Application. New York, John Wiley & Sons, 1974.
13. Golden CJ, Hammeke TA, Purisch AD. The Luria-Nebraska Neuropsychological Battery. Los Angeles, Western Psychological Services, 1980.
14. Strub RL, Black FW. The Mental Status Examination in Neurology. Philadelphia, F.A. Davis, 1977.
15. Byck R. Personal Communication. 1975.
16. McElroy SL, Pope, HG, Woods BT, et al. Brain electrical activity mapping (BEAM) in bulimia nervosa. *Ann Clin Psychiatry* 1991; 3:281–286.
17. Johnston J, Giannini AJ. Application of quantitive EEG/EP in psychiatry. *Psychiatric Ann* 1990; 20(7):405.
18. Trzepacz PT, Hertweek M, Starrett C, et al. The relationship of SPECT scans to behavioral dysfunction in neuropsychiatric patients. *Psychosomatics* 1992; 33(1):62–71.

9
Anorexia in the Elderly

A. James Giannini

The concept of fasting as a virtue originated in the Judeo-Christian tradition where it was utilized to scourge the flesh and thus purify the spirit. The early Passover rite gave birth to fasting during Lent, Ramadam and Yom Kippur, as well as the preparation for the Eucharistic sacrament are other Western fasting rituals that continue today. During the Middle Ages, the warrior class and the royal class fasted preparatory to being ennobled or enthroned. Anorectic symptoms were noted in the Italian Renaissance and depicted amoung young and old in the paintings of Florentine artists as Botticelli and della Francesca. These seem to be the first visual record of this condition in the modern West. The Judeo-Christian fasting rituals that were continued sought to purge the corrupt portion of Man's duality. Simultaneously, the rediscovered Greco-Roman ideal of a slim silhouette was pursued with the mental, philosophical, and pharmacological tools of this period.[1]

During this time, Giovanni Bocaccio described enforced anorexia in older men in his novel *II Decameron*. He noted that older men would employ a starvation-weakened state to protect them from carnal desires. Thus, both temporal and spiritual goals could be achieved by adults utilizing a fasting regimen. In 1668, Thomas Hobbes made the first medical notation of anorexia. Twenty-four years later, Richard Morton published the first account that described anorexia as a clinical entity. His patient was an adolescent girl whom he described as ". . . a skeleton clad only with skin."[2] One-hundred seventy-four years later, Sir William Gull described a similar condition in young women that he labelled "anorexia nervosa."[3] At about this time, Gull's contemporary, Henry Samuel Purdon, described "senile marasmus," an anorexia of the elderly. Significantly, the marasmus described by Purdon occurred in patients whose ages ranged from 69 to 92 years.[4]

Anorexia in the elderly is a problem that has continued to develop in the American milieu. Thousands of elderly patients are hospitalized each year with anorectic symptoms. In one-third of these patients, there was no discernable etiology for the anorexia.[5] Nearly 60 percent of Florida's nursing home residents have been documented to have some form of malnutrition.[6] The Health and Nutrition Examination Survey (HANES) of the U.S. Public Health Service has reported that 18 percent of American blacks and 16 percent of American whites over 60 living above the poverty line subsist on a daily intake of less than 1000 calories.[7]

There are multiple etiologies that manifest as geriatric anorexia. At the biochemical level, many neurotransmitters combine in a complex and interactive manner to regulate appetite. Peripherally, gustatory villi (taste buds) contain the transmitter, substance P, which relays complex taste information to the central nervous system. In the central nervous system, appetite itself is governed by the paraventricular nucleus (PVN) in the hypothalamus.[8] The biogenic amines exert a central effect. Norepinephrine increases craving for carbohydrates when injected into the PVN.[9] Serotonin may increase or decrease appetite depending upon whether the 1A or 1B receptors are stimulated.[10] The peripheral polypeptide cholecystokinin (CCK) also effects appetite. After it is secreted by the gastrointestinal tract, its messages are transmitted to the PVN via the vagal nerves and the nucleus tractus solitarius. Though CCK can, of itself, produce satiety it generally acts synergistically with other gastrointestinal hormones.[11]

These neurotransmitters, in turn, modulate an opioid-regulated "feeding drive" in the PVN.[12] Opioids appear to modulate intake of fatty and strongly flavored foods. They also appear to reduce perception of sweet and salty tastes while increasing aversive responses to bitter taste. The major opioid is dynorphin, which stimulates appetite.[12] Its action is modulated by zinc. Also important is "neuropeptide Y," which increases carbohydrate intake.[13]

It is of major clinical interest that all of the neurotransmitters that regulate appetite and intake decline with age.[14] Peripherally, there is an anatomical degeneration of the gustatory villi. As these villi degenerate, there is a marked decrease in the synthesis of substance P. Complex and subtle taste discrimination as well as gross taste sensation (e.g., salt, sweet, sour, and bitter) then decline. As a result the PVN receives less information about the food being chewed. Subjectively, food is then viewed as "tasteless." A higher threshold of taste sensation is therefore needed to carry information. This can be done by either increasing taste information or taste intensity. Foods that contains the alkaloid, capsaicin, increase the amount of taste information carried to the PVN. Capsaicin is a compound that decreases the rate of metabolism of substance P. It is found in such spices as basil, chile, coriander, cumin, curry, oregano, and red pepper. In addition to using spices, the intensity of flavoring can be increased. The use of meat stock and fish stock serves this purpose as does the commercial flavor enhancers.

CCK also increases appetite peripherally. Its action appears to be an indirect one, acting upon other neurotransmitters including the biogenic amines. It declines slowly throughout the aging process, accelerating somewhat after the sixth decade. The biogenic amines also decline. Centrally, there is a decline in noradrenergic activity with advancing age.[15] Norepinephrine inhibits release of corticotropin releasing factor (CRF), a peptide neurotransmitter. This CRF antagonism is responsible, in animals, for increasing the size of each meal.[16] Thus, decreasing levels of norepinephrine may produce anorectic symptoms in some elderly patients, especially those suffering from clinical depression.[17] Indeed, increased levels of CRF have been found in young anorectics.[18] The role of serotonin in producing geriatric anorexia is less clear but it appears that progressively decreasing levels of serotonin may disrupt overall regulation of food consumption and energy production.[19]

Central opioid transmitter levels and receptor densities are also reduced with age. Of possible clinical significance is the observation that older mice have an exaggerated anorectic response to morphine and other opiates as compared to younger mice.[20] Dynorphin levels also seem to experience overall decline leading to a progressive loss of overall appetite.[21] Neuropeptide Y usually decreases with age, but this decline is exaggerated in patients with Alzheimer's dementia.[22] Zinc levels also progressively decline with age.[23] This produces a positive feedback loop that accelerates the anorectic process. A zinc deficiency thus further reduces the activity of the opioid regulatory behavior.[23]

Because of biochemical and other factors the symptoms of anorexia nervosa can emerge for the first time in the seventh decade or later. Symptoms may include a conscious effort to reduce intake with no true comprehension of the magnitude of the actual weight loss achieved. In other cases, appetite wanes without conscious effort.[24] Weight loss in both of these cases often exceeds 15 percent of body mass.[25] Depression and anxiety appear to be common features.[26] There may be reverse satiety (i.e., the patient becomes less hungry when refraining from eating but increasingly hungry when he does eat) and the patient usually manifests some peculiar attitude towards food.[24] Patients have been reported to exaggerate their physician's warning to reduce fat intake and subsist solely on grains and leafy vegetables. Others have entirely avoided dairy products or other specific food groups. Harmful fad diets "tailored to the healthful senior" have also wreaked havoc on proper nutrition. In the elderly as well as other segments of the American milieu, there is often an intense fear of becoming fat.[23] This fear may be due to aesthetic reasons or just as likely to idiosyncratic health concerns. A physician's advice to "lose a little weight" after the appearance of hypertension or angina in the patient or family members can be amplified to the level of distortion.[24]

Bulimia may supplement anorectic behavior. Self-induced emesis is occasionally reported. Rarely, there is abuse of such homemade purgatives as mustard or soap-water. Most commonly laxative abuse and enema are noted. Laxatives can usually be detected by the presence of phenolphthalein in successive stool samples. Chronic digital insertion of soap (as a lubricant) also produces chronic effects similar to laxative abuse by irritation of rectal mucosa. This latter practice sometimes produces anal irritation which can be readily visualized. Both emesis and laxative abuse can produce malabsorption as well as the intended evacuation of the ingested food.

In addition to "true" or "apparent" (i.e., forme fruste) anorexia nervosa, this segment of the population may present with a depressive anorexia. While many of the symptoms of the disease "depression" are present, a complaint of the subjective feeling of "depression" may not ever be voiced.[25] In depressive anorexia, weight loss is associated with anergia and anhedonia. In contrast to the previous anorectic group there is less concern with body image though somatic complaints (i.e., "my bowels are plugged up") are often voiced.[26] Insomnia, decreased concentration, and subjective difficulties with concentration and memory are all part of the history of "geriatric depression with anorexia" but not "geriatric anorexia."[27,28]

The distinction is clinically significant. Both course and treatment differ greatly. Geriatric depression usually responds to low to moderate doses of tertiary tricyclic antidepressants while with primary anorexia, the results are mixed.[24,25] Imipramine or amitryptiline can increase food intake in the same manner it reverses other symptoms of the depression. In severe cases, electroconvulsive therapy may be employed.[29] Psychotherapeutically, in both cases, the focus is on loss and sometimes guilt.[26,27] In depressive anorexia, there can be loss of food's symbolism. In this group, anorexia can be viewed as an instrument of passive suicide. For the primary anorectic, issues such as mourning of a lost youth, waning sexuality, and exaggerated health concerns predominate. Many elderly patients respond to goal-directed short-term cognitive or behavioral therapy. Some, however, require longer-term, insight-oriented psychotherapy.

In a recent Finnish study of depression, a significant number of older men had gastrointestinal symptoms and complaints that could give rise to anorectic symptoms. Constipation and abdominal cramping was noted in 36 percent of the sample. Twenty-seven percent had nausea, 22 percent had loss of appetite, 20 percent had chronic diarrhea and 10 percent had bulimic symptoms.[30] In the United States, appetite suppression is the most common symptom among depressed geriatric populations.[31] Also, loss of appetite is a potential side effect among the geriatric patients receiving benzodiazepines and sedatives.[32]

Whether therapy is conducted on an inpatient or outpatient basis, a team approach is recommended. The therapeutic/administrative split allows one psychiatrist or other physician to focus on weight management and medication while a second psychiatrist resolves underlying conflicts. Other members of this treatment team should include both occupational therapists and dietitians. The occupational therapist can develop an environmental structures that reduce the importance of food intake. Dietitians can deal with nutritional care and meal planning.[33] On an inpatient basis, nurses can be utilized so that eating does not become a control issue in the therapeutic milieu.[34] It should be stressed, however, that in all cases a treatment protocol should not be established until an evaluation had been made by a physician experienced in the diagnosis and treatment of anorexia.

At any age, anorexia is usually established as a chronic condition by the time the psychiatrist sees the patient.[35] Since chronicity of eating disorders is associated with poor treatment outcome, it is of paramount importance that the psychiatrist actively considers the possible diagnosis of anorexia. Early intervention can reduce both the morbidity rate and the not inconsiderable mortality rate.[34]

References

1. Giannini AJ. Anorexia: A retrospective view. *Int J Psychiatry Med* 1981; 11:199–202.
2. Morton KI, Sor HC, Krupp JR. Involuntary weight loss: Diagnostic and prognostic significance. *Ann Int Med* 1981; 95:568–572.
3. Gull W. *Lancet* II 1968; 171.
4. Purdon HS. Statistical details of the diseases of advanced life. *Med Mirror* 1868; 5:662–664.
5. Morton KI, Sor HC, Krupp JR. Involuntary weight loss: Diagnostic and prognostic significance. *Ann Int Med* 1981; 95:568–572.
6. Pinckovsky-Devien GD, Kaninski MV. Correlation of pressure sores and nutritional status. *J Am Ger Soc* 1986; 34:435–440.
7. Abraham S, Carroll MD, Dresser CM, et al. Dietary intake of persons 1–74 years of age in the United States. *Vital and Health Statistics of the National Center of Health Statistics No. 6* Rockville, MD, Health Resources Admin, Public Health Services, 1977.
8. Nishimoto T, Akai M, Inagaki S, Shiizu K, Yamamoto E, Senba M. On the origin of substance P in the papillae: An experimental and histochemical study. *J Comp Neurol* 1982; 207:85–92.
9. Lesbowitz SF, Hamner NS, Chang K. Feeding behavior induced by central norepinephrine injection by central norepinephrine injection is attenuated by discrete lesions in the hypothalamic paraventricular nucleus. *Biochem Behav* 1983; 19:945–950.
10. Dourish CT, Huston PH, Kennet GA, Curzos G. 8-OH-DPAT induced hyperphagia: Its neurol basis and possible therapeutic relevance. *Appetite Suppl* 1986; 7:127–140.
11. Hinton V, Rosofsky M, Granger J, Geary N. Combined injection potentiates the satiety glucagon, cholecystokinin and bombesin. *Peptides* 1886; 17:615–619.
12. Morley JE, Levine AJ, Gosnell BA, Billington CJ. Which opioid receptor modulates feeding. *Appetite* 1984; 5:61–68.
13. Stanley BG, Leibowitz SF. Neuropeptide Y: Stimulation of feeding and drinking by injection into the paraventricular nucleus. *Life Sci* 1984; 33: 2635–2642.

14. Morley JE, Silver AJ. Anorexia in the elderly. *Neurobiol Aging* 1988; 9:9–16.
15. Kahlil T, Walker JP, Wiener J, Fagan CJ, Townsend CM, Greely GH, Thompson LC. Effect of aging on gallbladder construction and release of cholecystokinin-33 in humans. *Surgery* 1985; 98:423–429.
16. Krahn DD, Gosnell BA, Grace M, Levine AJ. CRF-antagonist partially reverses CRF- and stress-induced effects on feeding. *Brain Res Bull* 1986; 17:285–289.
17. Giannini AJ. Drug abuse and depression: Possible models for geriatric anorexia. *Neurobiol Aging* 1988; 9:26–27.
18. Hotta M, Shibasaki T, Masuda A, Imaki T, Demora H, Ling N, Shizume M. The responses of plasma adrenacorticotropin and cortisal to corticotropin-releasing hormone (CRH) and cerebrospinal fluid immunoreactive CRH in anorexia nervosa patients. *J Clin Endocrinol Metab* 1986; 62:319–324.
19. Blundell JE, Hill AJ. Serotonergic modulation of the pattern of eating and the profile of hunger satiety in humans. *Int J Obesity* 1987; 11:141–155.
20. Gosnell BA, Levine AJ, Morley JW. Effects of aging on opioid modulation of feeding in rats. *Life Sci* 1983; 32:2793–2799.
21. Hess GD, Joseph JA, Roth GS. Effect of age on sensitivity to pain and brain opiate receptors. *Neurobiol Aging* 1981; 2:49–55.
22. Missale CS, Giovoni S, Croce L, Bono A, Spano PF, Trabucchi M. Changes of B-endorphin and metenkephalin in the hypothalamus induced by aging. *J Neurochem* 1983; 40:20–24.
23. Essatera MD, Morley JE, Levine AS, Elson MK, McClain CJ. The role of endogenous opiates in zinc-deficiency anorexia. *Physiol Behav* 1984; 32: 475–478.
24. Giannini AJ, Telew N. Anorexia nervosa in geriatric patients. *Geriatric Med Today* 1987; 6:75–78.
25. Giannini AJ, Collins JI, Lewis D. Anorexia in the elderly—Case studies. *BASH* 1989; 8:126–130.
26. Price WA, Giannini AJ, Colella J. *J Am Geriatric Soc* 1985; 33:213–215.
27. Giannini AJ, Slaby AE. Dietary Management. NY, Elsevier (in press).
28. Cantwell D, Sturzenberger S, Burroughs J. Anorexia nervosa—an affective disorder. *Arch Gen Psychiatry* 1988; 34:1087–1089.
29. Bernstein IC. Anorexia nervosa: 94 year old women treated with electroshock. *Minn Med* 1972; 55:552–556.
30. Kivieda SL, Nissin A, Tuonilehto, Pevleanen J, Punsar S. Prevalence of depressive and other symptoms in elderly Finnish men. *Acta Psychiatr Scand* 1986; 73:93–100.
31. Zung WW. Depression in the normal ages. *Psychosomat* 1967; 8:287–292.
32. Giannini AJ. Un modello biopsichiatrico per riconoscere la tossicomania. *Ricerca e' Saluta* 2(3):4–9, 1990.
33. Giannini AJ. Treating anorexia and bulimia. In Taylor RB (ed): Difficult Medical Management. Philadelphia, Saunders, 1990.
34. Giannini AJ, Newman M, Gold MS. Anorexia and bulimia. *Am Family Physician* 1990; 41:1169–1176.
35. Ryle JA. Anorexia in an older population group. *Lancet* 1936; 893.

10
Depression and Eating Disorders

RUSSELL D. MARX

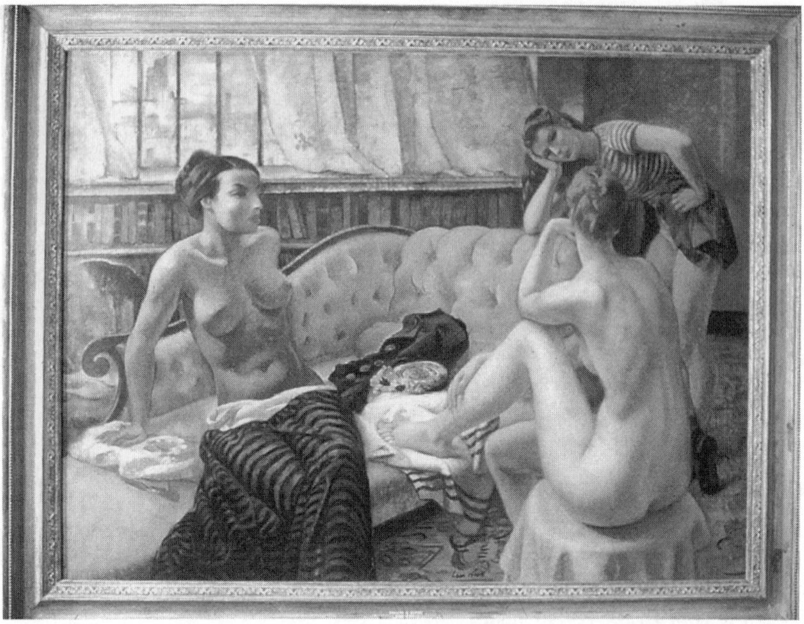

Kroll, Leon—*Dancers in Repose*—(Butler Institute of American Art, Youngstown, Ohio)

The relationship between eating disorders and affective disorders has intrigued psychiatrists for many years. Freud,[1] Brill,[2] Fenichel,[3] and Nemiah[4] have all commented on the connection between anorexia nervosa and depression. Abraham[5] has discussed the relationship between depression and binge eating seeing the latter as a substitute for a more direct libidinal gratification.

More recently this relationship has been examined from a scientific perspective. One hypothesis that has generated much speculation in recent years is the question of whether eating disorders are a variant of affective illness. Specific evidence regarding the relationship of eating disorder as affective illness can be looked at in a number of different areas:

1. prevalence of depressive symptoms and clinical depression in eating disorder patients;
2. family studies of affective illness in relatives of eating disorder patients;
3. antidepressant treatment research;
4. polysomnography;
5. positron emission tomography comparison of regional brain metabolism;
6. neuroendocrine research;
7. neurochemistry research.

Frequency of Depression

Strober and Katz,[6] looking at a broad range of studies, found a mild to moderate level of depression in anorexia nervosa and bulimia nervosa. Specific diagnostic instruments used in these studies included the Beck Depression Inventory, Minnesota Multiphasic Personality Inventory, Montgomery Asberg Depression Rating Scale, Raskin Three Factor Depression Index, Schedule for Affective Disorders and Schizophrenia, Hamilton Depression Rating Scale, Depression Symptom Index, Middlesex Hospital Questionnaire, Hopkins Symptom Checklist, Children's Depression Inventory, Present State Examination, and visual analog scales of depression. They found that while mean scores on these instruments exceeded normal controls, they tended to be lower than the average severity scores for primary depressives.

Standardized diagnostic interviews have also shown increases in affective illness in eating disorder patients with rates of major depressive disorders ranging from 25 to 80 percent. A recent study by Laessle et al.[7] of 52 patients with anorexia nervosa and bulimia nervosa showed that 44 percent had a lifetime diagnosis of DSM III major affective disorder. He found that abstaining anorectics had a lower rate of depression than those with bulimic symptoms. This agrees with the work of Garfinkel et al.[8] and Strober[9] although studies of Herzog[10] and Piran et al.[11] have not confirmed this finding. Laessle[7] also found that in the great majority of his cases the onset of the affective illness followed the onset of the eating disorder by at least one year. They also found that the rate of depressive symptoms were lower in those patients whose eating disorder was in remission as compared with those in the acute stage of their illness.

The question of whether depression generally precedes or follows the onset of an eating disorder is a controversial one. In contrast to the work of Laessle et al., Piran et al.[11] found that depressive symptoms preceded the onset of anorexia nervosa by at least one year in 44 percent of anorectic patients with a lifetime history of major depression. Among bulimic patients, a substantial prior history of depression has been found by Hudson et al.,[12] Lee et al.,[13] and Walsh et al.[14]

A large study by Eckert et al.[15] of 105 hospitalized female anorexia nervosa patients looked at the extent of depression in terms of symptoms and mood rather than looking at formal diagnostic criteria for affective disorder. In agreement with the findings of Laessle they found that improvement in the eating disorder (such as weight gain) was correlated with decrease in depressive symptoms. Their study also related more severe symptoms of depression with more disturbed eating attitudes and eating patterns, more disturbed body image, lower weight, greater denial about the severity of illness, more laxative abuse, a more disturbed relationship with her father, and more sexual disturbance. In summary, they found that severity of depression was associated with characteristics that have classically been considered signs of greater severity of anorexia nervosa.

Herzog[10] studied 82 female outpatients with anorexia nervosa and bulimia using a structured interview technique. Research Diagnostic Criteria for major depression were met by 56 percent of the anorexia patients and 24 percent of the bulimic patients. Similar results were found using the Extracted Hamilton Depression Rating Scale with moderate to severe depression seen in 41 percent of the anorectic patients and 24 percent of the bulimic patients. In this study significant differences were not found between restricting and bulimic anorectics.

Walsh et al.[14] looked at 50 female patients meeting DSM III criteria for bulimia. He found that 70 percent of patients met Research Diagnostic Criteria for major depression and 88 percent had met RDC for some affective disturbance at some point in their life.

Hudson et al.[12] looked at 90 patients with anorexia nervosa and bulimia and found that 77 percent of these patients had a lifetime diagnosis of DSM III major affective disorder. No significant differences were found in these rates between eating disorder subgroups but the lifetime rates of major affective disorder were significantly greater in inpatients compared with outpatients.

Piran et al.[11] looked at 47 female patients with anorexia nervosa and bulimia and found that 38 percent met criteria for a major depressive episode. No significant difference in these rates were found between bulimic and restrictive subgroups.

Viesselman et al.[16] looked at 95 patients diagnosed with anorexia nervosa or bulimia and found major depression by Feigner criteria in 80 percent of patients with lifetime suicide attempts in 20 percent of these patients. Russell,[17] looking at 30 patients with bulimia nervosa found 43 percent with severe depressive symptoms, a previous course of ECT, or a serious suicidal act.

Outcome studies also shed light on the relationship between eating disorders and affective illness. Cantwell et al.[18] looked at 26 patients with anorexia nervosa an average of 5 years after hospitalization. He found that 46 percent met Feighner criteria for affective disorder. Only one of the 26 patients was still possibly anorectic although other eating difficulties were noted in a substantial number of patients.

Not all follow-up studies are consistent with a high rate of depression in eating disorder patients. Swift et al.[19] looked at 30 bulimia patients using a time frame of two to five years follow-up and found only a small amount of depression using Beck and Hamilton ratings. A significant percentage of these patients continued to show bulimic symptoms.

In looking at outcome for 18 normal weight bulimic patients, Norman et al.[20] found significant improvement in eating attitudes and depressive symptoms at one and three year follow-up. Using a much shorter time frame of ten weeks Lacey[21] found in 30 women with severe bulimia, that as bulimic symptoms decreased, depressive symptoms increased.

Several points need to be made concerning this body of evidence linking eating disorders and affective illness.

First of all, as Levy et al.[22] point out, "While the prevalence of depression, as determined by non-blind investigators is much higher in bulimic persons than in the general population, the possibility of bias cannot be totally dismissed." He further states that "there have been no large studies investigating depression in bulimia and control (psychiatric and normal) subjects in which structured interviews were conducted by raters blind to diagnosis." Furthermore, "samples of bulimic subjects are generally drawn from patients seeking treatment, which may create a skew toward bulimic subjects with greater depression, and thus the results may not be generalizable to the bulimic population as a whole." There are other difficulties in determining the true relationship between eating disorders and affective illness. One factor related to an increased incidence of depressive symptoms in eating disorders is the nature of the DSM III criteria for bulimia which include "depressed mood and self-deprecating thoughts."[23]

Another area of confusion relates to the propensity of eating disorders to produce depressive symptoms themselves, rather than the depressive symptoms arising from a concurrent affective illness. As Strober, et al.[6] state "It is doubtful whether assessments of depression in eating disorder patients can have real significance without multiple follow-up ratings in which the independent and joint effects of starvation and related behavioral abnormalities (e.g., frequency of binge eating, nutrient content of diet, body weight, etc.) on degree and persistence of depression can be statistically discriminated."

Scientific studies of the effect of starvation on mood have existed for over forty years. In the famous study by Ancel Keys and colleagues[24] at the University of Minnesota, thirty-six healthy male volunteers, screened to be psychologically normal, had their food intake restricted by one-half during a period of six months so that they lost an average of 25 percent of their original body weight. (This degree of weight loss corresponds to the DSM III criteria for the degree of weight loss needed for anorexia nervosa.) Numerous changes were observed including preoccupation with food, unusual eating behaviors, decreased sexual interest, and social withdrawal.

Serious depressive symptoms were noted by many subjects with 20 percent having symptoms of such severity that their functioning was markedly decreased. Anxiety, irritability and anger significantly increased for most of the subjects. Minnesota Multiphasic Personality Inventory (MMPI) testing revealed significant increases in depression, hysteria, and hypochondriasis. During the refeeding period these depressive symptoms did not necessarily quickly improve but actually became worse for some of the subjects.

These findings are important not only in looking at patients with anorexia nervosa, but also in patients with bulimia nervosa. It has been demonstrated by Pirke et al.[25] that normal weight bulimic patients can evidence biological signs of starvation including elevated free fatty acid, reduced T-3 (triiodothyronine) levels and decreased peripheral noradrenergic response with orthostatic testing.

Another argument that some normal weight bulimic patients are in a state of semistarvation comes from the work of Garner and Fairburn.[26] They have shown that many bulimia nervosa patients presenting at a statistically normal weight have actually lost as much body weight as anorexia nervosa patients. They propose that these bulimia patients "may be genetically predisposed to higher than average "natural" weights, and it is their very attempt to lose weight from this initial level that sets into motion the vicious cycle of bulimia nervosa."

Finally, in addition to biological causes of depressive symptoms in eating disorders there are obvious psychological and behavioral connections. Loss of control resulting in such symptoms as the binging of bulimia can bring about feelings of guilt, shame, and low self-esteem. The secrecy that accompanies many cases of bulimia can increase social isolation and lead to loss of social supports which in turn can increase depressive symptoms.

Family Studies

There is much evidence that the prevalence rates of major af disorders are increased in first and second degree relatives of eating disorder patients. Winokur et al.[27] compared the relatives of 25 patients with anorexia nervosa to the relatives of 25 normal control subjects. Diagnoses were assigned by nonblind raters using Research Diagnostic Criteria. Using both direct family study and family history methods, 22 percent of the relatives of patients with anorexia nervosa had major affective disorder compared to only 10 percent of the relatives of the controls. Both unipolar and bipolar depressions were significantly increased in the anorexia nervosa relatives.

Hudson et al.[28] looked at 420 first degree relatives of 14 patients with anorexia nervosa, 55 patients with bulimia, and 20 patients with both disorders. These were compared to a control group of 499 first degree relatives of 33 patients with bipolar disorder, thirty-nine patients with schizophrenia, and 15 patients with borderline personality disorder. The family history method was used for a majority of families. The morbid risk for major affective disorder was 27 percent in the relatives of eating disorder patients compared to 12 percent in the relatives of bipolar patients and 1 percent and 3 percent in the relatives of patients with schizophrenia and borderline personality disorder. Significant differences in relatives' morbid risk for affective disorder were not found between the eating disorder subgroups.

Gershon et al.[29] looked at 99 first degree relatives of 24 patients with anorexia nervosa (of whom 11 were also bulimic). He compared these relatives by interview and family history with 265 relatives of 43 medically ill controls. He found a significant increase in unipolar depression, bipolar disorder and schizoaffective disorder in anorexia nervosa families. The increase in unipolar depression in families was not correlated with concurrent depression in the anorexia nervosa patients. No differences were seen comparing restricting and bulimic anorexics for family prevalence of affective disorders.

Rivinus et al.[30] compared 545 first and second degree relatives of 40 patients with anorexia nervosa and 217 first and second degree relatives of 23 normal controls. Family history method was used by nonblind raters. A significant increase in unipolar depression and substance abuse was found in anorexia nervosa families. One difference from previous studies was that bipolar disorders were not found in the first degree relatives of either group. Also it was necessary to pool diagnoses of depression and substance abuse to reach statistical significance.

The data in this study was reanalyzed by Biederman et al.[31] He separated the anorectic group into those with and without current nonbipolar major depression and looked at their first degree relatives. He found a morbid risk of 25 percent in the families of depressed anorexic patients versus only 6 percent in the families of nondepressed anorexia patients and 4.7 percent of the families of normal controls. These findings differed from Gershon's who did not find that the presence of a current episode of affective disorder in the patient predicted unipolar depression in the relatives.

A different result was found in the study of Stern et al.[32] He looked at the lifetime prevalence of affective disorder in the first and second degree relatives, excluding children of 27 bulimic women (who had never had anorexia nervosa) and 27 women with no history of an eating disorder. A family history method was used and raters were blind to probands diagnoses. No significant increase was found in bulimic families of either unipolar depression or bipolar depression or substance abuse. No significant difference was found in limiting the comparison to mothers, or first degree relatives or examining male and female relatives separately. Thus, Stern found that "contrary to our expectations, there was no significant difference between the relatives of bulimic and control probands with regard to the lifetime prevalence of affective disorder."

A recent study by Kassett et al.[33] using the more accurate family study method found results more consistent with the majority of family studies. She compared 185 adult first degree relatives of 40 bulimic subjects with 118 first degree relatives of 24 normal controls. She found a significantly higher morbid risk of 28 percent for major affective disorder among relatives of bulimic probands compared to 9 percent among relatives of normal controls. A significantly higher morbid risk for major affective disorder was found for the families of both bulimic probands with and without affective disorders. In the former group, there was a 35 percent morbid risk for major affective disorder among relatives, and in the latter group there was a 19 percent morbid risk compared to a 9 percent morbid risk in families of control subjects.

Other studies have looked at the differences between bulimics who have a family history of depressive illness compared with those who do not. Mitchell et al.[34] compared 164 bulimic patients with no family history of depression in first degree relatives to 111 bulimic patients who had at least one first degree relative with depression or manic-depressive illness. They found that patients in the positive family history group were significantly more likely to have been treated previously for depression. They also found more problems reported for functioning at work or socially in this group. The positive family history group was also more likely to give reasons for binge eating related to depressive symptoms such as unhappiness or tension. The two groups, however, did not differ as far as levels of depression measured by Hamilton Rating Scale or the severity of their eating problems.

In other studies, Lee et al.[13] looked at 56 bulimic patients of whom 59 percent reported first degree relatives with affective disorder. The positive family history group had an earlier onset of bulimia than those without such relatives. Wilson et al.[35] found that bulimic patients who were more depressed had a greater likelihood of a family history of depression.

Antidepressant Treatment

Numerous controlled studies have shown antidepressant medications to be effective in reducing symptoms of bulimia nervosa. These medications have not, on the contrary, been shown to be very helpful in the treatment of anorexia nervosa.

Pope et al.[36] conducted one of the first controlled trials looking at 22 bulimic patients studied for 6 weeks with 200 mg of imipramine. Nineteen patients completed the study with 8 of 9 patients on medication showing a positive response whereas none of the 10 placebo patients showed a positive response. These ten patients were then openly given imipramine and seven showed a positive response.

Hughes et al.[37] also conducted a six week trial with 22 bulimic patients using different doses of desipramine. Only nondepressed patients were studied. Patients receiving active drug had a much more significant reduction in bulimic symptoms than did patients receiving placebo and 68 percent of patients receiving desipramine were able to obtain symptomatic remission either during or after the study.

Mitchell et al.[38] conducted an 8 week trial using 150 mg of amitriptyline in which 16 patients received active drug and 16 patients received placebo. All patients received behavioral treatment during this study. Active drug patients showed a 70 percent reduction in binge frequency compared to a 52 percent reduction in the placebo group (not a significant difference). Of note, blood levels of antidepressant were below therapeutic levels for antidepressant efficacy in one-half of the patients who were tested. Also contributing to the high placebo response level may have been a high level of motivation among the subjects as well as the concurrent behavioral treatment.

Agras et al.[39] studied imipramine in a 16 week controlled trial in 20 bulimic women. After 16 weeks there was a 72 percent reduction of binge frequency in the active drug group compared to a 43 percent reduction in the placebo group.

Several controlled trials have also demonstrated the efficacy of monoamine oxidase inhibitor antidepressant treatment of bulimia. Walsh et al.[40] studied phenelzine in a double-blind, placebo controlled trial in 30 bulimic patients. In the active drug group 6 out of 14 patients were in remission at the end of the study compared to none out of 16 patients in the placebo group. The active drug group also scored significantly lower than the placebo group on the Eating Attitudes Test by the end of the study. Binging frequency, which was about ten times per week in each group at the beginning of the study, was reduced to 3.4 times per week in the active drug group compared to 9.1 times per week in the placebo group.

Kennedy et al.[41] looked at another monoamine oxidase inhibitor, isocarboxazid, in a controlled study with 18 bulimic women. They found a significant reduction in binge frequency after six weeks with the active drug group going from 7.0 binges to 2.7 binges compared to the placebo group reduction of 7.5 binges to 4.5 binges. There was also a significant reduction in scores on the Eating Attitudes Test.

One controlled study that did not find a significant advantage for antidepressant treatment was that of Sabine et al.[42] who studied Mianserin in 50 bulimic women for eight weeks. No significant difference was seen between the 20 patients on active drug compared to 30 patients on placebo. One possible reason for this negative finding is that the dose of Mianserin used, 60 mg, is lower than the doses generally used to treat depression. Although it has not been established that the antidepressant medication therapeutic blood levels shown to be effective for depression are the same as for bulimia there is some suggestive evidence. For example, in the study of Hughes et al. cited previously, when the desipramine dose was increased in six nonresponders who had subtherapeutic blood levels, four were able to achieve complete symptom remission.

Summarizing the results of nine controlled antidepressant trials, Mitchell et al.[43] found a mean reduction in binge eating of 73 percent with 29 percent of the patients in remission. But important questions remain about the mechanisms by which these medications are effective. The neurochemical systems that mediate mood are also quite important in central regulation of hunger and satiety. Desipramine, for example, has been shown to reduce hunger in the rat. A recent study by Blouin et al.[45] found independence of the antibulimic and antidepressant properties of desipramine. In a controlled study, desipramine was investigated in 24 normal-weight bulimic women. Although a significant reduction in weekly binging and vomiting was seen with medication, no effect was seen on depressive symptomatology measured either by the SCL-90 or the Profile of Mood States (POMS). This was in contrast to the findings of Pope et al. and Mitchell et al. in studies cited previously in which tricyclic anti-depressants were found to have a significant effect on the Hamilton Rating Scale for depression in their bulimic subjects. Of note in both these studies, however, is that the patients who were more depressed showed a worse response to medication in terms of their eating disorder compared with less depressed patients.

Polysomnography

Sleep EEG studies have demonstrated certain abnormal findings in patients with depression such as shortened REM latency, increased REM density, and decreased delta sleep.[22] However, as Hudson et al.[46] stated recently, "EEG sleep abnormalities are often not present, or present only to a modest degree, in younger outpatients with depression" and he suggests that this may be a better comparison group to patients with eating disorders.

Katz et al.[47] compared the sleep EEGs of 20 women with anorexia nervosa (17 of whom also had bulimic symptoms) with that of 10 control subjects. He found a significant difference in shortened REM latency for the anorectic group. He speculated that a subgroup of his anorectic patients had concurrent affective disorder and found that in the shortened REM latency group, Hamilton scores for depression averaged 38 compared to 20 for a group with long REM latency.

Most controlled studies, however, have not found significant abnormalities in the sleep EEGs of bulimic patients. Walsh et al.[48] compared the sleep EEG of 8 women with anorexia nervosa, 16 normal-weight bulimic women, and 14 normal controls. Although the patients with anorexia nervosa spent less time asleep and less of their sleep time in stage 1 the bulimic women showed sleep EEGs that were essentially similar to that of the control subjects. No sleep abnormalities characteristic of major depression were seen in these patients.

Levy et al.[49] looked at sleep EEGs of 9 anorectic women, 9 bulimic women, and 10 normal controls. He found results similar to those of Walsh in that the patients with anorexia nervosa had more sleep disruption but normal-weight bulimics did not show significant sleep EEG differences from control subjects.

Hudson et al.[46] compared 11 women with normal-weight bulimia to groups of 20 normal controls and 44 young outpatient women with depression. The bulimic women showed essentially normal sleep EEG characteristics.

Lauer et al.[50] recently compared sleep EEGs of 10 young depressed patients, 20 patients with anorexia nervosa, 10 patients with bulimia nervosa, and 10 normal controls. The only significant difference found was increased REM density in the depressed patients. No difference in EEG sleep was seen in eating disorder patients with a concomitant major depressive episode.

One recent study that seemed to find more of a relationship between the sleep EEGs of depressed and bulimic patients is that of Waller et al.[51] He compared 12 bulimic women with 20 normal controls and 61 subjects under 40 years of age with endogenous depression. Compared with normal controls, shortened REM latency was found in some bulimic patients without concurrent major depression. He suggests that there is a subgroup of bulimic patients whose eating disorder is more closely related to major depressive disorder.

Positron Emission Tomography

Hagman et al.[52] compared brain metabolism in 8 women with bulimia nervosa, 8 women with major affective disorder, and 8 normal women controls using positron emission tomography and 18-fluoro-2-deoxyglucose. She found that compared to normal women, the bulimic women lost the normal higher right than left cortical metabolic rates in certain areas. Similar to the normal women, the bulimic women retained active basal ganglia activity. The depressed women retained right hemisphere activation but showed decreased basal ganglia activity. She suggests that this evidence supports the position that the "pathophysiologic basis of bulimia differs from that of major affective disorder."

Neuroendocrinology

About 50 percent of patients with major depression secrete greater amounts of cortisol than do normal subjects.[53] A substantial number of these patients also show abnormalities in cortisol suppression after dexamethasone administration and this test has had some utility in the diagnosis of affective disorders.

In anorexia nervosa, similar abnormalities in hypothalamic pituitary-adrenal functioning have been found. These include elevated levels of plasma cortisol and abnormal dexamethasone suppression tests. However, these abnormalities also occur in other forms of starvation and weight restoration usually results in return of normal cortisol patterns.

Numerous studies have demonstrated abnormal DST responses in bulimia. Hudson et al.[54] found a 47 percent nonsuppression in bulimic patients compared to 9 percent of normal controls. Gwirtsman et al.[55] in an uncontrolled study found 67 percent abnormal results in 18 bulimic patients. Mitchell et al.[56] found 50 percent abnormalities among 28 bulimic patients in another uncontrolled study. Lindy et al.[57] in an uncontrolled study looked at 55 bulimics and found a 35 percent abnormality rate. In a controlled study, Kiriike et al.[58] found a 63 percent abnormality rate in the bulimic group compared with 11 percent of controls. Levy et al.[59] had 100 percent of 8 bulimic patients show abnormal results compared with no abnormal results in 8 patients with nonendogenous major depression. Perez et al.[60] had a 58 percent abnormal rate in 33 bulimic patients.

Findings are mixed concerning the relationship of these abnormal DST results with either concurrent depressive symptoms or a family history of depression. Perez found a significant relationship between abnormal DST and concurrent major depression but neither Gwirtsman nor Mitchell found such a relationship. Mitchell did find a relationship between DST abnormalities and a family history of depression but this was not found by Perez, Kiriike, or Hudson.

The significance of these abnormal DSTs is unclear. Abnormal DSTs have been seen in numerous physical and psychiatric conditions including dementia, mania, and acute psychosis.[53] Walsh et al.[61] reported normal cortisol secretions in bulimic women, as opposed to the elevated level in depressed patients.

Looking at another level of hypothalamic-pituitary-adrenal functioning, corticotropin releasing hormone (CRF) yields a blunted ACTH response in both low weight anorectics[62] and depressed patients.[63] In contrast to this finding, Gold looked at 8 bulimic patients who abstained from binging and purging for 10 days and found a normal ACTH response to corticotropin releasing hormone.[62]

In looking at the thyroid axis, 25 percent of patients with affective illness show a blunted thyrotropin (TSH) response to thyrotropin releasing hormone (TRH).[64] In low weight anorectics this response is usually normal although it may be delayed or blunted.[64] In bulimic patients three controlled studies (Norris,[65] Levy,[66] and Kaplan[67]) did not show a blunted TSH response to TRH.

TRH stimulation has also been shown to produce increased growth hormone (GH) levels[68] and decreased prolactin levels[69,70] in depressed patients. Underweight anorectics show impaired GH responses to TRH[71] but normal prolactin responses to TRH stimulation.[72] In contrast, Levy et al.[73] found increased prolactin and growth hormone responses to TRH stimulation in bulimic patients.

In depressed patients, Amsterdam et al.[74] show normal basal luteinizing hormone (LH) and follicle stimulating hormone (FSH) levels and normal LH and FSH response to luteinizing hormone-releasing hormone (LH-RH). In underweight anorectics low basal levels of LH and FSH were seen with decreased LH response to LH-RH but possible exaggerated FSH response.[75] Levy et al.[22] found decreased basal LH in bulimic patients but a greater increase in response to LH-RH stimulation than control subjects showed.

Neurochemistry

Understanding of the neurochemical abnormalities in the eating disorders and their relationship to neurochemical abnormalities in affective disorders remains preliminary. Kaye et al.[76] found that CSF and plasma norepinephrine concentrations tend to be low in normal-weight bulimia compared to normal or high levels in major depressive disorders. These researchers also found no relationship between CSF norepinephrine levels and depression in bulimic patients.

Anorectic patients tend to show lower than normal levels of urinary and plasma MHPG as well as CSF norepinephrine and MHPG.[77] While this often shows normalization with weight gain, Kaye et al.[78] has shown that weight-recovered anorectics had a 50 percent lower CSF norepinephrine level than normal control subjects.

In looking at other neurotransmitter systems Kaye et al.[76] found that normal-weight bulimic patients had normal CSF levels of the major serotonin metabolite, 5-hydroxyindoleacitic acid (5-HIAA), and of the major dopamine metabolite, homovanillic acid (HVA). Kaye et al. also found that more frequent binging was associated with significantly lower CSF HVA levels. On the other hand, depression has been related to low brain serotonin levels.[79] Also, suicidal patients have been shown to have significantly lower concentrations of CSF 5-HIAA and HVA than do nonsuicidal patients and normal control subjects.[80] Findings in anorectic patients are conflicting with Gerner et al.[81] finding normal CSF levels of 5-HIAA whereas Kaye et al.[78] found lower than normal CSF 5-HIAA levels that normalized after weight recovery. Studies of CSF HVA levels in anorectic patients have yielded similarly conflicting results with both normal levels found as well as lower than normal levels which normalized after weight recovery.[77]

Summary

The existence of a relationship between eating disorders and depression seems to be well established. Studies show substantial amounts of both depressive symptoms and diagnoses of depression in eating disorder patients. Similarly the vast majority of studies looking at families of eating disorder patients show significantly greater amounts of affective illness than in families of normal controls. Conflicting evidence exists about such basic questions as which eating disorder subgroups are more likely to have depression and whether the onset of depression tends to precede or follow the onset of the eating disorder. Other evidence about the relationship between eating disorders and affective illness presents a complicated picture. It is clear that antidepressants reduce symptoms of bulimia. However, similar neurochemical systems regulate hunger/satiety and mood. Thus, it is not clear what degree of the efficacy of medication is due to improvement in mood.

Sleep EEG studies allow conclusions that sleep of eating disorder patients is more similar to that of normal controls than to depressed patients except perhaps for a subgroup of eating disorder patients with significant depression. The one study of positron emission tomography comparison of regional brain metabolism also presents a distinct profile for bulimic patients compared with depressed patients, but this must be considered very preliminary.

Looking at neuroendocrine studies, generally distinct profiles are seen for eating disorders and affective illness. There is some similarity when underweight anorectics are compared with depressed patients but these tend to disappear with weight restoration. The significance of abnormal DST results in both bulimia and depressed patients is questionable for several reasons. Firstly, this test is abnormal in a large number of psychiatric and physical conditions. Secondly, other tests of hypothalamic-pituitary adrenal functioning, such as cortisol levels, are elevated in depressed patients but not in bulimic patients. Lastly, neurochemical research in eating disorders is at a preliminary stage, but at the present time no convincing pattern of similarity to depression has been shown.

One is left with speculation about the nature of the relationship between eating disorders and affective illness. The hypothesis that eating disorders are merely a variant of affective illness does not seem to fit with the evidence available. Rather, it seems more sensible to conceive of eating disorders as both heterogeneous in nature and having complex and variable biopsychosocial components of etiology.

Swift et al.,[82] Levy et al.,[22] Strober et al.,[6] Hsu,[75] and others have offered interesting speculations about different patterns of interactions between eating disorders and depression. One subgroup of eating disorder patients may be those with preexisting depression or a biological or psychological vulnerability to depression. In such a group, normal dieting might progress to an eating disorder due to a greater need for the personal sense of competence and social reinforcement that weight loss elicits in our society. Another variant involves the use of binging or purging to cope with dysphoric or anxious feelings.

A third possibility is that nutritional deficiencies associated with eating disorders could lead to abnormal neurochemical states. A fourth contributor, significant depression in the family of origin, could impact on psychological development in ways that could make an eating disorder more likely. A fifth possibility is that the negative psychosocial impact of an eating disorder could make depression more likely in vulnerable patients. And finally, there might be, as yet unknown, common biological risk factors for both eating disorders and depression. Perhaps one statement that can be made with certainty is that the complex interrelationship of these disorders will provide fertile ground for future discoveries.

References

1. Freud S. On the origins of psychoanalysis. Letters to Wilhelm Fleiss. New York, Basic Books, 1954.
2. Brill AA. In discussion following Pardoe I: "Cachexia Nervosa: A psychoneurotic simmonds syndrome." *Arch Neurolog Psychiatry* 1939; 41:842.
3. Fenichel O. The Psychoanalytic Theory of Neurosis. London, Routledge and Kegan Paul, 1945.
4. Nemiah JC. Anorexia nervosa. *Medicine* 1950; 29:225–268.
5. Abraham K. The first pregenital stage of the libido (1916). Selected Papers of Karl Abraham. New York, Basic Books, 1954; 262–285.

6. Strober M, Katz JL. Depression in the eating disorders: A review and analysis of descriptive, family and biological findings. In Garner DM, Garfinkel PE (eds): Diagnostic Issues in Anorexia Nervosa and Bulimia Nervosa. New York, Brunner/Mazel, 1988.
7. Laessle RG, Kittl S, Fichter MM, et al. Major affective disorder in anorexia nervosa and bulimia. *Br J Psychiatry* 1987; 151:785–789.
8. Garfinkel PE, Moldofsky H, Garner DM. The heterogeneity of anorexia nervosa: Bulimia as a distinct subgroup. *Arch Gen Psychiatry* 1980; 37:1036–1040.
9. Strober M. The significance of bulimia in juvenile anorexia nervosa: An exploration of possible etiologic factors. *Int J Eating Disord* 1981; 1:28–43.
10. Herzog DB. Are anorexic and bulimic patients depressed? *Am J Psychiatry* 1984; 141:1594–1597.
11. Piran N, Kennedy S, Garfinkel PE, et al. Affective disorders in eating disorders. *J Nervous Mental Disease* 1985; 173:395–400.
12. Hudson JI, Pope HG, Jonas JM, et al. Phenomenologic relationship of eating disorders to major affective disorder. *Psychiatric Research* 1983; 9:345–354.
13. Lee NF, Rush AJ, Mitchell JE. Depression and bulimia. *J Affective Disord* 1985; 9:231–238.
14. Walsh BT, Roose SP, Glassman AH, et al. Depression and bulimia. *Psychosomatic Medicine* 1985; 47:123–131.
15. Eckert ED, Goldberg SC, Halmi KA, et al. Depression in anorexia nervosa. *Psychological Medicine* 1982; 12:115–122.
16. Viesselman JO, Roig M. Depression and suicidality in eating disorders. *J Clin Psychiatry* 1985; 46:118–124.
17. Russell GFM. Bulimia nervosa: An ominous variant of anorexia nervosa. *Psychological Medicine* 1979; 9:429–448.
18. Gantwell DP, Sturzenburger S, Burroughs J, et al. Anorexia nervosa: An affective disorder? *Arch Gen Psychiatry* 1977; 34:1087–1093.
19. Swift WJ, Kalin NH, Wamboldt FS, et al. Depression in bulimia at 2- to 5-year follow-up. *Psychiatric Research* 1985; 16:111–122.
20. Norman DK, Herzog DB. A 3-year outcome study of normal-weight bulimia: Assessment of psychological functioning and eating attitudes. *Psychiatry Research* 1986; 19:199–205.
21. Lacey JH. Bulimia nervosa, binge eating, and psychogenic vomiting: A controlled treatment study and long term outcome. *Br Med J* 1984; 286:1609–1613.
22. Levy AB, Dixon KN, Stern SL. How are depression and bulimia related? *Am J Psychiatry* 1989; 146:162–169.
23. American Psychiatric Association; Diagnostic and Statistical Manual of Mental Disorders (third edition). Washington, DC, APA, 1980.
24. Keys A, Brozek J, Henschel A, et al. The Biology of Human Starvation. Minneapolis, University of Minnesota Press, 1950.
25. Pirke KM, Pahl J, Schweiger U, et al. Metabolic and endocrine indices of starvation in bulimia: A comparison with anorexia nervosa. *Psychiatric Research* 1985; 15:33–40.
26. Garner DM, Fairburn CG. Relationship between anorexia nervosa and bulimia nervosa: Diagnostic implications. In Garner DM, Garfinkel PE (eds): Diagnostic Issues in Anorexia Nervosa and Bulimia Nervosa. New York, Brunner/Mazel, 1988.

27. Winokur A, March S, Mendels J. Primary affective disorder in relatives of patients with anorexia nervosa. *Am J Psychiatry* 1980; 137:695–698.
28. Hudson JI, Pope HG, Jonas JM, et al. Family history study of anorexia nervosa and bulimia. *Br J Psychiatry* 1983; 142:133–138.
29. Gershon ES, Schreiber JL, Hamovit JR, et al. Clinical findings in patient with anorexia nervosa and affective illness in their relatives. *Am J Psychiatry* 1984; 141:1419–1422.
30. Rivinus TM, Biederman J, Herzog DB. Anorexia nervosa and affective disorders: A controlled family history study. *Am J Psychiatry* 1984; 141:1414–1418.
31. Biederman J, Rivinus T, Kemper K, et al. Depressive disorder in relatives of anorexia nervosa patients with and without a current episode of non-bipolar major depression. *Am J Psychiatry* 1985; 142:1495–1497.
32. Stern SL, Dixon KN, Nemzer E, et al. Affective disorder in the families of women with normal weight bulimia. *Am J Psychiatry* 1984; 141:1224–1227.
33. Kassett JA, Gershon ES, Maxwell ME, et al. Psychiatric disorders in the first-degree relatives of probands with bulimia nervosa. *Am J Psychiatry* 1989; 146:1468–1471.
34. Mitchell JE, Hatssukami D, Pyle RL, et al. Bulimia with and without a family history of depressive illness. *Comprehensive Psychiatry* 1986; 27:215–219.
35. Wilson GT, Lindholm L. Bulimia nervosa and depression. *Int J Eating Disord* 1987; 6:725–732.
36. Pope HG, Hudson JI, Jonas JM, et al. Bulimia treated with imipramine: A placebo-controlled, double-blind study. *Am J Psychiatry* 1983; 140:554–558.
37. Hughes PL, Wells LA, Cunningham CJ, et al. Treating bulimia with desipramine. *Arch Gen Psychiatry* 1986; 43:182–186.
38. Mitchell JE, Groat R. A placebo-controlled, double-blind trial of amitriptyline in bulimia. *J Clin Psychopharmacol* 1984; 4:186–193.
39. Agras WS, Dorian B, Kirkley BG, et al. Imipramine in the treatment of bulimia: A double blind controlled study. *Int J Eating Disord* 1987; 6:29–38.
40. Walsh BT, Stewart JW, Roose SP, et al. A double-blind trial of phenelzine in bulimia. *J Psychiatric Research* 1985; 19:485–489.
41. Kennedy S, Piran N, Garfinkel PE. Isocarboxazid in the treatment of bulimia. *Am J Psychiatry* 1986; 143:1495–1496.
42. Sabine EJ, Yonace A, Farrington AJ, et al. Bulimia nervosa: A placebo-controlled double-blind therapeutic trial of mianserin. *Br J Clin Pharmacol* 1983; 15(Suppl 2):195S–202S.
43. Mitchell JE, Psyle RL, Eckert ED, et al. A comparison study of antidepressants and structured intensive group psychotherapy in the treatment of bulimia nervosa. *Arch Gen Psychiatry* 1990; 47:149–160.
44. Blavet N, deFeudis FV. Inhibition of food intake in the rat. *Neurochemistry Research* 1982; 7:339–348.
45. Blouin J, Blouin A, Perez E, et al. Bulimia: Independence of anti-bulimic and antidepressant properties of desipramine. *Can J Psychiatry* 1989; 34:24–29.
46. Hudson JI, Pope HG, Jonas JM, et al. Electroencephalographic sleep in bulimia. In Hudson JI, Pope HG (eds): The Psychobiology of Bulimia. Washington, DC, American Psychiatric Press, Inc, 1987.
47. Katz JL, Kuperberg A, Pollack CP, et al. Is there a relationship between eating disorder and affective disorder? New evidence from sleep recordings. *Am J Psychiatry* 1984; 141:753–758.

48. Walsh BT, Goetz R, Roose SP, et al. EEG-monitored sleep in anorexia nervosa and bulimia. *Biol Psychiatry* 1985; 20:947–956.
49. Levy AB, Dixon KN, Schmidt H. Sleep architecture in anorexia nervosa and bulimia. *Biol Psychiatry* 1988; 23:99–101.
50. Laver CJ, Krieg J, Riemann D, et al. A polysomnographic study in young psychiatric inpatients: Major depression, anorexia nervosa, bulimia nervosa. *J Affective Disord* 1990; 18:235–245.
51. Waller DA, Hardy BW, Pole R, et al. Sleep EEG in bulimic, depressed and normal subjects. *Biol Psychiatry* 1989; 25:661–664.
52. Hogman JO, Buchsbaum MS, Wu JC, et al. Comparison of regional brain metabolism in bulimia nervosa and affective disorder assessed with positron emission tomography. *J Affective Disord* 1990; 19:153–162.
53. Kennedy S, Walsh BT. Drug therapies for eating disorders: Monoamine oxidase inhibitors. In Garfinkel E, Garner DM (eds): The Role of Drug Treatments for Eating Disorders. New York, Brunner/Mazel, 1987.
54. Hudson JI, Pope HG, Jonas JM, et al. Hypothalamic-pituitary-adrenal axis hyperactivity in bulimia. *Psychiatry Research* 1983; 8:111–117.
55. Gwirtsman HE, Roy-Byrne P, Yoger J, et al. Neuroendocrine abnormalities in bulimia. *Am J Psychiatry* 1983; 140:559–563.
56. Mitchell JE, Pyle RL, Hatsukami D, et al. The dexamethasone suppression test in patients with bulimia. *J Clin Psychiatry* 1984; 45:508–511.
57. Lindy DC, Walsh BT, Roose SP, et al. The dexamethasone suppression test in bulimia. *Am J Psychiatry* 1985; 142:1375–1376.
58. Kiriike N, Nishiwaki S, Izumiya Y, et al. Dexamethasone suppression test in bulimia. *Biol Psychiatry* 1986; 21:328–332.
59. Levy AB, Dixon KN. DST in bulimia without endogenous depression. *Biol Psychiatry* 1987; 22:783–786.
60. Perez EL, Blouin J, Blouin A. The dexamethasone suppression test in bulimia: Non suppression associated with depression and suboptimal weight. *J Clin Psychiatry* 1988; 49:94–96.
61. Walsh BT, Roose SP, Katz JL, et al. Hypothalamic-pituitary-adrenal-cortisol activity in anorexia nervosa and bulimia. *Psychoneuroendocrinology* 1987; 12:131–140.
62. Gold PW, Gwirtsman H, Augerimose PC, et al. Abnormal hypothalamic-pituitary-adrenal function in anorexia nervosa. *N Engl J Med* 1986; 314: 1335–1342.
63. Gold PW, Loriaux DL, Roy A, et al. Responses to corticotropin releasing hormone in the hypercortisolism of depression and Cushing's diseases. *N Engl J Med* 1986; 314:1329–1335.
64. Kaplan AS. Thyroid function in bulimia. In Hudson JI, Pope HG (eds): The Psychobiology of Bulimia. Washington, DC, American Psychiatric Press, Inc, 1987.
65. Norris PD, O'Malley BP, Palmer RL. The TRH test in bulimia and anorexia nervosa: A controlled study. *J Psychiatric Research* 1985; 19:215–219.
66. Levy AB, Dixon KN, Malarkey WB. Pituitary response to TRH in bulimia. *Biol Psychiatry* 1988; 23:476–484.
67. Kaplan AS, Garfinkel PE, Warsh JJ, et al. The DST and TRH stimulation test in normal weight bulimia. Presented at the 2nd International Conference on Eating Disorders, New York, April 1986.

68. Brambilla F, Smeroldi E, Sacchetti E, et al. Deranged anterior pituitary responsiveness to hypothalamic hormones in depressed patients. *Arch Gen Psychiatry* 1978; 35:1231–1238.
69. Linkowski P, Brauman H, Mendelwicz J. Prolactin secretion in women with unipolar and bipolar depression. *Psychiatry Research* 1980; 3:265–271.
70. Witschy JK, Schlesser MA, Fulton CL, et al. TRH-induced Prolactin release is blunted in females with endogenous unipolar depression. *Psychiatry Research* 1984; 12:321–331.
71. Gwirtsman HE, Hohlstein LA, Roy-Byrne P. New neuroendocrine findings in anorexia nervosa and bulimia. In Blinder B, Chaitin BF, Goldstein RS (eds): The Eating Disorders. New York, PMA Publishing Corp, 1988.
72. Casper RC, Frohman LA. Delayed TSH release in anorexia nervosa following injection of TRH. *Psychoneuroendocrinology* 1982; 7:59–63.
73. Levy AB, Dixon KN, Malarkey WB. Pituitary response to TRH in bulimia. *Biol Psychiatry* 1988; 23:476–484.
74. Amsterdam JD, Winokur A, Caroff S, et al. Gonadotropin release after administration of GHRH in depressed patients and healthy volunteers. *J Affective Disord* 1981; 3:367–380.
75. Hsu LKG. Eating Disorders. New York, The Guilford Press, 1990.
76. Kaye WH, Ballenger JC, Lydiard RB, et al. CSF monoamine levels in normal-weight bulimia: Evidence for abnormal noradrenergic activity. *Am J Psychiatry* 1990; 147:225–229.
77. Fava M, Copeland PM, Schweiger U, et al. Neurochemical abnormalities of anorexia nervosa and bulimia nervosa. *Am J Psychiatry* 1989; 146:963–971.
78. Kaye WH, Ebert MH, Baleigh M, et al. Abnormalities in CNS monoamine metabolism in anorexia nervosa. *Arch Gen Psychiatry* 1984; 41:350–355.
79. Kaye WH, Gwirtsman HE, Brewerton TD, et al. Serotonin regulation in bulimia. In Hudson JI, Pope HG (eds): The Psychobiology of Bulimia. Washington, DC, American Psychiatric Press, Inc, 1987.
80. Jonas JS, Stanley B, Mann JJ, et al. CSF 5-HIAA and HVA concentrations in elderly depressed patients who attempted suicide. *Am J Psychiatry* 1990; 147:1225–1227.
81. Gerner RH, Cohen DJ, Faibanks L, et al. CSF neurochemistry of women with anorexia nervosa and normal women. *Am J Psychiatry* 1984; 141:1441–1444.
82. Swift WS, Andrews D, Barteloge NE. The relationship between affective disorder and eating disorder: A review of the literature. *Am J Psychiatry* 1986; 143:290–299.

11
Sexual Abuse and Its Relationship to Eating Disorders

ROBERT H. LOISELLE

Early childhood abuse and its influence on eating disorders has tended to be limited to sporadic case reports and a few systematic studies. Its importance is exemplified by the fact that sexual abuse in general and incest in particular have occurred in all societies and taboos against them exist in every known culture. The attitude towards these activities is conveyed by the origins of the words. Incest comes from the Latin, incestus, meaning impure, immodest, or bad. It may also be derived from the latin incestare, meaning stained or defiled.[1] Incest generally implies sex between blood relatives or step relatives, even though no blood relationships exist. Sexual abuse leads to confusion on the part of children, because of the abrogation of responsibility by the adult, especially the protective responsibility. Historically, incest has also been sanctioned by law, tradition, and religion. The definition has varied at different times by various societies. The strongest and most universal taboo is against mother-son incest.

Sexual abuse is similar to physical abuse. It is more likely to escape detection because customarily it does not result in conspicuous physical injury.

Sexual abuse occurs when the child is maliciously used to gratify an adult's sexual needs or desires. Girls are ten times more likely to be victims of sexual abuse than boys. In girls, it generally takes the form of exhibitionism; fondling; genital contact; or vaginal, oral, or anal intercourse. In boys, it most often involves fondling, mutual masturbation, fellatio, or anal intercourse. Sexual abuse is the detrimental, intentional exploitation or misuse of a child by a parent, caretakers, or stranger. It is more common than expected. Twenty to 35 percent of women report forced sexual contact at some time. Sexual abuse is probably more common than this since it is only occasionally reported but more commonly found incidentally.

As a consequence of the guilt and shame experienced by the victim and perpetrator, it is difficult to elicit information on sexual abuse. Information actually obtained must be evaluated as to its validity, to separate the factual from fantasy. The mental status of the patient has to be assessed since that obtained from a psychotic, hysterical, angry, or borderline patient is subject to question. Also, behavior perceived by someone as incestuous or sexual may not be so intended. Examples might include the family sauna among the Finnish people, family bathing among Japanese, and "skinny-dipping" among vacationing Americans.

If a physical examination is required, it must be conducted with the utmost sensitivity.[2] The child may otherwise perceive it as a repetition of the assault. Procedures should be explained in detail to the child and parents. Much information can be obtained from a simple inspection of the mouth, anus, and genitalia for signs of trauma. In the male child, the penis should be examined for evidence of injury and for blood in the urine.

The high incidence of sexual abuse in children emphasizes that a complete and thorough history is essential. Due to the longstanding taboos against intrafamilial sexual abuse and the shame, guilt, and rage associated with this, the parent and child may be resistant to revealing data during the interview and history. It may also be legally dangerous. Consequently, the parents and child should be interviewed separately, especially to avoid coercion by the parent.

Establishing rapport is critical. The child or parent may hesitate because he or she fears that the interviewer will object to something in the history. In addition, the child or parent may not want to stir up memories of old fears, old hurts, or old losses that are associated with his or her sexual life.

The sympathetic interviewer is aware of things other than the spoken word that are nonetheless readily understood by most people. These include a change in facial expression, a slight tensing of muscle, a flick of an eye, and a change in voice. If the interviewer's manner expresses surprise, disapproval, condemnation, or even cold disinterest, the interviewer will not get the whole record.

The victim or parent is likely to be uneasy during the interview. The interviews should be held in places that are appropriate to the subject's social background. The physician's office or examining room may offer confidentiality that the emergency room lacks, but is missing in familiarity.

To help assure privacy, the interview room should be reasonably soundproof and there should be no unexpected interruptions such as other people entering the room. The interview should begin with everyday affairs that are far removed from anything that is sexual and lead gradually to things more difficult to discuss. Leave topics that produce more cover-up and blockage to the end of the interview. Avoid questions phrased in a way to bias the subject's responses. Tone of voice and choice of words should not give clues to get answers the interviewer expects.

When it becomes important to ask direct questions, it should be done without embarrassment or uncertainty. Euphemisms should not be used as substitutes for frank terms. The latter may easily lead to misinterpretations.

With children twelve or older, it is usually feasible to adapt the interview to their vocabulary. With younger children, especially those eight years or less, the interview becomes a social session involving participation in the child's ordinary activity. This may include looking at dolls, playing with toys, joining in games, telling stories, and drawing pictures. Many small children cannot describe anatomical differences between males and females but they can draw pictures of boys and girls that make this distinction.

The child should never be forced to describe the molestation in detail or graphically. There are inevitably consequences as a result of sexual abuse. These might include mistrust, poor self-image, depression, hysterical symptoms and character traits, substance abuse, increased sexual arousal, and sexual avoidance. This kind of information can often be obtained from parents without stress to the child.

Multiple examples exist of biological or gut responses to emotions. Idioms such as "butterflies in my stomach," "makes me want to throw up," etc. are common. In fact, there is likely to be a biologic response to every emotion and vice versa. For example, when one is embarrassed, blushing occurs—a cardiovascular response to an emotion. There are many other illustrations of involuntary nervous system control being influenced by stress and emotions. Anorexia, bulimia, nausea, vomiting, and dysphagia are believed by some to be forms of conversion disorders.[3] There are many physiological disturbances associated with mood disorders. Appetite increases significantly in neurological disorders involving the hypothalamus, temporal lobes, and bulimic syndromes.

Mood disorders and syndromes of drug and alcohol dependence as well as anorexia nervosa are accompanied by decreased appetite and changes in taste and olfactory response.

Anorexia involves a refusal to eat because of an intense fear of becoming obese, disturbance in body image, severe weight loss, refusal to maintain body weight, and amenorrhea.[4]

Bulimia implies binge eating with some attempt to avoid weight gain, usually by self-induced vomiting or laxative abuse. It is generally limited to individuals who display frequent eating binges. Bulimia is exhibited primarily in young women although approximately 5 percent of bulimics are men.

Many attempts have been postulated to explain the etiology of anorexia and bulimia. Psychodynamically, anorexia has been explained initially as a fear of oral impregnation. Currently, family dynamics are believed to play a more important role. Overcontrol of the anorectic by the family prevents the child from becoming emotionally congruent with bodily needs.

Sociocultural explanations include the emphasis placed on thinness among women. This emphasis is apparent in the media, professional models, style magazines, and fashions. The innumerable and expensive weight control programs that "guarantee" thinness are confirmation of this.

Biological approaches rely on complex neuroendocrine and neurochemical abnormalities. Attention is placed on the findings that anorexia and bulimia are present in patients with mood disorders or a prevalence of mood disorders in first degree relatives. Implicit in this is a belief that these mood disorders have a genetic predisposition and neurochemical basis.

Although sexual conflicts have long been recognized in the pathogenesis of eating disorders, actual cases of sexual trauma or incest have been relatively neglected in the literature. There are, however, some well controlled studies that demonstrate this relationship. Sloan and Leichner[5] observed that five of six patients on an inpatient unit for eating disorders revealed an early history of sexual abuse or incest.

Scott and Thoner[6] report that ego deficits are a frequent theme for patients of anorexia nervosa and victims of incest, using the Minnesota Multiphasic Personality Inventory to examine this relationship. Thirty women were used in each of three groups: 1) hospitalized anorectics, 2) women victims of father-daughter rape, and 3) women controls. They found remarkable similarities between the first two groups which both differed from controls. There included elevations in five clinical scales and a decrease in Barron's ego strength scale.

Oppenheimor et al.[7] examined 68 patients with eating disorders. These patients were questioned systematically about any history of adverse sexual experiences. The researchers found that two-thirds of the women gave such a history. Women with a history of anorexia or bulimia, as defined by the DSM III, completed a Sexual Life Events Questionnaire. Adverse sexual experiences were identified and met the criterion. The girl had to be less than 13 years of age and the other participant older than 16 years of age, or if the women was between 13 and 16 years of age the other participant had to be at least five years older. In 8 percent of the women with a history of adverse sexual experiences, these had occurred in childhood or adolescence. In addition, most involved significantly older males who were known by the subject.

Among the cases reported by Sloan and Leichner[5] a 42-year-old woman whose body weight was below average for her age and height had experienced the death of both parents within a 12 month span. She was left to take care of her elderly uncle who was intrusive and domineering. Between the ages of 12 and 16 her uncle had forced incest and she began binge eating, self-induced vomiting, and laxative abuse.

Another case was a 24-year-old anorectic health worker who was 5 feet 6 inches tall and weighed 87 pounds. Her mother was domineering and controlling; her father was a passive alcoholic. Her history revealed that she had been raped by her older brother. Now she avoids sexual feelings and inflicts superficial wounds on herself.

A 28-year-old woman with a history of bulimia and self-induced vomiting came from an overcontrolling family. Her father used his uncontrollable temper, and her mother used "guilt trips." The only praise she received was from her father in regard to her athletic abilities. She was competitive and bright with masculine traits. She tried to keep her body boylike, and eating helped her maintain a masculine, preadolescent, boylike body. Bulik et al.[8] studied the environments and psychiatric histories of 35 bulimic women. The authors found that over 34 percent had been sexually abused.

These examples and others[9,10,11] are given to emphasize the fact that regardless of the patient's presenting symptoms or chief complaints especially involving anorexia or bulimia, a thorough history is essential to help determine the etiology of these symptoms. Antecedent sexual traumas may produce or contribute significantly to symptoms seemingly unrelated to the trauma. Memories of these events may not be readily available to the patient because of the guilt, shame, or anger associated with them. Repression of strongly aversive memories may also prevent their recollection. A meticulous and sensitive inquiry is therefore essential.

References

1. Sadock VA. Normal human sexuality and sexual disorders. In Kaplan HI, Sadock BJ (eds): Comprehensive Handbook of Psychiatry, Vol. 1. Baltimore, Williams and Wilkins, 1989.
2. Green AH. Physical and sexual abuse of children. In Kaplan HI, Sadock BJ (eds): Comprehensive Textbook of Psychiatry, Vol. 2. Baltimore, Williams and Wilkins, 1989.
3. Engel GL. Psychological aspects of gastrointestinal disorders. In Reiser MF (ed): American Handbook of Psychiatry, Vol. 4. New York, Basic Books, 1975; 53.
4. Diagnostic and Statistical Manual of Mental Disorders (third edition revised). Washington, DC, American Psychiatric Association. 1990.
5. Sloan G, Leichner P. Is there a relationship between sexual abuse or incest and eating disorders? *Can J Psychiatry* 1986; 656–660.
6. Scott R, Thoner G. Ego deficits in anorexia nervosa patients and incest victims, an MMPI comparative analysis. *Psychol Rep* 1986; 839–846.
7. Oppenhelmer R, Howells K, Palmer RL, Chaloner DA. Adverse sexual experience in childhood and clinical eating disorders: A preliminary description. *J Psychiatric Research* 1985; 357–361.
8. Bulik CM, Sullivan PF, Rorty M. Childhood sexual abuse in women with bulimia. *J Clin Psychiatry* 1989; 460–464.
9. Tice L, Hall RC, Beresford TP, Quinones J, Hall AK. Sexual abuse in patients with eating disorders. *Psychiatric Medicine* 1989; 257–267.
10. Kumar A, Agarwal M. Incest and anorexia nervosa (letter).
11. Hambridge DM. Incest and anorexia nervosa: What is the link. *Br J Psychiatry* 1988; 145–146.

12 Males with Eating Disorders

BARBARA ELLER

Diagnosticians have typically been taught that if you do not consider it, you will not diagnose it. The resultant index of suspicion, while important in the diagnosis of any disorder, is all the more important in the case of males with eating disorders. First, the preponderance of studies show that the female-to-male ratio of anorexia nervosa lies in the range of 10–20 to 1. Second, most clinicians do not even see significant numbers of female eating-disordered patients. Thus there clearly remain those who do not even realize that anorexia nervosa and bulimia nervosa can be diagnosed in the male. A study done in 1979 found that 40 percent of internists and 25 percent of psychiatrists believed that anorexia nervosa only occurs in the female sex.[1] A 1983 survey found that at least one-quarter of psychiatrists and psychologists considered femaleness as fundamental to anorexia nervosa.[1]

Therefore, the overriding objective of this chapter is to familiarize the reader with the slowly emerging mosaic of males with eating disorders. It is our hope that this will lead to quicker diagnosis—and thus quicker treatment of males so afflicted.

It is interesting that although one of the first patients diagnosed with anorexia nervosa was actually a male,[2] for many decades the male with anorexia nervosa was either forgotten, shrouded in confusion, or nullified. Besides the sheer rarity of presentation in the male, there was also the thinking that males could not possibly develop a disorder whose diagnosis then required amenorrhea or which historically was associated with the psychodynamic fear of oral impregnation.[3]

Yet, through the years case histories of males gradually made their way into the literature, and these echoed the physical and psychological concomitants found in females with eating disorders. These case histories were few and far between but were not cast aside. Researchers and clinicians struggling with the diagnosis of anorexia nervosa variantly have opted for a host of different diagnostic criteria (Feighner's criteria, modified Feighner's criteria, Russell criteria, DSM-III, and DSM-III-R criteria, etc.). Yet regardless of the specific criteria selected, it had become clear that anorexia nervosa (and later bulimia nervosa) do exist in the male.

The impressionistic case histories far outnumber the scientific studies, so only slowly are we learning the specifics of presentation, course of illness, prognosis, and treatment of males with eating disorders. Similarly we are slowly looking at what factors might be etiologically responsible for bringing out these disorders in males—a group not typically found to be eating-disordered. Unfortunately, due to the small numbers of males diagnosed with eating disorders, a seemingly sluggish interest in the topic, and inherent methodological problems with such studies, large-scale studies yielding more definitive conclusions have not been completed.

How do we explain the relative rarity of males with eating disorders? This might be explained in part by a protective factor afforded by maleness itself. With boys reaching puberty slightly later than girls, males are by nature granted more time to emotionally adjust to the biological, psychological, and social vicissitudes of puberty. Another partial protective factor for males is that society does not place upon them as pressured an ultimatum to be thin. Rather society emphasizes masculinity, which it translates into aggressiveness and an analogously strong, well-muscled, mesomorphic body build.[4]

Of relevance here is that there are certainly distinct subgroups of the male population who are theoretically not as protected from the possible development of eating disorders. Examples are groups that either place a premium on thinness for occupational reasons, for example, athletes, male models, and entertainers,[4] or homosexual males whose aesthetics and sexual values place svelteness at a higher priority.[5] In addition to the lesser likelihood for clinicians to diagnose eating disorders in the male, there is also a lesser likelihood for the male to present for its treatment. The media has taught the public that these are female problems, and it is believed that many males are embarrassed to admit their affliction. It is sometimes the general practitioner who incidentally discovers the male with an eating disorder during a visit for an unrelated medical reason. It may even be the dentist or dental hygienist who first identifies the patient with bulimia who rather suddenly and inexplicably develops extensive and profound tooth decay.[6] It should be recalled that these disorders tend to be secretive disorders; this places a particular onus on the clinician to do the case-finding.

The first and most outward requisite for the diagnosis of anorexia nervosa is a marked weight loss or failure to make an expected weight gain during a period of growth. The DSM-III-R adult threshold for anorexia nervosa is a body weight 15 percent below that expected.[7] As males may be able to conceal their weight loss a bit easier than females, the physician's physical examination should always screen both visually and by weighing the patient and measuring his height. Obviously it is more challenging to detect anorexia nervosa in its earlier stages.

If cachexia or significant weight loss is found, it is the physician's foremost duty to rule out an organic etiology. One major psychiatric center has noted that they have never seen a patient with the psychological features of an eating disorder (i.e., distorted body image, intense fear of becoming fat, and the relentless pursuit of thinness) who in addition had an organic reason for the weight loss.[8] However, another psychiatrist described the case of a male with the typical anorexia nervosa psychological profile who was discovered to have a brain tumor.[9]

Of note is that the state of severe malnutrition brings along with it structural, biochemical, and physiological stigmata, so that these features must not a priori be taken as certain evidence that the patient has anorexia nervosa. For example, bradycardia can be seen in anorexia nervosa, but it can also be seen in starvation secondary to esophageal stenosis.[10]

Confirmation of the psychological criteria for both anorexia nervosa and bulimia nervosa requires some expertise in interviewing the patient. This can be difficult at times, and a referral to a psychiatrist is frequently in order. Clearly, there are multiple reasons for weight loss. The psychiatrist needs to determine whether food refusal is a result of, for example, fear of gaining weight although underweight; a schizophrenic delusion; or a fear of choking in public (panic disorder with agoraphobia).[8] It also must not be automatically assumed that a patient's weight loss is a neuro-vegetative sign of depression. Asking the patient pertinent questions to discern these distinctions is key.

We will now explore the clinical presentation of anorexia nervosa in the male and will afterwards examine bulimia nervosa in the male.

Anorexia Nervosa

The relative frequency of male and female cases of anorexia nervosa has been cited as 1 in 10 to 20 cases.[3] That is to say that 5 to 10 percent of cases are males. By looking at specific studies, however, we see varying frequencies: 9 percent by Burns and Crisp;[11] as low as a 1 percent rate by Crisp, Burns, and Bhat;[12] and as high as a 20 percent rate by Sheppard's group.[13]

Relative frequency relies in part on the case acceptance policy of each research facility with typically the "interesting" male case being accepted for evaluation but a certain number of female cases being r[illegible]rred elsewhere. In addition there are the issues of decreased [illegible] diagnosis in the male and less self-referral of male an[illegible] reluctance to admit to having a typically female disorder [illegible]

Age of Onset

Especially in some of the earlier literature, the age of onset of anorexia nervosa in the male was noted to be prepubertal. Bruch found that each of the 5 boys with primary anorexia nervosa that she studied had an onset at ages 12 to $13\frac{1}{2}$ years. She reasonably added that this was her finding but should not be considered conclusive.[14] Taipale also studied 5 boys and found that the age of onset ranged from 10 to 15 years of age.[15] Sheppard's group found a range of 13 to 25 years of age with a mean of 18.4, and they noted that 2 out of 9 were prepubertal.[13] Margo studied 13 patients and found a range of 13.8 to 35.1 years with a mean of 20 (7 were under 17; 3 were from 18 to 25; and 3 were over 25 years of age).[16]

Vandereycken et al. noted that the mean age of onset for the male anorectic was 15.6 and that this was not significantly different from the female statistic. They concluded from their study that male anorexia nervosa begins in (pre)puberty, adolescence, or early adult life.[1] Beumont concurs with this conclusion.[17]

Of importance is the observation that a few studies eliminate the possibility of finding older-onset male cases of anorexia nervosa by a priori utilizing diagnostic criteria which preclude them. For example, one of Vandereyckens et al. criteria is that the maximum age for illness onset be 25 years old.[1] Similarly Fichter and Daser used Feighner's criteria, which stipulate that the age of onset must be prior to 25.[18] It is prejudicial to automatically eliminate older males, just as it would be to eliminate postmenopausal females from carrying the diagnosis of anorexia nervosa.

Given that the majority of the studies do not eliminate older-onset cases, it appears that the mean age of onset lies somewhere in the mid to late teens; however, it is not at all unusual to have an onset prepubertally, in early puberty, or in young adulthood.

Eating Behaviors

Beumont found that weight control behaviors in male anorectics ran the gamut from food refusal, purging, strenuous exercise, subterfuges to dispose of food, and selection of a diet low in fattening food. He indicates that this is similar to the weight-control behaviors found in female anorectics.[17]

Although the range of weight-control behaviors appear to be similar, some researchers have looked for a typically male profile of weight control methods. Crisp and Burns note that although purging and laxative abuse were found marginally less often than in their female series, they were well within the range of other female series.[11] Margo notes that the frequency of bulimia was not statistically different in their male and female groups.[16] Crisp, Burns, and Bhat note that the frequency of purging was similar, but that regular laxative abuse was found significantly more among the females.[12]

Using a structured interview, Fichter's group found that males had significantly higher pathological scores on preoccupation with food, weight, and eating. Overall they found that the global severity of the anorexia nervosa was not significantly different between the male and the female.[10]

Fichter and Daser noted that somatic complaints were more often found in males than in females and that this was statistically significant.[18] Dally noted that males gave various somatic reasons for not eating which included: feeling nauseated; not being hungry; and food making them tired and interfering with their concentration.[19] Beumont noted that some males complained of epigastric discomfort upon eating.[17]

It is known that the female anorectic is not always forthcoming about her weight phobia and weight control behaviors. Crisp and Toms stated that males usually conceal or initially deny the eating disorder. It has been noted that some patients will submit to extensive medical investigations first rather than admit to their disorder.[20]

It has been emphasized in the literature that males with eating disorders do not always use the same language and/or have the same focus as females with regard to their physique. Women are more concerned with exactly what size clothing they wear and about specific body parts such as their hips and face. This is in contrast to males who tend to speak about muscle definition and being in shape and lean.

Some note that anorexia nervosa in the male may begin after the athletic male sustains physical injury preventing him from pursuing sports; he has a consequent fear of gaining weight while sedentary, and then embarks on a diet, which to the extreme develops into anorexia nervosa.[11]

Some researchers believe that dieting itself is the fundamental prerequisite for the development of anorexia nervosa in the predisposed male. Some point to a high incidence of premorbid obesity in the male;[4] a false belief on his part that he is fat; and/or comments made to him that he is overweight to which the predisposed male then responds by relentless dieting.

Premorbid Obesity

Anderson and Mickalide found that on the average anorectic males were mildly obese before their weight loss as compared to the females whose average weight before dieting was within 10 percent of their ideal body weight. They do not state whether this reached statistical significance.[8] Margo found that almost one-third of her 13 male anorectics were premorbidly obese, which was much higher than the 10 percent found in the female group; this did not, however, reach statistical significance.[16] Herzog's group found that 39 percent of males versus 36 percent of females had been previously overweight, but this did not reach statistical significance either.[21] Crisp, Burns, and Bhat found that males were significantly more overweight at the onset of the illness than females; the females were on the average about 99 percent MPMW (mean population matched weight), whereas the males were about 109 percent MPMW.[12] Crisp and Toms noted their male anorectics were an overweight population premorbidly with a mean weight of 114 percent MPMW and that they had been sensitive about their obese condition and had sometimes been teased about it.[20] On the other hand, Crisp and Burns found that although 5 of 36 patients were greater than 115 percent MPMW and one was 156 percent MPMW, for the series as a whole the mean weight at onset was only about 101 percent MPMW.[11]

Overactivity and Athleticism

There are two basic concepts to be differentiated here: 1) generalized motor activity and restlessness, and 2) marked athletic activity. Unfortunately these concepts are sometimes confused in the literature.

Bruch noted that hyperactivity was remarkable in all her male anorectics,[14] and Taipale noted that 3 of 5 males were "overactive motorically."[15] Hasan and Tibbetts noted restlessness and overactivity beyond normal expectations.[22] Crisp and Burns noted that 44 percent were overactive and stated this was usually a generalized "rushing around sorting things out."[11]

Margo noted that 62 percent of males had a strong tendency to exercise compared to 26 percent of females, and this was statistically significant.[16] Crisp and Burns noted that 42 percent were judged to be premorbidly active in sports.[11] Bruch noted that there was an interest in athleticism in 4 of 5 male anorectics studied.[14] Crisp, Burns, and Bhat found that males had more interest in sports (23% vs. 39%) and that this was significant.[12] Oyebode found a tendency for males to excessively exercise, but this did not reach statistical significance.[23] Fichter's group noted that males were more physically active and overvalued physical fitness and muscle strength.[10] Hall noted that 6 of 9 male anorectics studied over-exercised to reduce weight.[24]

Family History and Relationships

Hasan and Tibbetts impressionistically commented that a family psychiatric history was "moderately prominent but not invariable."[22] Crisp and Toms found that 25 percent of 24 fathers and mothers had a history of severe chronic psychiatric illness (e.g., alcoholism, agoraphobia, suicide, depression, disabling anxiety[20]). Sheppard et al. noted that there was parental alcoholism in 3 of their 9 male anorectics' families,[13] and Taipale noted paternal alcoholism in 2 of their 5 male anorectics' families.[15]

Comparing family history of male and female anorectics, Margo found that about 38 percent of the male anorectics had a first degree relative with a history of mental illness as compared to about 23 percent for a group of female anorectics.[16] Crisp, Burns, and Bhat found that 25 percent of both their male and female anorectic groups had at least one parent with a history of psychiatric illness: depressive disorder, bipolar disorder, agoraphobia, alcoholism, or neurotic depressive illness.[12]

Some authors have looked at the history of eating disorders in the families of male anorectics. Crisp and Toms found that in 3 cases more than one sibling had anorexia nervosa.[20] Dally noted that one out of 12 anorectics had a sister who later developed anorexia nervosa and that one patient's mother had a history of severe anorexia nervosa.[19] Crisp, Burns, and Bhat found weight disorders (anorexia nervosa and marked obesity) in the families of both male and female anorectics.[12] Screenivason found that 2 of 3 male anorectics feared resembling an obese father. He also found that their parents were generally overweight (especially the fathers).[25]

In addition to looking at family history, some authors have examined relationships in the family of the male anorectic. Some studies have pointed out that the mothers of male anorectics tend to be overinvolved with and overprotective of their sons.[13,20,25] Some studies have found that the male anorectic and his father tend to have a poor relationship. Sheppard noted that the father tends to be absent, unavailable, or clearly rejecting,[13] and Screenivason noted "overt hostility" between them.[25] Taipale found 5 of 5 boys had a remote relationship with their father. Taipale noted that all his male anorectics instead had close relationships with a substitute mother such as a grandmother.[15]

Regarding the relationship between the male anorectics' parents, some studies noted that the mother tended to be the dominant partner.[18,19,22] Fichter and Daser found that 9 of 29 male anorectics had an absent father either due to divorce, separation, death, or illegitimacy.[18] Many studies have noted significant marital discord among the parents of male anorectics.[15,16,19,20,25]

Of note is that several authors found that the families initially presented as harmonious[13,14] and that it was only with intensive psychotherapeutic work that significant underlying discord was detected.

Sexuality

It is clear that male anorectics have decreased libido during the course of the illness. Beumont noted that patients who had already passed through puberty lost their recently acquired interest in sex during their illness.[17] Crisp and Burns noted that the loss of libido was marked during the illness and few objected; often there was a cessation of masturbation and morning erections.[11] This picture of diminished sexuality during the illness parallels that described about the female anorectic.

Thus the more interesting question is the premorbid sexual functioning of the male anorectic. There is continuing controversy in the literature as to whether males with eating disorders have sexual peculiarities. A number of deviations from the sexual norm have been hypothesized and these include: 1) homosexuality or past history of homosexual practices, 2) gender identity confusion or dysphoria, 3) asexuality or relative asexuality, and 4) avoidance of females due to low self-esteem and rejection hypersensitivity.

The scientific word is not yet out on these issues due to a number of shortcomings in the literature coupled with inherent methodological problems in doing these types of studies. There is a paucity of controlled studies with sufficiently large numbers of subjects. Some studies do not collect hard data, and some do not even examine these issues. Some studies collect data on the male but disregard the female. Another problem is that eating-disordered males are of various ages, and each age group has different age-appropriate sexual norms which need to be taken into account. Another difficulty relates to the need for longitudinal outcome studies to determine the development or resolution of any prior sexual problems. Finally it is possible that an artificially inflated male eating-disordered homosexual rate could be found, since homosexual males may be more likely to present for treatment compared to heterosexual males.

Herzog's group found that eating-disordered males (anorectics and bulimics were considered together) were more likely than female anorectics to have reported being homosexual ($p < .01$). They found a 26 percent homosexual rate in the males as compared to only a 4 percent lesbian population in their clinic. They also found that 5 of the 7 homosexuals felt conflicted about their homosexuality.[21]

Burns and Crisp, to the contrary, found in their outcome study of male anorectics that not one patient was living in an established homosexual relationship. (They did not address these male anorectics' sexuality at initial assessment.)[26]

Fichter and Daser found 25 percent (5 out of 20 male anorectics) had homosexual "contacts" (in 3 cases with sexual intercourse). Three had a negative reaction to the experience; one had a positive reaction; and one was indifferent.[18] We emphasize "contacts," because it is known that some male adolescents have brief homosexual experimentation and then later go on to be exclusively heterosexual. Also with regard to the Herzog group's finding of a 26 percent homosexual rate, we wonder what part of this group, if any, consists of such experimenting adolescents who are worrying that they are homosexual.

Pope et al. studied male bulimics and found only a 7.1 percent homosexual rate; they advised that a study be performed with age-matched male controls with another problem of a medical nature (at the same research facility).[27] This would control for that particular research population's male homosexuality rate.

Another possible explanation for having a history of homosexual contacts without necessarily being homosexual was pointed out by Fichter and Daser. A male who has a lack of confidence with women and who is passive is more likely to be approached by a homosexual man for sex.[18]

Dally noted that 50 percent of their male anorectics were clearly heterosexual, while the remainder appeared to have little interest in either sex.[19] Hasan and Tibbetts noted no firm evidence of homosexuality but rather a notable lack of assertive masculinity or identification. Only 2 of their subjects were married and the others had virtually no history of sexual intercourse.[22] Herzog's group found that eating-disordered males (anorectic and bulimic males were considered together) were more likely to have had no sexual relationship ($p < .05$) and were less likely to be in a current heterosexual relationship ($p < .001$) than the female anorectic group.[21]

Crisp, Burns, and Bhat noted that out of 36 male anorectics "premorbid sexual activity" was absent in 13; marked but fantasized in 4; and remarkable or high in 19. They state there was no significant difference between this and the female anorectic statistics. They state that one-third of the males found sexual activity pleasurable, as compared with only one-fifth of the females (significant at the .025 level).[12]

Fichter and Daser found that the male anorectics had sexual anxieties about both heterosexual and homosexual behavior. They also noted that they tended to be shy and lacked confidence with women. They found that 95 percent of their male anorectics had tried to suppress their sexual drive. Of importance is that 21 of 29 male anorectics (72 percent) were 18 years of age or older at the time of assessment. Only 6 patients (30 percent) had ever had intercourse with a woman and only 5 additional cases had ever experienced "petting." At least 11 and probably 16 patients (80 percent) had not had a genuine relationship with a girl. Fifteen patients (75 percent) reported a very high degree of anxiety and disgust with regard to heterosexual relationships and intercourse.[18]

Fichter's group found by using the Freiburger Personality Inventory that the male and female profiles were very much the same except the males were more "sociable" and scored "super-feminine."[10] Fichter and Daser state in a later study that 65 percent of their male anorectics preferred cooking, sewing, and playing with dolls in childhood; that 85 percent reported being "anything but a dare-devil" in childhood; and that 20 percent would have preferred to be a girl. They conclude that males with atypical gender role behavior have an increased risk for developing eating disorders in adolescence.[18]

Further studies are certainly needed to delineate the role sexuality plays in the development of anorexia nervosa in males. I will discuss my recommendations for such studies at the end of this chapter.

Bulimia Nervosa

Compared to anorexia nervosa, there are even fewer studies examining bulimia nervosa's relative presentation in males and females. As with anorexia nervosa, again, the sample sizes are unfortunately small. This must be kept foremost in mind, as with studies with a small number of subjects, the conclusions may not be representative of the general population of male bulimics.

Age of Onset

Herzog noted that the mean age of onset was somewhat older in the male bulimic (20.7 years vs. 17.7 years). This did not reach statistical significance.[21] Pope et al. found that the age of onset in the male was slightly older than the female (25.8 vs. 20.2), but this barely reached statistical significance.[27] On the other hand, Mitchell and Goff found the age of onset for males and females to be "roughly similar."[28]

Thus the age of onset may be slightly older in the male bulimic as compared to the female bulimic. Larger studies could help to determine this.

Eating Behaviors

Robinson and Holden noted in their study of 9 male bulimics that either a history of anorexia nervosa and/or obesity was present in 100 percent of their sample. Four of their 9 male bulimics who did not have a history of anorexia nervosa had a history of premorbid obesity.[29] Pope et al. noted that about 29 percent of their 15 male bulimics had a history of anorexia nervosa, which was not statistically significant compared to their sample of female bulimics.[27]

Regarding premorbid obesity, Herzog found that 64 percent of his bulimic males had a history of obesity compared to 37 percent of his bulimic females. This did not, however, reach statistical significance.[21] Schneider and Agras found that their male bulimics' highest previous weight was 129 percent IBW (ideal body weight); whereas for the female bulimics it was only 111 percent IBW. In addition the average weight at assessment was 110 percent IBW for the males and about 98 percent IBW for the females. These differences were not statistically significant.[30] Anderson and Mickalide noted that on the average both anorectic and bulimic males were mildly obese before weight loss compared to the females who before dieting were within 10 percent IBW.[8]

In summary, it appears that two conditions that may be precursors to bulimia nervosa are anorexia nervosa and/or premorbid obesity. Whether male bulimics actually have a higher prevalence of premorbid obesity than female bulimics has not been proved. Larger studies would be needed to explore this.

Regarding the prevalence of weight-reducing behaviors such as binging and purging, Carlat and Camargo, Jr. reviewed the literature and found that the female-to-male prevalence ratio for binge eating varied from 0.2 to 2.8 and clustered in the 1.54 to 2.0 range. Nonetheless it is quite possible that the prevalence among males may be roughly the same; females tend to exaggerate binging, and males may underestimate binging. Males realize that society deems it less inappropriate for males to food binge than for females to do so.[31]

Their review of the literature regarding the prevalence of self-induced vomiting among males showed a female-to-male prevalence ratio from 0.9 to 9.7 with the majority clustering around 4 to 5. It is possible that men may be at lower risk for purging, as they may react to binge eating with less remorse and self-deprecation.[31]

Male bulimics may use laxatives, diuretics, and diet pills less than female bulimics according to Mitchell and Goff[28] and Schneider and Agras.[30]

Psychiatric Disorders and Family History

An important hypothesis being looked at in female bulimia is a relationship between major affective disorder and bulimia. Several of the male bulimic studies have noted the frequency of major affective disorder in male bulimics. Pope et al. notes that about 68 percent of their male bulimics had a history of major affective disorder, and that 57 percent of them had a first-degree relative with major affective disorder. This was not statistically different from their female bulimic series.[27] Mitchell and Goff noted that 3 of their 12 male bulimics suffered from depression, and 4 of the 12 families also had a history of depression.[28] Robinson and Holden noted that depression and suicide gestures (overdose and cutting) occurred in 4 of 9 of their male bulimics.[29] As suicide gestures certainly occur in diagnoses other than major affective disorder (e.g., borderline personality disorder, schizophrenia, and alcoholism), this finding does not specifically address the issue of major depression.

Studies have also reported a substantial prevalence of substance abuse among male bulimic patients. Schneider and Agras reported that their sample had drug and alcohol problems more often than did female bulimics. This was not statistically significant.[30] Mitchell and Goff noted 5 of their 12 male bulimics had problems with substance abuse along with a fairly strong family history of substance abuse in their sample.[28]

Sexuality

As with anorexia nervosa there is the same hypothesis that bulimic males have sexual deviances that run the gamut from asexuality to homosexuality to gender identity confusion and dysphoria to sexual avoidance due to abysmally poor self-esteem. As mentioned earlier, Herzog et al. reported in their study of 14 male bulimics and 13 male anorectics that males with eating disorders were significantly more likely to have reported homosexuality, and were less likely to be in a current sexual relationship and to have had no sexual relations. They found that 26 percent of their eating-disordered males were homosexual as compared to only 4 percent in the total female population of their clinic (bulimic-specific statistics were not reported).[21] Robinson and Holden found that 3 of their 9 male bulimics were homosexual.[29] All 15 of Schneider and Agras' female bulimics were heterosexual; whereas, there were 4 male homosexuals, 4 male bisexuals, and 7 male heterosexuals.[30]

In stark contrast to the previous findings, Pope et al. in their study of 15 male bulimics found that only one had reported any homosexual activity, which represents about 7 percent of the sample. They point out that the rest of the patients had age-appropriate sexual behavior except for 4 persons who were sexually inactive while bulimic, two of whom had normalized sexually after responding to antidepressant medication.[27]

In order to arrive at more definitive conclusions regarding the sexuality of male bulimics and anorectics the following would be in order: 1) large case-control studies using appropriately matched control groups of anorectic and bulimic females and nonanorectic and nonbulimic males, 2) long-term longitudinal follow-up of these patients to help clarify the evolving nature of their sexual functioning and preferences, 3) thorough psychological evaluation (using both interviews and psychological instruments) to select out those males, who while appearing asexual or even homosexual at first glance, may truly suffer from abysmally poor self-esteem with consequent avoidance of females (this is the type of man who may be propositioned by male homosexuals who sense his lack of sexual assertiveness towards females; furthermore, a number of adolescents suffer a period of confusion regarding sexual preference and many of these boys go on to become actively and exclusively heterosexual), and 4) well-designed studies that control for the prevalence of male homosexuals in that particular study population's locale. (Clearly if a study is done in a community with a high proportion of male homosexuals, then finding a high percentage of male homosexual bulimics in a sample would not assume the same significance.)

Conclusion

Anorexia nervosa and bulimia nervosa *do* exist in the male. Furthermore, they both present similarly in the male and in the female. The factors that are etiologically responsible for bringing out these disorders in males—a group that is usually not found to have a high prevalence of eating disorders—are by no means fully elucidated. Further studies are needed to look at such factors as sexuality; comorbid psychiatric illness and substance abuse problems; family history of same; family pathology, etc. to determine if and how these may be scientifically implicated in the development of eating disorders in males. Studies are needed that utilize far larger numbers of subjects; that examine hard data rather than speak impressionistically; and that follow patients longitudinally and long term. There needs to be more education of both clinicians and the public regarding the existence and presentation of eating disorders in males. Hopefully this would lead to greater comfort for afflicted individuals to facilitate their presentation for treatment. In addition this would hopefully lead to a higher rate of diagnosis and then treatment of eating disorders in males. If future studies confirm male subgroups that we already feel may be at higher risk for eating disorders, then educational campaigns and therapeutic programs will be able to target these groups with more clout. With more investigation and long-term studies we also hope that outcome measures will be delineated. The ultimate goal would be tailoring eating disorders treatment programs to the special needs of the particular group—in this case males.

Lastly, it would be helpful for diagnosis if the DSM-III-R criteria were amended so that it states outright that males can carry diagnoses of anorexia nervosa and bulimia nervosa. Perhaps future endocrinological investigations may even uncover a biological male analogue to amenorrhea that could be amended to the DSM criteria at a later time.

References

1. Vandereycken W, VandenBroucke S. Anorexia nervosa in males. A comparative study of 107 cases reported in the literature (1970 to 1980). *Acta Psychiatr Scand* 1984; 70:447–454.
2. Morton R. Phthisiologia. London, Princes Arms Press, 1694.
3. Andersen AE. Practical Comprehensive Treatment of Anorexia Nervosa and Bulimia. Baltimore, The Johns Hopkins University Press, 1985.
4. Andersen AE. Males with eating disorders. In Larocca FEF (ed): Eating Disorders. New Directions for Mental Health Services, no. 31. San Francisco, Jossey-Bass, Fall 1986; 39–46.
5. Silberstein LR, Mishkind MS, Striegel-Moore RH, Timko C, Rodin J. Men and their bodies: A comparison of homosexual and heterosexual men. *Psychosomatic Medicine* 1989; 51:337–346.
6. Andrews FFH. Dental erosion due to anorexia nervosa with bulimia. *Br Dental J* 1982; 152:89–90.
7. Diagnostic and Statistical Manual of Mental Disorders (third edition revised). Washington, DC, The American Psychiatric Association, 1987.
8. Andersen AE, Mickalide AD. Anorexia nervosa and bulimia. Their differential diagnoses in 24 males referred to an eating and weight disorders clinic. *Bulletin of the Menninger Clinic* 1985; 49(3):227–235.
9. Swann I. Anorexia nervosa—A difficult diagnosis in boys. *Practitioner* 1977; 218:424–427.
10. Fichter MM, Daser C, Postpischil F. Anorexic syndromes in the male. *J Psychiatric Research* 1985; 19(2):305–313.

11. Crisp AH, Burns T. The clinical presentation of anorexia nervosa in males. *Int J Eating Disord* 1983; 2(4):5–10.
12. Crisp AH, Burns T, Bhat AV. Primary anorexia nervosa in the male and female: A comparison of clinical features and prognosis. *Br J Med Psychology* 1986; 59:123–132.
13. Sheppard NP, Malone JP, Jackson A. Male anorexia nervosa: A review of nine patients. *Irish Med J* 1984; 77(1):4–8.
14. Bruch H. Anorexia nervosa in the male. *Psychosomatic Medicine* 1971; 33(1):31–47.
15. Taipale V, Larkio-Miettinen K, Valanne EH, Moren A, Aukec M. *Psychosomatics* 1972; 13:236–240.
16. Margo JL. Anorexia nervosa in males. A comparison with female patients. *Br J Psychiatry* 1987; 151:80–88.
17. Beumont PJV, Beardwood CJ, Russell GFM. The occurrence of the syndrome of anorexia nervosa in male subjects. *Psychological Medicine* 1972; 2:216–231.
18. Fichter MM, Daser C. Symptomatology, psychosexual development and gender identity in 42 anorexic males. *Psychological Medicine* 1987; 17:40–44.
19. Dally PJ. Anorexia Nervosa. London, Heinemann, 1969.
20. Crisp AH, Toms DA. Primary anorexia nervosa or weight phobia in the male: Report on 13 cases. *Br Med J* 1972; 1:334–338.
21. Herzog DB, Norman DK, Gordon C, Pepose M. Sexual conflict and eating disorders in 27 males. *Am J Psychiatry* 1984; 141(8):989–990.
22. Hasan MK, Tibbetts RW. Primary anorexia nervosa (weight phobia) in males. *Postgraduate Med J* 1977; 53:146–151.
23. Oyebode F, Boodhoo JA, Schapira K. Anorexia nervosa in males: Clinical features and outcome. *Int J Eating Disord* 1988; 7(1):121–124.
24. Hall A, Delahunt JW, Ellis PM. Anorexia nervosa in the male: Clinical features and follow-up of nine patients. *J Psychiatric Research* 1985; 19(2/3): 315–321.
25. Screenivason U. Anorexia nervosa in boys. *Can Psychiatric Assoc J* 1978; 23:159–162.
26. Burns T, Crisp AH. Outcome of anorexia nervosa in males. *Br J Psychiatry* 1984; 145:319–325.
27. Pope HG, Hudson JI, Jonas JM. Bulimia in men: A series of fifteen cases. *J Nervous Mental Disease* 1986; 174(2):117–119.
28. Mitchell JE, Goff GG. Bulimia in male patients. *Psychosomatics* 1984; 25(12): 909–913.
29. Robinson PH, Holden NL. Bulimia nervosa in the male: A report of nine cases. *Psychological Medicine* 1986; 16:795–803.
30. Schneider JA, Agras WS. Bulimia in males: A matched comparison with females. *Int J Eating Disord* 1987; 6(2):235–242.
31. Carlat DJ, Camargo Jr. CA. Review of bulimia nervosa in males. *Am J Psychiatry* 1991; 148(7):831–843.

13 The Medical Care of the Patient with an Eating Disorder

Joel R.L. Ehrenkranz

Introduction

This chapter reviews the clinical evaluation and treatment of medical aspects of both anorexia and bulimia. It is not intended to be a comprehensive review of all aspects of the medical consequences encountered as a result of these psychiatric disorders. It does not review the care of osteoarthritis even though this is a frequent complication of obesity nor does it discuss the role of parenteral nutrition in the treatment of anorexia. However this chapter is intended to be a practical guide for handling most of the medical complications frequently encountered or commonly due to anorexia or bulimia. The medical complications of eating disorders are discussed in terms of acute and chronic complications. These in turn are divided into organ systems.

Although anorexia and bulimia are considered two distinct clinical entities,[1] experience teaches that this distinction is blurred. Considerable overlap occurs between the two eating disorders in terms of both behavioral manifestations and medical complications. Patients with eating disorders may alternate between anorexia and bulimia, and also may exhibit select symptoms of each disorder simultaneously.

It is generally accepted that anorexia and bulimia nervosa represent primary psychiatric disorders. Nonetheless, the initial evaluation of the patient with a presumptive eating disorder requires that a physician perform a thorough, detailed history and physical exam to exclude a medical cause for the weight loss, amenorrhea, vomiting, and mood disorder that are commonly encountered in patients with anorexia nervosa. Endocrine, metabolic, gastrointestinal, neurologic, hematologic, oncologic, and infectious etiologies must be excluded before arriving at a diagnosis of anorexia nervosa. Certain diseases, such as Type I diabetes mellitus, are so frequently associated with eating disorders[2] that the physician caring for patients with Type I diabetes should always consider whether a patient with diabetes and poorly controlled blood sugars or irregular menses may have a concomitant eating disorder. Once the diagnosis of anorexia or bulimia nervosa has been confirmed, the patient must be evaluated for the medical complications that can result from significant weight loss. These include the direct pathophysiologic effects of the catabolic state, as well as the complications that occur if purging, laxative or diuretic abuse, or other weight loss adjuvants, such as sympathomimetic abuse, are employed. Because the medical consequences differ if weight loss is rapid or excessive (i.e., less than 80% ideal body weight), patients must be individually evaluated at the time of presentation.

Endocrine and Metabolic Complications

The most acute and life-threatening complication of anorexia nervosa is a cardiac arrhythmia in association with an electrolyte abnormality. Hypokalemia is a common finding in patients with anorexia, resulting from volume contraction, vomiting, diarrhea, and diuretic use. The anorectic heart is often at increased risk for a rhythm disturbance because of a cardiomyopathy due to vitamin B1 deficiency (i.e., wet beriberi) or ipecac use. Hyponatremia is also commonly encountered in patients with anorexia, due to both GI losses and excessive free water ingestion. Hypochloremia due to GI losses and alkalosis secondary to volume depletion or diuretic use are also frequently encountered and contribute to the myopathy and general feeling of malaise that accompanies significant weight loss. Electrolyte concentrations must be expediently measured in patients with a history of significant weight loss, vomiting, diarrhea, or laxative or diuretic use. If there is a history of significant diuresis, either due to water loading, primary polydipsia, or diuretic abuse, serum magnesium levels must also be checked.

As a rule, electrolyte disturbances can be treated by oral replenishment. Hypokalemia can be corrected by p.o. supplementation as long as the patient is willing to take medication by mouth. Administration of potassium salts, that is KCl, will also correct hypochloremia and intravascular volume contraction alkalosis. Hypomagnesemia is treated by the administration of parenteral $MgSO_4$. Electrolyte levels must be checked during therapy to prevent overtreatment.

Recent studies reported on 39 inpatients at Fair Oaks Hospital suggest that mineralocorticoid metabolism is affected in patients with both anorexia and bulimia and may represent a common link between volume contraction due to purging; laxative, diuretic, or sympathomimetic use; and hypokalemia.[3] Plasma aldosterone levels measured in supine patients were found to be elevated in subjects who purged, no matter what method of purging was used. The highest levels of aldosterone were seen in patients who both vomited and used laxatives. Patients with elevations in aldosterone were at increased risk for developing edema following intravascular volume repletion. Edema has been reported in up to 20 percent of patients with eating disorders. The constellation of hyperaldosteronism and hypokalemic alkalosis in these patients may mimic Conn's and Bartter's syndromes and require additional endocrine evaluation to exclude these treatable metabolic diseases. Patients who exhibit significant refeeding edema associated with dyspnea or compression neuropathies may benefit from a short treatment course with an aldosterone antagonist such spironolactone.

Polyuria and polydipsia are frequently encountered in patients with anorexia nervosa. Patients with eating disorders tend to exhibit excessive drinking behavior. Additionally, hypokalemia and hypomagnesemia can impair the kidney's ability to concentrate the urine through free water resorption. One study suggests that the defect in water metabolism represents a CNS defect in ADH metabolism, as secretory dynamics of ADH in spinal fluid are disrupted in anorectics and this defect persists after correction of fluid and electrolyte status.[4,5] Consequently, altered water metabolism are common in patients with an eating disorder. This is readily monitored by following the serum sodium concentration. If hyponatremia occurs, fluid restriction is generally indicated.

In addition to a defect in ADH secretion seen in up to 44 percent of anorectic patients, other disorders of hypothalamic function are commonly encountered in anorexia nervosa. These include abnormal thermoregulation,[5] hypercortisolism,[6] and hypothalamic amenorrhea.[7] Hypothermia is commonly encountered in patients with anorexia. Clinical investigation, using environmental chamber ambient temperature exposure, demonstrates alterations in thermoregulatory reflexes.[8] Loss of subcutaneous fat and intracellular glycopenia contribute to the depression in core body temperature commonly encountered. Using a calibrated urinary basal body thermometer (OvuDate^R, Franklin Diagnostics, Morristown, NJ) that uses a peak detecting temperature sensor in an insulated collecting cup (Figure 13-1) to precisely measure core body temperature from a freshly voided urine specimen,[9] Jonas et al. studied changes in core temperature regulation that occurred during treatment in 23 hospitalized anorectic patients.[10] Using an established clinical cutoff for hypothermia, 36.1°C,[11] 10 of 23 anorectic patients were hypothermic upon admission to the hospital. These subjects showed a rise in core temperature, as measured by urinary basal body temperature, that paralleled their weight gain. Hypothermic individuals were also more likely to gain weight with treatment than nonhypothermic subjects. Additionally, 9 of the 10 hypothermic patients experienced oligomenorrhea or amenorrhea prior to the onset of any weight loss or weight loss behavior. The normothermic subjects, who tended to be older than the hypothermic individuals, were less likely to gain weight with treatment and uniformly experienced amenorrhea after the onset of weight loss. Measurement of urinary basal body temperature with a calibrated urinary thermometer appears to be an integral part of the evaluation of all patients with eating disorders. Urinary thermometry, because it is noninvasive, precise, yet resistant to manipulation, appears to be the temperature-taking method of choice for the physical assessment of patients with eating disorders as well as other psychiatric diseases.

Anorectic and bulimic patients often exhibit hypercortisolism of varying degrees. This may be manifest as increased urinary free cortisol, or 17-hydroxysteroid excretion, or lack of suppression to overnight dexamethasone. These patients will, however, show an intact, although exaggerated response to i.v. corticotropin releasing hormone (CRH), and also demonstrate appropriate suppression to formal low dose dexamethasone testing. There are no recognized complications from the degree of hypercortisolism encountered in patients with eating disorders although some investigators have suggested that this may account for the osteoporosis commonly encountered in anorexia nervosa[12] (see below). Both the pattern of hypersecretion and lack of apparent sequelae encountered in patients with eating disorder is very similar to the hypercortisolism that is seen in patients with endogenous depression.[13]

The most frequently encountered endocrine defect in anorexia nervosa is amenorrhea. This appears to be secondary to a lack of hypothalamic luteinizing hormone releasing hormone (LHRH) secretion; however what underlies this defect has yet to be determined. Although amenorrhea is commonly thought to result from weight loss per se, it is not uncommon for amenorrhea to precede the onset of weight loss. Additionally, patients with the onset of amenorrhea prior to commencing weight loss usually are younger and tend to be hypothermic; they tend to respond to traditional antidepressant therapy. This suggests that amenorrhea is not a simple result of body weight being less than the presumed critical threshold required for regular ovulation. It also implies that the hypothalamic defect in LHRH release may represent a separate and distinct clinical entity in the anorectic syndrome.

The lack of pituitary stimulation by LHRH results in low gonadotropin (i.e., LH and FSH) levels. This in turn yields low circulating estrogen levels, anovulation, and an absence of circulating progesterone. Ovarian size tends to be reduced and ovarian cysts are not uncommon.[14] Prolactin levels tend also to be low, and if prolactin is found to be elevated, other causes such as medication, structural pituitary disease, or seizures should be ruled out. Breast size tends to decrease because of both weight loss and lack of estrogen stimulation. Recently, considerable attention has been directed towards determining whether osteoporosis occurs in anorectic patients as a result of estrogen deficiency. Many studies have demonstrated decreased bone mineral density in patients with anorexia. In patients with pathologic fractures, bone biopsy has confirmed the diagnosis of osteoporosis. Surprisingly, the degree of bone loss does not correspond to the degree of estrogen deficiency. There have been no studies documenting that exogenous estrogen administration can reverse this apparent loss of bone. Additional studies have shown that alterations in vitamin D, parathyroid hormone, and calcium metabolism also do not appear to account for the loss of bone observed, but that exercise, often compulsively performed, can protect certain skeletal parts, such as the femur, from losing bone.[15,16,17]

Two treatment options exist for correcting the sex steroid deficiency of anorexia. These are sex steroid replacement using either sequential estrogen and progesterone or oral contraceptive administration or the use of LHRH analogues.[18] Administration of sex steroids will correct the target organ deficiencies and prevent irregular bleeding. Exogenous estrogen may have antidepressant effects. To achieve ovulation, however, LHRH analogues must be used. These require around the clock, pulsatile subcutaneous administration and represent an inconvenient, invasive, and expensive therapy whose only indication is ovulation induction in order to achieve fertility.[19]

The final endocrine disturbance that is frequently encountered in anorexia is that of the thyroid function. Undernutrition, no matter what the cause, almost invariably produces the euthyroid sick syndrome.[20] This is characterized by low levels of circulating T3, low or normal levels of circulating T4, normal thyroid binding globulin levels, and normal to slightly elevated concentrations of TSH. It can be distinguished from primary hypothyroidism by the lack of dramatically increased TSH levels in the setting of low T3 levels and from secondary hypothyroidism by an intact TSH response to thyrotropin releasing hormone (TRH). The thyroid hormone deficiency, particularly the low T3 levels, corrects within a matter of days of refeeding. Elevations in reverse T3 levels are also common in the euthyroid sick syndrome. However, there is usually little need to perform the expensive measurement of reverse T3. Unfortunately, the constellation of thyroid hormone values encountered in the euthyroid sick syndrome is frequently misdiagnosed, particularly by inexperienced physicians, as representing hypothyroidism and patients are commonly treated with exogenous thyroid hormone because of this diagnostic error. This inappropriate treatment can result in exacerbation of the underlying psychiatric disease if the patient is undertreated or in thyrotoxicosis medicamentosia if the patient is overmedicated.

The most common metabolic and nutritional deficiencies encountered in anorexia nervosa are B1 and B6 deficiencies. Both B1 and B6 deficiencies can present as a peripheral neuropathy. B1 deficiency, additionally, may produce a cardiomyopathy and be associated with atrial fibrillation. Rarely, however, are pure syndromes of a single vitamin deficiency encountered. A common and rational practice is to treat all anorectics with fat and water soluble vitamins, folic acid, and supplemental doses of additional cofactors or minerals, such as iron, if clinically indicated.

Cardiac Complications

Clinical and experimental studies conducted over the past 50 years document the pathologic effects of starvation on the heart. Anatomic studies demonstrate a decrease in cardiac size and left ventricular mass, associated with myofibrillar atrophy, interstitial edema, and mitochondrial swelling.[21] Vital signs generally demonstrate relative hypotension and bradycardia. The murmur of mitral valve prolapse is frequently noted and echocardiographic evidence for mitral valve prolapse is encountered in up to 37 percent of patients with eating disorders.[22] ECG findings commonly seen include sinus bradycardia (as well as a number of other less commonly encountered rhythm disturbances), a right axis deviation, ST-T wave changes, prolonged Q-T intervals, and U waves.[23] As mentioned previously, sudden death due to an arrhythmia is a common cause of death in anorectic patients.

Congestive heart failure can occur as a consequence of anorexia nervosa, but paradoxically may also be seen during refeeding.[24] Although poorly understood, the so-called refeeding syndrome probably results from intravascular volume expansion as well as a further depression of stroke volume brought on by hypophosphatemia associated with carbohydrate refeeding. No specific therapy, beyond correction of nutritional deficiencies, has been demonstrated effective in treating the refeeding syndrome.

Although studies are limited, weight gain in anorectics is associated with a recovery of heart size, wall thickness, and ventricular mass.[25] Anecdotal evidence suggests that mitral valve prolapse may also remit with cardiac repletion.

Gastrointestinal Complications

Patients with eating disorders frequently have a number of gastrointestinal complaints. They commonly present to a physician with the belief that the self-imposed anorexia, induced vomiting, diarrhea and constipation, or abdominal pain are the cause rather than the consequence of their eating disorder. Nonetheless, it is essential to rule out underlying gastrointestinal pathology as a cause for a patient's complaints and to assess each patient with an eating disorder for any gastrointestinal complications that can result from anorectic or bulimic behavior.

It is traditionally thought that patients with self-induced vomiting may develop a loss of enamel and dentin on the lingual surface of the teeth, termed permolysis, due to excessive carbohydrate ingestion, increased salivary gland secretions, and regurgitated gastric acid.[26] Milosevic and Slade, working in Liverpool, England, performed psychological and dental assessments on 106 individuals referred from a clinical psychology evaluation unit. Patients were characterized as anorectic or bulimic using A.P.A. DSM-III revised diagnostic criteria. Dental characteristics in age, sex, and socioeconomic matched controls were also assessed. Of the 106 patients referred from the psychology service, 58 were found to have an eating disorder and 33 gave a history of induced vomiting. One hundred percent of the eating disorder patients showed increased dental wear, compared to a 6 percent incidence of tooth wear in the control group. However, plaque and gingival pathology were not increased in the eating disorder patients; additionally there did not appear to be any direct relationship between induced vomiting and increased tooth wear.[27]

A number of studies have described esophageal complications in eating disorders, most often associated with bulimia, and characterized by mucosal irritation, erosion, bleeding, and stricture formation due to gastric acid reflux.[28] Two types of esophageal laceration can occur with self-induced vomiting: Boerhaave's Sydrome, named after an eighteenth century bulimic Dutch sea captain, and Mallory Weiss Syndrome. Both can present with hematemesis; physical examination may reveal a Hammon's crunch if air has dissected through the mediastinum into subcutaneous tissues. H2 receptor antagonists are well-tolerated and effective therapy for esophageal reflux.

A number of anecdotal reports and case studies have described disorders of gastrointestinal motility in both anorexia and bulimia. These generally show delayed gastric emptying and decreased motility in patients with eating disorders. Acute gastric dilatation has also been reported in anorexia and bulimia nervosa. This, however, appears to occur during the refeeding period and has also been described during refeeding of emaciated prisoners of war.[29] This suggests that gastric dilatation is a manifestation of refeeding a starved and shrunken stomach and is not specific to eating disorders. Additionally, electrolyte imbalances, particularly hypokalemia, may interfere with smooth muscle function in the G.I. tract. Metoclopramide, a cholinergic smooth and CNS dopamine agonist used to facilitate gastric emptying, has been reported to correct the delay in gastric motility encountered in anorexia nervosa.[30]

Colonic manifestations of eating disorders are primarily due to laxative abuse. Patients who abuse laxatives will complain of alternating periods of diarrhea and constipation. The barium enema may show a dilated and atonic colon, lacking haustrations. These radiographic abnormalities may be confused with those of inflammatory bowel disease. Colonoscopy may reveal melanosis coli if the patient is abusing anthraquinone laxatives, nonspecific inflammation, or stigmata of the "cathartic colon," such as mucosal atrophy and cyst formation, superficial hemorrhage, and mononuclear cell inflammation.[31] Normalization of bowel habits and reversal of large bowel pathology occurs with conservative therapy.

Two digestive glands, the parotids and the pancreas, may be involved in eating disorders. Parotid gland enlargement is a common finding on physical examination and has been associated with obesity and fatty infiltration, hypoproteinemia, and pellagra.[32] Interestingly, parotid hypertrophy has also been reported in individuals with a history of excess starch consumption. This is presumably due to chronic stimulation of salivary gland secretion.[33] Hyperamylasemia is frequently encountered in patients with an eating disorder and may originate from the parotids or the pancreas. Protein calorie malnutrition alone can produce chronic pancreatitis as well as exocrine and endocrine insufficiency. Furthermore, acute pancreatitis can occur with refeeding and following induced vomiting.[34]

Malnourished patients often exhibit hepatic abnormalities including decreased bilirubin synthesis, hepatomegaly, and fatty infiltration of the liver. Hepatic transaminases may be elevated. These findings are reversible and not associated with cirrhosis. Because patients with eating disorders often abuse alcohol and illicit drugs, liver toxicity due to alcoholic and viral hepatitis is frequently encountered.

Renal disease is rarely encountered as a complication of an eating disorder, although dehydration and prerenal azotemia are not infrequent. Pulmonary complications include aspiration pneumonitis due to induced vomiting. Common dermatologic abnormalities include alopecia if there has been significant starvation, and increased lanugo hair. A loss of public and axillary hair suggests pituitary disease; Simmond's cachexia and hypothalamic tumors can masquerade as anorexia nervosa in this fashion. The anorectic's skin is often cold, coarse, and dry, perhaps due to decreased circulating levels of thyroid hormone or due to vitamin deficiencies (e.g., pellagra). Anorectic patients often demonstrate leukopenia, but absolute neutropenia is not common and the low circulating white count does not appear to increase the risk for opportunistic infection. Other hematologic abnormalities include anemia, often secondary to iron, B12 or folic acid deficiency, and coagulopathy in association with vitamin K deficiency.

Overweight bulimic patients exhibit a number of dermatologic signs, including hirsuitism, skin tags, acanthosis nigricans, and intertrigo. Direct renal, pulmonary, and hematologic complications secondary to bulimia have not been described.

Neurologic complications of anorexia include metabolic encephalopathy and peripheral neuropathy secondary to vitamin (e.g., B12, B6) deficiencies, Wernicke's Syndrome associated with hyperemesis, and pressure neuropathies due to loss of subcutaneous fat. Bulimic patients, if obese, are predisposed to pseudotumor cerebri and vascular disease, especially if hypertension and hypercholesterolemia are also present.

In summary, the internal medicine of eating disorders consists of first evaluating the patient who presents with symptoms of anorexia or bulimia to ensure that there is no underlying medical condition to account for the mood disorder, weight change, amenorrhea, or gastrointestinal abnormalities that are often the present complaints. Once the diagnosis of an eating disorder has been made, the patient must be assessed for medical complications due to weight loss, binging, and purging. Acute, life-threatening complications of starvation must be detected and immediately corrected. As these patients are treated, they must be monitered for additional medial complications such as refeeding edema and hypophosphatemia that may occur. The eating disorders are potentially life-threatening illnesses. A systematic approach to the medical evaluation of these patients and the medical complications associated with this group of illnesses will decrease the likelihood of an unfavorable outcome.

References

1. Diagnostic and Statistical Manual of Mental Disorders (third edition revised). Washington, DC, American Psychiatric Association, 1987; 65–69.
2. Steel MJ, Young RJ, Lloyd GG, Clarke BF. Clinically apparent eating disorders in young diabetic women: Associations with painful neuropathy and other complications. *Br Med J* 1987; 294:859–862.
3. Jonas JM, Ehrenkranz JRL, Gold MS. Elevation of serum aldosterone in subjects with eating disorders: A marker for purging behaviors. *Endocrinology* 1990; Vol. 124(Suppl): 314.
4. Gold PW, Kaye W, Robertson GL, et al. Abnormalities in plasma and cerebrospinal arginine vasopressin in patients with anorexia nervosa. *N Engl J Med* 1983; 314:1117.
5. Nishita JK, Knopes KD, Ellinwood EH, Rockwell WJK. Hypothermia and abnormalities in thermoregulation in patients with anorexia nervosa. *Int J Eating Disord* 1986; 5(4):713–725.
6. Bliss E, Migeon CJ. Endocrinology of anorexia nervosa. *J Clin Endocrinol Med* 1957; 17:766.
7. Boyar RM, Katz J, Finkelstein JW, Kapen S, Weiner H, Weitzman ED, Hellman L. Anorexia nervosa; Immaturity of the 24-hour luteinizing hormone secretory pattern. *N Engl J Med* 1974; 291:861–865.
8. Vigersky R, Loriaux DL. Anorexia nervosa as a model of hypothalamic dysfunction. In Vigersky RA (ed): Anorexia Nervosa. New York, Raven Press, 1977; 112–113.
9. Ehrenkranz JRL. A new method for measuring basal body temperature. *Endocrinology* (Suppl) 1985; 116:312.
10. Jonas JM, Ehrenkranz JRL, Gold MS. Urinary basal body temperature in anorexia nervosa. *Biol Psychiatry* 1989; 26:289–296.
11. Halmi KA, Golderg SC, Eckert E, Casper R, Davis JM. Pretreatment evaluation in anorexia nervosa. In Vigersky RA (ed): Anorexia Nervosa. New York, Raven Press 1977; 43–54.

12. Newman MM, Halmi KA. Relationship of bone density to estradiol and cortisol in anorexia nervosa and bulimia. *Psychiatry Research* 1989; 29: 105–112.
13. Gold PW, Gwirtsman H, Avergerinos PC, et al. Abnormal hypothalamic-pituitary-adrenal function in anorexia nervosa. *N Engl J Med* 1986; 314:1335.
14. Weiner H. Psychoendocrinology of anorexia nervosa. *Psychiatry Clin NA* March 1989; Vol. 12(1):187–206.
15. Rigotti NA, Nussbaum SR, Herzog DB, Neer RM. Osteoporosis in women with anorexia nervosa. *N Engl J Med* 1984; 311(25):1601–1606.
16. Joyce JM, Warren DL, Humphries LL, Smith AJ, Coon JS. Osteoporosis in women with eating disorders: Comparison of physical parameters, exercise, and menstrual status with SPA and DPA evaluation. *J Nuclear Medicine* 1990; 31:325–331.
17. Prior JC, Vigna YM, Schechter MT, Burgess AE. Spinal bone loss and ovulatory disturbances. *N Engl J Med* 1990; 323(18):1221–1227.
18. Santor N, Wierman ME, Filocori M, Waldstreicher J, Crowley Jr WF. Intravenous administration of pulsatile gonadotropin-releasing hormone in hypothalamic amenorrhea: Effects of dosage. *JCEM* 1986; 62:109–116.
19. Martin K, Santoro N, Hall J, Filicori M, Wierman M, Cowley Jr WF. Management of ovulatory disorders with pulsatile gonadotropin-releasing hormone. *JCEM* 1990; 71(5):1081A–1081G.
20. Leslie BDG, Isaacs AJ, Gomez J, et al. Hypothalamic-pituitary-thyroid function in anorexia nervosa; influence of weight gain. *Br Med J* 1978; 2:526.
21. Schocken DD, Holloway D, Powers PS. Weight loss and the heart. *Arch Intern Med* 1989; 149:877–891.
22. Johnson GL, Humphries LL, Shirley PB, Mazzoleni A, Noonan JA. Mitral valve prolapse in patients with anorexia nervosa and bulimia. *Arch Intern Med* 1986; 146:1525–1529.
23. Arik TH, Desser KB, Benchimol A. Cardiac complications of intensive dieting and eating disorders. *Arizona Medicine* 1985; 42(2):72–74.
24. Powers PS. Heart failure during treatment of anorexia nervosa. *Am J Psychiatry* 1982; 139:1167–1170.
25. Heymafield SB, Bethel RA, Analey JD, et al. Cardiac abnormalities in cachectic patients before and during nutritional repletion. *Am Heart J* 1978; 95:584–594.
26. Hellstrom I. Oral complications in anorexia nervosa. *Scand J Dental Research* 1977; 85:71–86.
27. Milosevic A, Slade PD. The orodental status of anorexics and bulimics. *Br Dental J* 1989; 167:66–70.
28. Cuellar RE, Van Thiel DH. Gastrointestinal consequences of the eating disorders: Anorexia nervosa and bulimia. *Am J Gastroenterol* 1986; 81(12): 1113–1124.
29. Keys A, Brozek J, Henschel A, Mickelsen O, Taylor HL. The gastrointestinal tract. In The Biology of Human Starvation. Minneapolis, U. of Minnesota Press, 1950; 587–600.
30. Salwh JW, Lebwohl P. Metoclopramide-induced gastric emptying in patients with anorexia nervosa. *Am J Gastroenterol* 1980; 74(2):127–132.
31. Oster JR, Materson BJ, Rogers AL. Laxative abuse syndrome. *Am J Gastroenterol* 1980; 74:451–458.

32. Sandstead HR, Koeh CJ, Sessions SM. Enlargement of the parotid gland in malnutrition. *Am J Clin Nutrition* 1955; 3:198–214.
33. Merkatz IR. Parotid enlargement resulting from excessive ingestion of starch. *N Engl J Med* 1961; 265:1304–1306.
34. Marano AR, Sangree MH. Acute pancreatitis associated with bulimia. *J Clin Gastroenterol* 1984; 6:245–248.
35. Wiele R. Anorexia nervosa and the hypothalamus. *Hospital Practice* 1977; 12:45–51.

14
Pediatric Management of Eating Disorders

KURT J. WEGNER and JAMES A. NARD

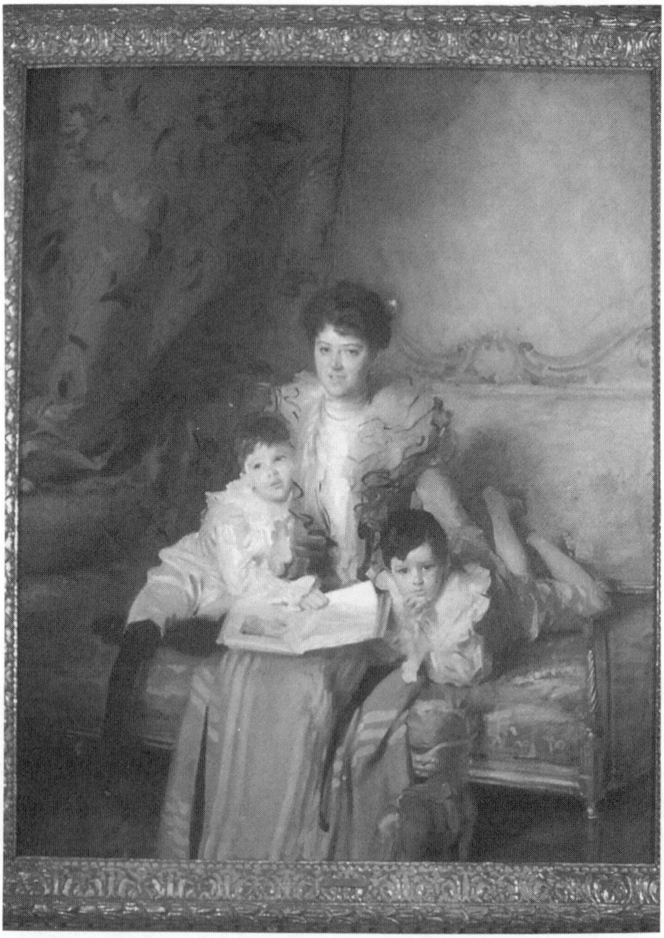

Sargent, John Singer—*Mrs. Knowles & Children*—(Butler Institute of American Art, Youngstown, Ohio)

Anorexia Nervosa and Bulimia

Eating disorders such as anorexia nervosa and bulimia are recognized with increasing frequency among the adolescent and preadolescent populations. This has led to voluminous expansion of literature in both medical journals and the lay press. Although diagnosis and treatment of these disorders are usually under the auspices of child psychiatry, these children and young adults frequently have serious, even life-threatening, medical complications.

Mortality rates from anorexia nervosa range from a low of 2 percent up to 18 percent[1] in various studies. A large review of 15 series over a 20 year period calculated a mortality rate of 5 percent.[2] The death rate is highest when the disease is present for more than 5 years.[3] While significant medical complications may occur as a result of involvement of almost any organ system, suicide,[4,5] electrolyte imbalances,[6,7] and starvation are the main causes of death.

Significant medical instability secondary to profound weight loss or binging and purging is found in the majority of patients with anorexia nervosa and bulimia.[9] Frequently the early physiologic aberrations are asymptomatic, but they may eventually progress and lead to the patient's demise.

Most of the literature and research has been on anorexia nervosa. The majority of the medical complications described below will pertain to this entity. Specific bulimic medical complications as well as overlapping problems will also be included in this chapter.

Specific Organ System Involvement

Major physiologic derangements may occur in any organ system in patients with severe eating disorders. Specific organ system abnormalities are described in the following sections.

Cardiopulmonary

The cardiovascular system is often affected by anorexia nervosa. Cardiovascular instability is frequently noted among inpatient anorectics whose vital signs are routinely monitored.[9] Postural hypotension, a decrease of systolic BP greater than 20 mmHg or reflex tachycardia when changing from supine to standing are frequently noted.[9]

EKG changes may commonly be seen, with abnormal T-wave morphology or ST segment depression in as many as one-half of cases of anorexia nervosa reported.[10,11] Bradycardia (pulse less than 60 BPM) is seen in greater than 90 percent of anorectic patients or patients who vomit and purge.[9] The bradycardia is thought to be secondary to decreased metabolism and not superior physical fitness which some anorectic patients possess, since this sign is also seen in other forms of severe malnutrition.[12] Other EKG abnormalities include prolonged corrected QT interval, ectopic atrial rhythm, bradycardia with nodal escape beats, ventricular ectopy, atrial fibrillation, atrial flutter, first and second degree AV block, intraventricular conduction disturbances, right bundle branch block,[5] ventricular escape with sinus arrest, and short runs of ventricular tachycardia.[9] Although many of these disturbances may be attributed to electrolyte imbalances, arrhythmias have also been documented in patients with normal electrolytes.[13]

With echocardiography anatomic changes are readily documented. Gottdiener et al.[14] demonstrated a decrease in cardiac chamber dimensions that are out of proportion to the body surface area in patients with anorexia nervosa. Other abnormalities include left ventricular contractility impairment, increased aortic dimension, and pericardial effusion.[15,16]

Congestive heart failure (CHF) has been reported during the weight gain recovery phase.[16–18] The cause is unexplained although it is thought that increased metabolic demands accompanying refeeding may predispose this set of patients to CHF.[17] A slow weight gain program (0.1–0.4 kg/d) may protect against this complication.[9] No cardiac impairment has been noted in nonanorectic bulimic patients.

Pulmonary complications have been limited to a few case reports of pneumomediastinum in anorectics with self-induced vomiting.[19,20] Overby and Litt[19] stress the need to differentiate benign causes of pneumomediastinum, that is, alveolar rupture, from the potentially life-threatening esophageal rupture which can be seen in the same group of patients. These authors suggest prompt radiographic evaluation of the upper GI tract.

Endocrine

The endocrine system has been a field of much research in patients with anorexia nervosa and bulimia. Areas of concern involve changes in the hypothalamic-pituitary axis, thyroid, and adrenal glands.

Amenorrhea is virtually universally found in anorexia nervosa and may be primary or secondary. Secondary amenorrhea is a more common pattern although a significant percentage of anorexia nervosa, 47 percent in one study,[9] had never menstruated. At times the amenorrhea may precede the weight loss by several months, leading to the hypothesis that anorexia nervosa may be of hypothalamic origin.[21] Menstruation usually resumes after the patient gains weight.[21] Regular menses may not begin until psychologic rehabilitation accompanies the weight gain.[22]

Menstrual irregularity rather than amenorrhea is a more common phenomenon in bulimia, especially at lower weights.[9]

Delayed puberty (greater than 2 SD from the mean age of attainment of Tanner Stage) was seen in 12 percent of strict dieters.[9] No pubertal delay was documented in patients who vomit and purge or those with bulimia in the study by Palla and Litt.[9]

Studies of gonadotropins have routinely demonstrated hypofunctioning of the hypothalamic-pituitary-ovarian axis in patients with anorexia nervosa. Usually low levels of LH and FSH are seen in these patients.[23–25] A few reports have documented normal or even elevated levels.[9,26] LH and FSH normalize with weight gain.[21] LH release after provocation with LHRH is also impaired. This improves with weight gain or with LHRH priming.[27,28] The authors believe this may reflect a deficit in endogenous stimulation of the pituitary by LHRH in low weight patients.[26–30] The LH secretory pattern in low weight patients is immature resembling the premenarchal female.[31] This pattern normalizes with weight gain and symptomatic improvement.[32]

LH and FSH are normal or low normal in bulimic patients, especially those with at least 90 percent of ideal body weight.[9]

Abnormally low levels of estrogen may be seen along with a shift from estradiol to estrone.[33–35] This is opposite of the pattern seen in obese women. Low testosterone levels are seen in a few of the male patients with anorexia nervosa.[37,38]

Alterations in thyroid hormone levels and abnormal response to TSH stimulation are commonly seen in patients with anorexia nervosa.[39] Normal or low T_4 levels with low T_3 levels are commonly found.[40,41] The reverse T_3 may be elevated. This reflects decreased peripheral conversion of T_4 to T_3.[40–43] In addition, reverse T_3 is a less active form of the hormone. These changes are an adaptation to starvation.[44] TSH is usually normal.[40] Changes in the patterns of TSH release following TRH stimulation have been demonstrated. These include delays in the peak[40] and fall[45] of TSH and blunting[46] of the TSH response to TRH. Similar thyroid functioning is seen in bulimic patients.[9]

Other endocrine alterations described include increases in baseline growth hormone, occasionally elevated prolactin levels,[25,40] low fasting blood sugars,[33,34] and elevated cortisol levels.[47–48]

Renal

Renal changes are frequently found in patients with anorexia nervosa and bulimia. BUN greater than 20 mg% may be found as often as 40.5%, reflecting the dehydrated state.[49] Creatinine values are therefore usually normal. Decreased concentrating capacity has been reported on the basis of partial diabetes insipidis.[33,50] A common finding on urinalysis is pyuria (greater than 5 WBC/HPF) or hematuria (greater than 5 RBC/HPF).[9] Urine cultures are usually negative. Both of these abnormalities resolve with hydration and improved nutrition.[9]

Hematologic

Multiple hematologic changes have been described in patients with anorexia nervosa and bulimia. Bone marrow hypoplasia is a common finding.[51,52] This may manifest itself as leukopenia (less than 4,000 WBC), often with a relative lymphocytosis.[53] Anemia (hemoglobin less than 12G%)[9] and rarely thrombocytopenia (less than 150,000/mm^3) may be seen.[51,52] The hematologic changes resolve with weight gain.[54]

Although these patients may be leukopenic, immunologically they appear to be intact. There is normal cell-mediated immunity and T lymphocyte populations, and actually hyper-responsive T-cell mitogen proliferation studies have been reported.[55] Patients with anorexia nervosa have reduced granulocyte killing activity against Staphylococcus aureus and E coli.[56,57] Despite this defect, patients remain immunocompetent until severely emaciated.[58] There are no conclusive studies showing an increased rate of infection in patients with anorexia nervosa; however, this remains controversial.[52,58]

Thermo-regulatory

Hypothermia is a common finding in both anorexia nervosa and bulimia patients. Body temperatures less than 36.3°C were noted in all anorectic patients, with marked hypothermia (less than 35.5°C) being found in 52 percent of strict dieters and 33 percent of patients who vomited and purged.[9]

Low core temperatures were found in 83 percent of bulimic patients. This finding was noted in overweight and underweight bulimic patients.[9]

Gastrointestinal

The gastrointestinal system is invariably affected in patients with anorexia nervosa and bulimia. Complications occur secondary to starvation, binging, or vomiting.[9]

Complications due to starvation include constipation, delayed gastric emptying, and superior mesenteric artery syndrome. Laxatives are used by these patients to relieve constipation. Delayed gastric emptying may manifest itself as postprandial bloating and fullness.[59] Dublis and associates[59] demonstrated a decreased functional emptying rate and hyposecretion of hydrogen ions in patients with anorexia nervosa compared to controls. Metoclopramide may be useful in treatment of this complication.[60]

Superior mesenteric artery (SMA) syndrome involves vascular compromise of the third portion of the duodenum. Compression results from pressure caused by structures in the root of the mesentery, especially the superior mesenteric neurovascular bundle, upon the duodenum. This syndrome may occur in extreme weight loss of any cause.[61] Symptoms include vomiting, abdominal pain, and weight loss.[61] These may be acute or chronic. Clinically, SMA syndrome may mimic or be secondary to the profound weight loss in anorexia nervosa.[39] Treatment is usually medical but surgery may be required.

Another serious complication of anorexia nervosa and bulimia is gastric dilatation.[62,63] Occasional gastric rupture may result from the dilatation with fatal consequences.[63] Saul[63] reviewed 66 cases of spontaneous rupture of the stomach; one-half of the cases were felt to be related to the ingestion of large amounts of food with or without acute gastric dilatation. Most of the cases were undergoing refeeding on an inpatient basis. In Saul's reference patient, the mechanism appeared to be gastric dilatation with obstruction at the cardioesophageal junction, since the obstruction was relieved by placement of a gastric tube. The patient infarcted and perforated the stomach, succumbing to irreversible shock.

Painless bilateral swelling of the salivary glands, mainly the parotid, is seen in patients with anorexia nervosa who vomit or purge and bulimic patients who vomit.[64] The mechanism of the swelling is unclear; various theories include high carbohydrate diets, alkalosis, and malnutrition.[65]

Other GI complications include esophagitis,[9] esophageal rupture,[66] Mallory-Weiss tears,[66] pancreatitis,[67] and mild elevations in liver function tests.[9]

Electrolytes

Mechanisms for the electrolyte derangements seen in patients with anorexia nervosa and bulimia are related to the chronic vomiting, water loading (before being weighed), and abuse of laxatives, diuretics, and ipecac.[9]

Hypokalemia (less than 3 meq/L) is most often seen. This occurs in 13.7 to 25 percent of patients who vomit and purge or abuse laxatives and diuretics.[9,39] Hypochloremia (less than 98 meq/L) associated with metabolic alkalosis is found in approximately 25 percent of patients.[9,39] Hypocalcemia and hyponatremia (most often seen with water loading) are infrequently seen.[9] Hypokalemia and alkalosis may cause weakness, constipation, and tiredness mimicking depression.[68] Correction of these abnormalities is important to prevent sudden cardiac arrhythmias and death.

Dental

Dental problems are commonly seen in patients with anorexia nervosa who vomit and purge and in bulimics.[69,70] Severe dietary deficiencies may affect periodontal tissue.[69] Dental caries are found in 69 percent of bulimics.[70] Perimyolysis develops secondary to chronic regurgitation.[71]

When this is found on the lingual surfaces of the maxillary anterior teeth as well as the buccal surfaces of the maxillary canines, premolars, and incisors, a diagnosis of bulimia is likely. Since amalgam is acid resistant, fillings look like islands in eroded enamel. These unique patterns are easily seen on routine dental examination.

Central Nervous System (CNS)

Studies in the area of CNS disease in eating disorders have centered around three main areas: 1) EEG abnormalities, mainly abnormal background activity and paroxysmal dysrhythmias, and the effect of phenytoin on these abnormalities;[72–74] 2) anatomic evaluations, looking for a primary brain lesion etiologic of anorexia nervosa or bulimia;[75,76] and 3) alterations in CSF neurochemistry.[77]

Further studies will be required before conclusions can be reached. New methods of imaging, for example, MRI and PET scanners, may help to elucidate any possible association of CNS disease with anorexia and bulimia.

Obesity

Obesity is the most prevalent and serious nutritional disease in children in the United States.[78] The very real and significant psychosocial impact of obesity in the pediatric age group is discussed in detail elsewhere in this book. There are, in addition, clearly defined medical associations and consequences of childhood obesity that have a significant impact on these youngsters.

In the following discussion, obesity refers to so-called exogenous obesity, and rare diseases and syndromes such as the Prader-Willi, Lawrence-Moon-Bardet-Biedl, Froehlich, and Alstrom are not considered. The latter account for less than 1 percent of child obesity cases.

Influence on Adult Obesity

Perhaps the most significant risk of overweightness in childhood is that of maturing into an obese adult. Quantitatively, this risk is not well defined. However, the obese child is nearly twice as likely to become an obese adult as is his nonobese cohort. Conversely, 60 to 70 percent of obese children do not become obese adults. Obese girls are slightly more likely than obese boys to remain obese.[79] Other factors influencing the probability of adult obesity in these children include the presence of other obese family members and the severity and duration of the weight excess. Thus the chance of the extremely obese child remaining obese is considerably higher than that of the moderately obese child. Maintaining obesity into adolescence from early childhood also increases the risk. Eighty percent of obese adolescents become obese adults.[80] Should adult obesity develop, then the well established adult health risks, including premature coronary artery disease, hypertension, diabetes mellitus, and certain malignancies, come into play.[81]

Growth

The development of obesity is a complicated process that may be oversimplified by assuming a consumption of energy greater than that needed for the resting metabolic state, dietary thermogenesis, physical activity, and average growth. It might be anticipated that this excess energy consumption would lead to an increased growth rate, and this does indeed occur. Repeated observations of obese children who do not have endocrine, genetic, or acquired conditions indicate that they are tall and have increased lean body mass for age and sex. In fact, this observation has been used diagnostically to differentiate exogenous obesity with its associated tallness from obesity associated with endocrine problems and genetic syndromes.[79]

Sexual Maturation

The occurrence of sexual maturation is related to growth. With increasing adiposity, there is earlier puberty. However, growth ceases earlier because of earlier sexual maturation, and the obese youngsters who had been taller than their peers prior to maturation tend to terminate their statural growth at a normal adult height distribution. Thus the icreased linear growth is eventually lost. Obese girls reach menarche, as a group, at an earlier age than the nonobese. It is not clear whether the accumulation of a certain amount of body fat triggers menarche, or whether girls with early onset menarche become fatter than those with a later onset.[82,83] Early maturers are fatter than late maturers and tend to remain heavier for many years.

Hypertension

The association of hypertension with obesity in adults has been recognized for many years. A similar association with childhood obesity is a more recent concern. Much of the hypertension recorded in obese children, however, is erroneous, the abnormally high blood pressures being secondary to the use of blood pressure cuffs that are too small.[79] To obtain accurate pressures, the cuff must be sufficiently large that the rubber bladder completely encircles the arm. Such cuffs are rarely found in pediatric medical facilities. In some very obese children, an adult thigh cuff has to be used. However, even when allowances are made for these technical problems, there is an increased risk of hypertension in the obese childhood population.[88] Data from the National Health Examination Survey and the National Health and Nutrition Examination Survey indicate that obese children are about $2\frac{1}{2}$ times as likely to be hypertensive as their normal-weight cohorts. The comparable ratio for superobese children is $3\frac{1}{2}$.[89] Obese children account for one-third to one-half of all children with hypertension. Obese adolescents account for a similar proportion in that age group. Of interest is the fact that weight loss results in decrease of blood pressure, and this result is more marked when the weight loss results from combined diet and exercise than from diet alone.[90] Other cardiovascular risk factors tend to be associated with hypertension in very fat children. However, obesity is apparently not related to premature atherosclerosis.[91]

Endocrine Factors

Endocrine factors associated with childhood obesity include changes in insulin, growth hormone, and prolactin levels.[92] Basal insulin levels tend to be higher, and growth hormone and prolactin responses to insulin tend to be lower. Impaired glucose tolerance occurs in about one-quarter of obese children. These changes tend to be reversed following weight loss.

Orthopedic Conditions

Both slipped femoral epiphysis and Blount's disease (tibia vara) tend to be associated with obesity. However, the relationship is not as clear as previously believed.[79]

Respiratory Disease

There have been studies suggesting an increased frequency of respiratory infections in obese infants. These studies have, however, not been verified, and the association is not well established.[84,85]

The association of hypoventilation, the Pickwickian Syndrome, with obesity is well recognized. During mild exercise or sleep in some extremely obese children, there is insufficient respiratory effort to maintain normal ventilation. The resulting elevation of pCO2 leads to drowsiness and somnolence. Obstructive apnea occurs. Snoring, daytime somnolence, and hypertrophied tonsils and adenoids are prominent features. Untreated, this complication can lead to cor pulmonale, cardiac failure, and death in as many as 25 percent of this group. The exact mechanism of this rare syndrome is not clear, but small tidal volumes, decreased compliance of the lungs, and lowered ventilatory response to a rise in pCO2 all appear to play a significant role.[86,87]

Burns and Accidents

A study in 1972 reported that fat boys were more likely to sustain burns than normal boys.[93] There is suggestive evidence that other accidents also tend to be more frequent in obese children. This association appears, however, not to be of major significance.

Skin Conditions

Obviously, morbid obesity makes the maintenance of cutaneous cleanliness difficult, and rashes related to excessive perspiration and skin maceration are relatively common. Acanthosis nigricans is a fairly uncommon condition in which skin markings are accentuated, and the surface is velvety, rugose, and furrowed. The color varies from tan to black. Sites of predilection are areas of friction and maceration, including the neck, axillae, groin, and elbows. This condition is frequently associated with internal malignancies in adults, but the association is almost unheard of in childhood. In about one-third of children with acanthosis nigricans, there are endocrine abnormalities, such as Cushing Syndrome, thyroid disease, diabetes, or gigantism. In the rest of these youngsters, obesity is a common association. Acanthosis nigricans is a chronic condition that improves or remits when the obesity or endocrinopathy is corrected.[94]

Risk to Future Generations

The epidemiology of obesity is complex, and both environmental and genetic/familial factors have significant impact. As mentioned previously, there is a significant risk that the obese child or adolescent will become an obese adult. The risk in the case of adolescents is about 80 percent. As these adolescents become obese adults and parents, they tend to have obese children. The risk of a child becoming obese is about 40 percent when one parent is obese, nearly 80 percent when both parents are affected.[78]

Summary

Although the list of complications and associations of childhood obesity may appear imposing, they have rather low prevalence and pose a relatively low risk to health during the pediatric years. However, it is reasonably clear that the risk of complications and persistence into adulthood rises with increasing severity, and weight reduction prior to or during adolescence is essential to prevent lifelong disease.[78]

References

1. Theander S. Long-term prognosis of anorexia nervosa: A preliminary report. In Darby PL, Garfinkel PE, Garner DM, et al. (eds): Anorexia Nervosa, Recent Developments in Research. New York, Alan R. Liss, Inc, 1983.
2. Maillot S, Porot M, Coudert AJ, et al. La Mort des anorexiques mentales. *Encephale* 1981; 7:113–21.
3. Crisp AH. Prevalence of anorexia nervosa. *Br Med J* 1978; 2:500.
4. Garfinkel PE, Moldofski H, Garner DM. Prognosis in anorexia nervosa as influence by clinical features, treatment and self perception. *Can Med Assoc J* 1977; 2:1041–1045.
5. Bruch H. Perils of behavior modification in treatment of anorexia nervosa. *JAMA* 1974; 230:1419–1422.
6. Mars DR, Anderson NH, Riggall FC. Anorexia nervosa: A disorder with severe acid base derangements. *South Med J* 1982; 75:1028–1042.
7. Cellerino R, Frezza M. Anoressia mentale associata ad ipopotassiemo ed, iperaldosteronismo secondario. *Minerva Med* 1974; 65:73–77.
8. Garrow JS. Underfeeding and overfeeding and their clinical consequences. *Proc Nutr Soc* 1976; 35:363–368.
9. Palla B, Litt I. Medical complications of eating disorders in adolescents. *Pediatrics* 1988; 81:613–623.
10. Thurston J, Marks P. Electrocardiographic abnormalities in patients with anorexia nervosa. *Br Heart J* 1974; 36:719–723.
11. Palossy B, Oo M. ECG alterations in anorexia nervosa. *Adv Cardiol* 1977; 19:280–282.
12. Nudel DB, Gootman N, Nussbaum MP, et al. Altered exercise performance and abnormal sympathetic responses to exercise in patients with anorexia nervosa. *J Pediatr* 1984; 105:34–37.
13. Mitchell JE, Gillum R. Weight-dependent arrhythmia in a patient with anorexia nervosa. *Am J Psychiatry* 1980; 137:377–378.
14. Gottdiener JS, Gross HA, Henry WL, et al. Effects of self-induced starvation of cardiac size and function in anorexia nervosa. *Circulation* 1958; 58:426–433.
15. Silverman JA, Krongrad E. Anorexia nervosa: A cause of pericardial effusion? *Pediatr Cardiol* 1983; 4:125–127.
16. Hemymsfield SB, Bethel RA, Ansley JD, et al. Cardiac abnormalities in cachectic patients before and during nutritional repletion. *Am Heart J* 1978; 95:584–594.
17. Powers PS. Heart failure during treatment of anorexia nervosa. *Am J Psychiatry* 1982; 139:1167–1170.
18. Schocken D, Holloway D, Powers P. Weight loss and the heart: Effects of anorexia nervosa and starvation. *Arch Intern Med* 1989; 149:877–881.
19. Overby K, Litt I. Mediastinal emphysema in an adolescent with anorexia nervosa and self-induced emesis. *Pediatrics* 1988; 81:134–136.
20. Chatfield WR, Bowditch JDP, Forrest CA. Spontaneous pneumomediastinum complicating anorexia nervosa. *Br Med J* 1979; 1:200–201.
21. Garfinkel PE, Brown GM, Darby PL. The psychoendocrinology of anorexia nervosa. *Int J Mental Health* 1981; 9:162–193.
22. Falk JR, Halmi KA. Amenorrhea in anorexia nervosa. Examination of the critical body weight hypothesis. *Biol Psychiatry* 1982; 17:799–806.

23. Vigersky RA. Anorexia nervosa as a model of hypothalamic dysfunction. In Vigersky RA (ed): Anorexia Nervosa. New York, Raven Press, 1977.
24. Brown GM, Garfinkel PE, Jeuniewic N, et al. Endocrine profiles in anorexia nervosa. Ibid.
25. Garfinkel PE, Brown GM, Stancer HC, et al. Hypothalamic-pituitary function in anorexia nervosa. *Arch Gen Psychiatry* 1975; 32:739–744.
26. Wiegelman W, Solbach HG. Effects of LH-RH on plasma levels of LH and FSH in anorexia nervosa. *Horm Metab Tes* 1972; 4:404.
27. Nillius SJ, Wide L. The pituitary responsiveness to acute and chronic administration of gonadotropin-releasing hormone in acute and recovery stages of anorexia nervosa. In Vigersky RA (ed): Anorexia Nervosa. New York, Raven Press, 1977.
28. Warren MP. Weight loss and responsiveness to LH-RH. Ibid.
29. Warren MP, Jewelewicz R, Dyrenfurth I, et al. The significance of weight loss in the evaluation of pituitary response to LH-RH in women with secondary amenorrhea. *J Clin Endocrinol Metab* 1975; 40:601–611.
30. Isaacs AJ, Leslie RDG, Gomez J, et al. The effect of weight gain on gonadotropins and prolactin in anorexia nervosa. *Acta Endocrinol* (Copenh) 1980; 94:145–150.
31. Boyar RM, Katz J, Finkelstein JW, et al. Anorexia nervosa—Immaturity of the 24-hour luteinizing hormone secretory pattern. *N Engl J Med* 1974; 291:861–865.
32. Morimoto Y, Oishi T, Hanasaki N, et al. Interrelations among amenorrhea serum gonadotropins and body weight in anorexia nervosa. *Endocinal Jpn* 1980; 27:191–200.
33. Mecklenburg RS, Loriauz DL, Thompson RH, et al. Hypothalamic dysfunction in patients with anorexia nervosa. *Medicine* 1974; 53:147–159.
34. Hurd HP, Palumbo PJ, Gharib H. Hypothalamic-endocrine dysfunction in anorexia nervosa. *May Clin Proc* 1977; 52:711–716.
35. Beumont PJV, Carr PJ, Gelder MG. Plasma levels of luteinizing hormones and of immunoreactive oestrogens (oestradiol) in anorexia nervosa: Response to clomiphene citrate. *Psychol Med* 1973; 3:495–501.
36. Fishman J, Boyar RM, Hellman L. Influence of body weight on estradiol metabolism in young women. *J. Clin Endocrinol Metab* 1975; 41:989–991.
37. McNab D, Hawton K. Disturbances of sex hormones in anorexia nervosa in the male. *Postgrad Med J* 1981; 57:254–256.
38. Wesselius CL, Anderson G. A case study of male with anorexia nervosa and low testosterone levels. *J Clin Psychiatry* 1982; 43:428–429.
39. Mitchell J. Medical Complications of Anorexia Nervosa and Bulimia. *J Psych Med* 1984; 1:229–255.
40. Miyai K, Yamamoto T, Azukizawa M, et al. Serum thyroid hormones and thyrotropin in anorexia nervosa. *J Clin Endocrinol Metab* 1975; 40:334–338.
41. Moshang T, Parks JS, Baker L, et al. Low serum triiodothyronine in patients with anorexia nervosa. *J Clin Endocrinol Metab* 1975; 40:470–473.
42. Suda AK, Pittman CS, Shimizu T, et al. The production and metabolism of 3,5,3′-Triiodothyronine and 3,3,′5′-Triiodothyronine in normal and fasting subjects. *Clin Endocrinol Metab* 1978; 47:1311–1319.

43. Gardner DF, Kaplan MM, Stanley CA, et al. Effect of triiodothyronine replacement on the metabolic and pituitary responses to starvation. *N Engl J Med* 1979; 300:579–584.
44. Vagenakis AG. Thyroid hormone metabolism in prolonged experimental starvation in man. In Vigersky RA (ed): Anorexia Nervosa. New York, Raven Press, 1977.
45. Casper RC, Frohman LA. Delayed TSH release in anorexia nervosa following injection of thyrotropin-releasing hormone (TRH). *Psychoneuroendocrinology* 1982; 7:59–68.
46. Macaron C, Wilber JF, Green O, et al. Studies of growth hormone (GH), thyrotropin (TSH) and prolactin (PRL) secretion in anorexia nervosa. *Psychoneuroendocrinology* 1978; 3:181–185.
47. Boyar RM, Hellman LD, Roffwarg H, et al. Cortisol secretion and metabolism in anorexia nervosa. *N Engl J Med* 1977; 296:190–193.
48. Walsh BT, Katz JL, Levin J, et al. Adrenal activity in anorexia nervosa. *Psychosomatic Medicine* 1978; 40:499–506.
49. Warren MP, Van de Wiele RL. Clinical and metabolic features of anorexia nervosa. *Am J Obstet Gynecol* 1973; 117:435–449.
50. Vigersky RA, Loriaux DL, Anderson AE, et al. Anorexia nervosa: Behavioral and hypothalamic aspects. *Clin Endocrinol Metab* 1975; 5:517–535.
51. Amrein PC, Friedman R, Kosinski K, et al. Hematologic changes in anorexia nervosa. *JAMA* 1979; 241:2190–2191.
52. Bowers TK, Eckert E. Leukopenia in anorexia nervosa: Lack of increased risk of infection. *Arch Intern Med* 1978; 138:1520–1523.
53. Carryer HM, Berkman JM, Mason HL. Relative lymphocytosis in anorexia nervosa. Staff meetings of the Mayo Clinic. 1959; 34:426–432.
54. Pearson HA. Marrow hypoplasia in anorexia nervosa. *J Pediatr* 1967; 71:211–215.
55. Golla JA, Larson LA, Anderson CF, et al. An immunological assessment of patients with anorexia nervosa. *Am J Clin Nutrition* 1981; 34:2756–2762.
56. Gotch FM, Spry CJF, Mowat AG, et al. Reversible granulocyte killing defect in anorexia nervosa. *Clin Exp Immunol* 1975; 21:244–249.
57. Palmblad J, Fohlin L, Lundstrom M. Anorexia nervosa and polymorphonuclear (PMN) granulocyte reactions. *Scand J Hematol* 1977; 19:334–342.
58. Pertschuk MJ, Crosby LO, Barot L, et al. Immunocompetency in anorexia nervosa. *Am J Clin Nutrition* 1982; 35:968–972.
59. Dubios A, Gross HA, Ebert MH, et al. Altered gastric emptying and secretion in primary anorexia nervosa. *Gastroenterology* 1979; 77:319–323.
60. Saleh JW, Lebwohl P. Metoclopramide-induced gastric emptying in patients with anorexia nervosa. *Am J Gastroenterol* 1980; 74:127–132.
61. Akin JT Jr, Gray SW, Skandelakis JE. Vascular compression of the duodenum: Presentation of ten cases and review of the literature. *Surgery* 1976; 79:515–522.
62. Mitchell JR, Pyle RL, Miner RA. Gastric dilatation as a complication of bulimia. *Psychosomatics* 1982; 23:96–97.
63. Saul SH, Dekkar A, Watson CG. Acute gastric dilatation with infarction and perforation. *Gut* 1981; 22:978–983.
64. Brady, JP. Parotid enlargement in bulimia. *J Family Practice* 1985; 20: 496–502.

65. Bernard JD, Shearn MA. Psychogenic pseudo-Sjogren's syndrome. *West J Med* 1974; 120:247–248.
66. Harris RT. Bulimarexia and related serious eating disorders with medical complications. *Ann Intern Med* 1983; 99:800–807.
67. Rampling D. Acute pancreatitis in anorexia nervosa. *Med J Aust* 1982; 2:194–195.
68. Webb WL, Gehi M. Electrolyte and fluid imbalance: Neuropsychiatric manifestations. *Psychosomatics* 1981; 22:199–203.
69. Roberts M, Tylenda C. Dental aspects of anorexia and bulimia nervosa. *Pediatrics* 1989; 16:178–184.
70. Jones R, Cleaton-Jones P. Depth and area of dental erosions, and dental caries, in bulimic women. *J Dental Research* 1989; 68:1275–1278.
71. House RC, Grisius R, Bliziotes MM, et al. Perimolysis: Unveiling the surrepitious vomiter. Oral Surg 1981; 51:152–155.
72. Crisp AH, Fenton GW, Scotton I. A controlled study of the EEG in anorexia nervosa. *Br J Psychiatry* 1968; 114:1149–1160.
73. Green RS, Rau JH. Treatment of compulsive eating disturbances with anticonvulsant medication. *Am J Psychiatry* 1974; 131:428–432.
74. Wermuth BM, Davis KL, Hollister LE, et al. Phenytoin treatment of the binge-eating syndrome. *Am J Psychiatry* 1977; 134:1249–1253.
75. Lewin K, Mattingly D, Millis RR. Anorexia nervosa associated with hypothalamic tumor. *Br Med J* 1972; 2:629–643.
76. Weller RA, Weller EB. Anorexia nervosa in a patient with an infiltrating tumor of the hypothalamus. *Am J Psychiatry* 1982; 139:824–826.
77. Gerner RH, Cohen DJ, Fairbanks L, Anderson GM, Young JG, Scheinin M, Linnoila M, Shaywitz BA, Hare TA. CSF neurochemistry of women with anorexia nervosa and normal women. *Am J Psychiatry* 1984; 141:1441–1444.
78. Dick WH. Childhood obesity: Susceptibility, cause and management. *J Pediatrics* 1983; 103:676–686.
79. Walker WA, Durie PR, Hamilton JR, Walker-Smith JA, Watkins JB. Pediatric Gastrointestinal Disease. Philadelphia, Toronto, B.C. Decker, Inc., 1991.
80. Lloyd JK, Wolff OH, Whelan WS. Childhood obesity. *Br Med J* 1981; 2: 145.
81. Kissebah AH, Freedman DS, Peiris AN. Health risks of obesity. *Med Clin NA* 1989; 73:111–138.
82. Frisch RE. Fatness and fertility. *Perspect Biol Med* 1985; 28:611–633.
83. Garn SM, LaVelle M, Rosenberg KR, Hawthorne VM. Maturational timing as a factor in female fatness and obesity. *Am J Clin Nutrition* 1986; 43: 879–883.
84. Tracey VV, De NC, Harper JR. Infantile obesity and respiratory infections. *Nutr Rev* 1971; 29:112–113.
85. Hutchinson-Smith B. Obesity and respiratory infection in children. (Letter) *Br Med J* 1971; 1:460–461.
86. Riley DJ, Santiago TV, Edelman NH. Complications of obesity-hypoventilation syndrome in childhood. *Am J Dis Child* 1976; 130:671–674.
87. Wittes EH, Thompson S. Obstructive sleep apnea and obesity. *Otolaryng Clin NA* 1990; 23:751–760.

88. Rames LK, Clark WR, Conner WE, Reiter MA, Lauer RM. Normal blood pressures and the evaluation of sustained blood pressure elevation in childhood: The Muscatine study. *Pediatrics* 1978; 61:245.
89. Gartmaker SL, Dietz WH, Sobol AM, Wehler CA. Increasing pediatric obesity in the United States. *Am J Dis Child* 1987; 141:535–540.
90. Rocchini AP, Katch V, Anderson J, Hinderliter J, Becque D, Martin M, Marks C. Blood pressure in obese adolescents: Effect of weight loss. *Pediatrics* 1988; 82:16–23.
91. Newman WP, Freedman DS, Voors AW, Gard PD, Srinivasan SR, Cresanta JL, Williamson GD, Webber LS, Berenson GS. Relation of serum lipoprotein levels and systolic blood pressure to early atherosclerosis. *N Engl J Med* 1986; 314:138–144.
92. AvRuskin TW, Pillai S, Juan C. Decreased prolactin secretion in childhood obesity. *J Ped* 1985; 106:373–378.
93. Wilmore DW, Pruitt BA. Fat boys get burned. *Lancet* 1972; ii:631–632.
94. Rudolph AM. Ed Pediatrics (eighteenth edition). Norwalk and LosAltos, Appleton and Lange, 1987.

15 The B.A.S.H. Approach

FELIX E.F. LAROCCA

"The first form of 'training' which seems to have induced professionals to become interested in mutual help groups or 'the strength in us'[1] has been professional defection of one kind or another."

—O. Hobart Mowrer, 1984[2]

"The goals of all psychologically help are to give people tools which enable them to cope with and alleviate distress they are experiencing . . . The quality of life of any individual is affected by the nature and quality of the helping networks or exchanges in which he participates."

—Phyllis R. Silverman, 1978[3]

Call it self-help, mutual aid, support, mutual support, face-to-face, encounter, consciousness-raising, linkage, peer therapy, natural support, share and care, personal help; the noun after these modiliers may be system, network, or, most often, group. There are a great many such organizations—around half a million of them in the United States, with 15 million members, according to an estimate in the *Directory of National Self-Help/Mutual Aid Resources* (1987). They address an enormous variety of problems. Many groups are small and ephemeral. Many more flourish. The oldest and largest, Alcoholics Anonymous, began in 1935 and has an international constituency in the millions.

Ostomates, wives of impotent men, stutterers, parents of a child with dystrophic epidermolysis bullosa, and people with hundreds of other afflictions all have self-help organizations. Whatever the differences among them, they rest on a common foundation. Their members find benefit in repeated encounters to discuss, fully and candidly, a shared predicament.

People who meet regularly under those conditions find company in their misery, but if the meetings are purposefully guided, more happens than commiseration. Participants see that they are not alone. Their feelings of guilt and despondency begin to lift. They learn new things about themselves and about others. They witness in their peers the benefits of changed behavior. Helped by the group, they are further reinforced when they find they can in turn help others. Passive acceptance to treatment—

the doctor's prescription—is displaced by self-motivation and active participation in healing. The whole, it appears, amounts to more than the sum of its parts.

The same nuclear principle underlies group therapy as administered by medical professionals. It is a principle especially appropriate, as we shall see later, to the treatment of eating disorders. Whether the group is conceived by a psychiatrist as part of a structured treatment program, by an expatient in rebellion against the mental-health "establishment," or by persons who feel oppressed by public attitudes toward their status (e.g., as convicts or homosexuals), in puts to work certain dynamics that have long been evident when people meet to bring about some change in their lives.

The processes that comfort, reassure, instruct, and strengthen people when they discuss a shared affliction have been described from the psychotherapist's point of view by Yalom[4] and Bloch and Crouch.[5] A brief summary of these processes is supplied by Gelder, Gath, and Mayou:[6] ". . . the feeling of belonging to the group (cohesiveness), learning from the successes and mistakes of others (interpersonal learning), discovering that other people have similar problems (universality), regaining hope through being valued and helped by others (altruism), learning from other members' reactions to one's own social behavior, copying the behavior of others (modeling), and the opportunity to express strong emotions (catharsis)." Yalom[4] adds to these a category of self-understanding, and observes that in a survey by himself and colleagues of group participants, the item regarded by them as having been most helpful to their progress was "Discovering and accepting previously unknown or unacceptable parts of myself."

Levy[7] offers a somewhat more empirical, treatment-oriented formulation of the therapeutic forces generated in groups. He finds four behavioral processes: 1) social reinforcement for desirable behaviors and the elimination or control of problematic behaviors; 2) training, indoctrination, and support in self-control behaviors; 3) modeling (i.e., imitation) of ways to cope with stress; and 4) providing an agenda for changing members' social environment. Levy follows these with seven cognitive processes: increased expectancy of change and help; guidance as to suitable norms and means; expanded awareness of one's problems and circumstances; heightened recognition of key stimuli and contingencies in one's life; support for changed attitudes toward oneself and environment; social comparison and consensual validation that reduce one's feelings of isolation, and redefinition of one's personal identity and self-esteem throught participation in an alternative or substitute culture—the "reference group," that the self-help organization itself may come to represent in the lives of its members.

Narrow etiological constructs to account for anorexia and bulimia nervosa have not withstood rigorous testing, and researchers now generally agree that a number of causative factors are present, in combinations and proportions that vary from case to case. The most important factor is mediated by our culture—a yearning for thinness expressed in German by die Magersucht, with a corresponding abhorrence of fat. This powerful sentiment, first documented in letters of Lord Byron,[8] has become pervasive over the last two centuries in developed Western nations, especially in their more educated and affluent classes. Magersucht is the primary motive for food restriction behavior that, in anorectics and bulimics, assumes pathopsychological character.

Further, the great preponderance of young females among the patients we see suggests that girls are particularly vulnerable to doubts and conflicts concerning their physiological and sexual development in adolescence, their stature among peers, their place in the family, their fitness for professional career achievement, and their identity as persons in the adult world. Self-starvation not only promises to many girls the extreme slenderness that is held up as a model in the ambient culture, but also offers them a tool for manipulating and controlling their environment.

Eating-disordered patients are often found to have symptoms of other common psychological disorders, such as depression and chemical abuse. They are more likely than controls to have close relatives who are depressed or alcoholic. A predisposition to develop an eating disorder may be to some extent genetically transmitted, but pharmacotherapy has not been found to have specific application to anorexia or bulimia. When depression is present, as often happens, we use medications to relieve it. For the disordered eating behavior itself, however, cognitive/behavioral therapy and psychotherapy are the preferred approaches. Because of the abnormal or dysfunctional relationships that are often found in the households of young anorectics and bulimics, emphasis is placed by some clinicians on family therapy.

Thus, depending on the point of view from which we observe them, the eating disorders are at the same time coherent and fragmented. Deliverance from anorexia nervosa, bulimia nervosa, and obesity alike is achieved through the establishment of normal eating behavior. The anorectic who quits starving herself to the point of amenorrhea and maintains a Body Mass Index at around 20 is quite slender but has become, for all practical purposes, no longer anorectic. She may not be an entirely happy, well-adjusted person, but with a small change in behavior, manifested inconspicuously at the dining table, her "caseness" has vanished. Likewise the bulimic who breaks out of a cycle of gorging and purging, and the obese person who maintains a suitable ratio of energy intake versus output, have achieved remission; so has the alcoholic who quits drinking.

To get patients to establish those desired behaviors is, of course, not so simple. Therapists must work their way attentively through a maze of sociocultural, psychological, familial, and perhaps genetic influences that seem to precipitate a morbid intensification of dieting in certain persons, and after treatment for the disorder, to press them toward relapse. William Ryan[9] wrote eloquently about the gulf between neat diagnostic labels and the sprawling, unruly messes that we so often find in patients' lives:

"... consider the case of a depressed and defeated working-class housewife turning to someone for help with a multitude of problems that are overwhelming her: an alcoholic husband who disappears for days at a time; the piling up of pressing debts; an eviction notice from the landlord; two children in diapers and a third who is enuretic; a sickly daughter and a neglected oldest son whose school work is worsening daily; headaches and stomach-aches; increasing trouble with her neighbors as she becomes more and more short-tempered; and a growing sense of guilt as she finds that she herself is turning more and more to liquor for consolation.

"If this woman were to be viewed in a narrow mental-health context, it is possible that she would be diagnosed as suffering from depression [and] referred for psychiatric treatment ... possibly she would ... then be referred for marital counseling ... One must consider the question of whether it is even appropriate to make such a referral—to abstract, as it were, a 'disease' from this complex of problems. Her 'depression' is a condition that might seem quite natural in view of what is happening to her. To call her situation a marital problem seems ... a glaring understatement ... Her emotional disturbance, her marital difficulties, are discovered in the context of serious social disturbance and are only parts of an interlocking system of problems. It may be that these realistic problems should be considered and dealt with as they exist—that is, as a total unit, without any attempt artificially to pull out one or another of the problems for separate treatment or to squeeze a complex situation into a diagnostic mode which does not fit it."

Here Ryan was commenting on the imperfections of public mental-health care in Boston in the 1960s, despite a high level of funding and treatment facilities. He objected specifically to a referral system that sorted patients, like letters at the post office, into narrowing channels of specialization. Instead, he contended, more people should be involved, with psychologists, counselors, nurses, schoolteachers, social workers, and ministers brought into a broad-based community mental-health team, collaborating with physicians and psychiatrists.

Ryan had in mind a sweeping interdisciplinary alliance of professionals; but in fact, effective attention to the problems he cited in 1969 was already coming from the self-help movement. For many years before Ryan wrote, signs had been evident of public dissatisfaction with the performance of professional healers.

The great technological advances in medical care after World War II brought with them higher cost, professional specialization, and the concentration of treatment in hospitals. At the same time there were sharply increased demands on the time physicians had to spend in professional consultation, paperwork, and study to keep up with the flow of new knowledge, Patients were getting better care, but less personal attention from the caregiver.

I think it fair to say that in the psychiatric branch of medicine, public expectations had never been very high, or feelings toward the provider very warm. The introduction of chlorpromazine in 1952 transformed the treatment of acute psychotics, not by curing them but by making most of them manageable at home—an outcome that not all families welcomed as liberating.

Although much can be said for the pharmacological innovations that have made it possible to shut down state mental hospitals, and restore depressed patients in significant numbers of near-normal activity, that progress has not made it easier for a great many psychiatrically ill people to get the continuing attention they need. It is significant that a large national self-help network, the Manic Depressive Association, has grown up around the very disorder which responds so reliably to medication that lawsuits have been filed (for the purpose of medical insurance claims) to label it a physical, rather than a mental, illness. The support organization is needed nonetheless because so many patients, although fully aware that the prescribed medicine controls their symptoms, neglect after a while to take it—either because of adverse collateral effects (e.g., weight gain and frequent urination in the case of lithium carbonate), or belief that the illness has gone away, or because the "high" of incipient mania is so attractive. In short, bipolar illness can be diagnosed, treatment prescribed, and serum levels checked within days by a psychiatrist; yet the patient may need a lifetime of support and vigilance by those around him to secure compliance and forestall a ruinous recurrence of mania.

In the course of treating dozens of anorectics and bulimics in the 1970s, it became clear to me that while the immediate course of action was relatively simple—to establish healthy, regular eating behavior during a hospital stay of several weeks—I could do little to reshape or redirect the various factors in the patient's family, school, and social environment that seemed to nourish the eating disorder. An hour-long predischarge interview with the parents was helpful, of course, but was no substitute for the long-term support and cognitive/behavioral rebuilding that I believed were needed in the family circle. Nor was any resource available to educate people about the signs of an incipient eating disorder among their family members or friends, that is, prevention.

It struck me that a solution to the problem of providing the comprehensive attention my patients needed—a solution that both they and my modest private practice could afford—might be found in the self-help organizations that were proliferating at the time. Autonomous support groups for eating-disorder patients began to appear in 1972. In devising BASH, I was chiefly guided not so much by the experiences of those groups as by Yalom's[4] formulation of group therapy processes, and to some degree by the published history of AA (1975).

Program Structure

From its beginning in April 1981, BASH has operated under professional tutelage, as a component in a hospital-based eating-disorders treatment program. Patients, parents, other family members, friends, and any interested persons were invited to attend free all-day meetings on the third Saturday of each month, in various hospital conference rooms. At the outset there is an informal period for socialization, light refreshment, and perusal of the meeting schedule; staff (nurses, dietitians, caseworkers) are present to answer questions and steer newcomers to appropriate activities on the schedule.

The morning and afternoon periods usually begin with hour-long general sessions led by guest speakers. These are medical professionals who speak with authority on various subjects according to their field of specialization—menstrual disturbances, bone disease, obesity, nutrition, etc.—and are prepared to answer questions from the lay audience.

For the ensuing self-help meetings and workshops, the whole body of attendees—it has often been more than 500—is subdivided into a number of smaller groups. Generally we take care to separate patients from parents, and to guide the information-seeking public, that is, teachers and others interested in the recognition of eating-disorder signs and symptoms, into groups of their own. Weekly meetings were added to the monthly meetings, and hospital inpatients have small groups of their own. Groups are added, subtracted, and modified with changes in the numbers and needs of the member constituency.

The frequency with which we found unipolar depression in our bulimic patients led to the development of meetings concerned primarily with affective disorders. Another condition I had often dealt with in my practice as a child psychiatrist was attention deficit-hyperactivity disorder. We arranged for mutual-support meetings for the parents of these boys and girls, and they proved very helpful in the long-term management of the illness.

Leadership of the groups presented a problem. From the beginning only one resident psychiatrist has participated, and as director of the program I thought it better on several counts not to participate directly in the groups. Following the model of autonomous self-help organizations, we started by encouraging stabilized patients or expatients to guide the discussion. These "facilitators" sat, and still sit, in a circle to parity with other participants. Six or eight of these circles of chairs may be scattered around the floor of the hospital gymnasium-auditorium; a few yards of intervening space between the circles is ample to procure intimacy and privacy for the various discussions.

I preferred not to impose a highly structured format but to let the facilitator's and participants' experiences direct the talk into the helpful lines that Yalom postulated. My supervisory function in this respect consisted of interviewing the facilitators at length after each meeting, suggesting ways to overcome obstacles encountered, casually collecting remarks by participants about how the meeting had gone, and watching attendance from month to month.

We soon learned that therapeutic efficacy in the meetings could easily be derailed by manipulators who sought to justify themselves with clever argument, or narcissists who would monopolize the hour with their own vehement interpretations of what was going on. In these cases, disillusionment would set in and attendance would drop off sharply after a couple of meetings. Other groups stayed together amicably but proved not to be making the progress we wanted. We saw, for example, that restricting anorectics tend to draw together in a sort of clubbish aristocracy. Some bulimics were even learning new ways of purgation and concealment from peers at the meetings.

In 1983 I wrote a training manual for the facilitators. By degrees we moved toward tighter structure and firmer direction in the meetings. Facilitators were urged to write a summary immediately after each meeting—not from notes or audiotape, which would have inhibited the discussion, but from memory. These "minutes" served them and me in understanding the attendees' circumstances and problems, and in keeping track of what sort of changes, if any, were taking place in them.

As training for the facilitators grew more rigorous and the demands on their time increased, the volunteers dropped out one by one and their places were taken by staff members. The training manual was revised to reflected the somewhat more structured program.[10]

The "Significant Other"

Group therapy proved a most useful instrument for cognitive input and output between the clinic and persons close to eating-disordered patients—family members, spouses, and close friends. In a treatment program it is of high importance to inform "significant others" as fully as possible of the nature of the illness, to explain the plan of therapy, and to enlist their cooperation in providing a home environment conducive to the patient's recovery.

In a conventional practice this can often be accomplished by the therapist in conference with those close to the patient; in any event a thorough, unhurried, face-to-face discussion should be scheduled at the outset of treatment, with the patient taking part unless her condition precludes it. In many other households, however, the stress of living with an eating-disordered person is such that family members welcome continuing exchanges with others in the same predicament. Kapoor[11] suggests that support groups for the "significant others" of bulimics may yield benefits analogous to those for wives of alcoholics; she summarizes research relevant to programs of the latter kind, and describes a structured 5-week program of her own called "Helping the Bulimic Get Better."

Religion

Religious beliefs in relation to mental illness and its treatment constitute a subject that most medical people deal with in a gingerly way, if they deal with it at all, because of the indistinct boundaries among "good" religion, "false" religion ("cults"), folk beliefs, and psychopathological delusions. Religious beliefs are present, however, in a large majority of the general population and in a significant minority of mental-health professionals. Galanter et al.,[12] from questionnaires completed by 193 of 260 U.S. psychiatrists who belong to the Christian Medical and Dental Society, gathered that the respondents were in the main quite selective in their application of the Bible and prayer to treatment, preferring conventional therapies for certain illnesses and for patients who are not devout Christians.

The issue is hard to avoid in an appraisal of self-help groups because of the eminence of Alcoholics Anonymous (AA), the oldest (1935), largest (around a million current members), and probably most influential of those organizations. From the beginning, AA members have subscribed to a 12-step program, and that program has been adopted by many other organizations working against addiction, including Overeaters Anonymous. Six of the 12 steps affirm submission to "a Power greater than ourselves . . . God . . . Him." This religious or spiritual element in AA recently drew critical attention,[13] with four authors presenting vigorous rebuttals of that criticism in the same publication.

In our own application of group techniques we have never employed the 12 steps or otherwise introduced religious elements into treatment. Neither have we tried to suppress religious issues when they are raised for discussion by group participants, or to discourage patient/participants from turning to spiritual guidance when they are inclined to do so. I have not met in our own program an eating-disordered patient whose religious convictions were such as to interfere with treatment and recovery.

Evaluation

How effective has our self-help or mutual-aid application been in the treatment of eating disorders? The difficulties of evaluation in this field are discussed by Lieber and Bond[14] and Levy.[15] Yalom[4] observes "the nature of our data is so rich, complex, and highly subjective that, to a large degree, it makes scientific methodology impossible." The methodological problems are similar to those that encumber research into the comparative efficacy of psychotherapy in general.

There are two main obstacles: formulation of a group-therapy procedure well enough defined and structured that it may be reproduced for comparison studies, and provision of a matched patient control group from whose treatment the group-meeting element might be withheld without the awareness of patients and staff. From the sketch of our program given earlier one can see that from the start we did not think of BASH as an element in a course of treatment, but as a coherent, comprehensive program in which self-help or support meetings had several important functions. Not least in importance was that of making us as caregivers aware of the full range of strengths, weaknesses, and dysfunctions in the patient's domestic environment.

Our own informal evaluation studies or surveys, like those described by Yalom, have been directed at "successful" participants, that is, those who as inpatients routinely attended a substantial number of group sessions within the hospital unit and who were willing, months or years later, to fill out a mailed questionnaire. These respondents exhibit a high degree of approval of their experience with the program. Obviously, such results cannot speak for hundreds of outpatients, "significant others," and casual or ephemeral attendees, as well as for patients who did not return the questionnaire. Furthermore, the questions did not try to segregate self-help from other psychotherapeutic and pharmacotherapeutic aspects of treatment.

In practical terms, however, it has been a sufficient measure of group-therapy performance for us that over a decade, nobody involved in our program—patients, nurses, caseworkers, volunteer facilitators, relatives, friends—has suggested that our free public self-help or support meetings be dropped, or converted into, say, a structured course of day-patient group therapy like the Canadian program described by Piran and Kaplan.[16] The BASH groups soon came to have a life of their own, creating a "family" wherein members can find reassurance at any time, at no cost to them. A telephone "crisis line" is answered at all hours; a nurse on the hospital unit takes time from her duties to counsel the caller, typically a bullmic who feels a "binge" coming on.

Conclusion

My intention here is not to set forth our own organization as a model. It keeps evolving in accordance with changing patient population trends and with the skills and attitudes of our facilitators. Changes in the administrative circumstances of the sponsoring hospital also affect our program. I do hope, however, to stimulate colleagues toward their own syntheses of self-help/mutual aid with clinical treatment, I have not met a colleague who believes patients are harmed by attendance at self-help meetings and tries to dissuade them from doing so. Giannini[17] encourages such participation, and I have the impression that many others do likewise. With this approving but detached posture, it seems to me that the therapist passes by a valuable opportunity to open a "window" into the patient's emotional and social resources. From reactions and interactions within the group we have often learned useful particulars about a patient that have eluded the diagnostic interview, social history taker, and self-report questionnaires.

Uneasiness is evident among physicians (e.g., Vandereycken et al.,[18] Goldsmith[19]) who sense that by incorporating group therapy or less formal self-help modalities into their clinical practice they lose full control, enter on processes that resist statistical measurement, and may have to deal at times with heterodox or "alternative" healing ideas, notably religion.

On the other side of the fence there is reluctance among leaders in autonomous groups to seeing themselves medicalized, "co-opted," and subjected to professional licensure requirements.[2] The first and greatest of the self-help organizations triumphed, after all, because of the failure of medicine and psychiatry to deal effectively with the great surge of alcoholism that ensued on repeal of Prohibition, Many physicians belong to AA and refer alcoholic patients to it; in some large cities there are enough alcoholic physicians and dentists to constitute AA chapters of their own.

Antze[20] emphasizes the ideologies, or systems of teachings, that some of the organizations cultivate, and which distance them from group therapys as most professionals employ it. He believes that they constitute ". . . the very feature of these groups that their members take most seriously." The examples he holds up for extended scrutiny, however, are eminently distinctive ones: AA with its 12 steps; Synanon, which attacks drug addiction with dramatic communal rites of denunciation and reconciliation; and Recovery, Inc., founded in 1937 by a psychiatrist of unconventional views, Abraham Low.

I do not expect an institutional rapprochement, yet professional medicine has the responsibility, I believe, to learn from the self-help people. Physicians in all fields should be introduced in medical school to the processes of group therapy and self-help/mutual support groups. Psychologists, nurses, school counselors, and social workers likewise have excellent reason to study a phenomenon that has been comforting afflicted people and producing impressive, if unquantifiable, therapeutic results for more than half a century.

Further reason to do so is presented by health-care economics. The cost of care, particularly in hospitals, continues to rise far faster than the inflation rate; the resistance of insurors has grown with it, particularly with respect to claims for psychiatric hospitalization. In the eating disorders, care-management companies now dole out by days inpatient treatment that a few years ago was measured in weeks.

Even in cases where money is not a factor, the physician's time is. A member of Overeaters Anonymous, Virginia Goldner, wrote poignantly[21] about belonging to a class of low-yield patients that tend to frustrate, and exasperate, their doctors. She might have been speaking for alcoholics, or bulimics, or anorectics:

"I can think of no better alternative [than OA]. Chronicity is, by definition, exhausting. Professionals don't have the time, and quickly lose interest in the tedious business of managing a lifelong disorder. The impulse, after a while, is to blame the victim, since relapses are practically inevitable, and progress, at best, is fitful. Moreover, the whole project is built out of small moments and trivial details. The victories are modest, epiphanies are rare—hardly the dramatic rewards that sustain a professional career."

References

1. *Katz A*, Bender E. The Strength in Us: Self-Help Groups in the Modern World. New York, Franklin-Watts, 1976.
2. Mowrer OH. The mental health professions and mutual help programs. In Gartner A, Riessman F (eds): *The Self-Help Revolution*, New York, Human Sciences Press, 1984.
3. Silverman PR, Mutual Help Groups: A Guide for Mental Health Workers. Washington, DC, NIMH monograph, DHEW Publication No. ADM 78–646, 1978.
4. Yalom ID. The Theory and Practice of Group Psychotherapy (third edition). New York, Basic Books, 1985 (previous edns 1970 & 1975).
5. Bloch S, Crouch E. Therapeutic Factors in Group Psychotherapy, New York Oxford University Press, 1985.
6. Gelder M, Gath D, Mayou R, Oxford Textbook of Psychiatry (second edition). New York Oxford University Press, 1989.
7. Levy LH. Processes and activities in groups. In Lieberman MA, Borman DL (eds): Self-Help Groups for Coping with Crisis. San Francisco, Jossey-Bass Publishers, 1979.
8. Brumberg J. Fasting Girls, Cambridge, Harvard University Press, 1988.
9. Ryan W (ed). Distress in the City, Cleveland, Case Western Reserve University Press, 1969.
10. Larocca FEF, Facilitator's Training Manual (second edition revised). St. Louis, BASH, 1989.
11. Kapoor S, Treatment for significant others of bulimic patients may be beneficial. *J Am Dietetic Assoc* 1988; 88:349–350.
12. Galanter M, Larson D, Rubenstone E. Christian psychiatry: the impact of evangelical belief on clinical practice. *Am J Psychiatry* 1991; 148:90–95.
13. Ellis A, Schoenfeld E. Divine intervention and the treatment of chemical dependency. *J Substance Abuse* 1990; 2:459–468.
14. Lieber L, Bond G. Self-help groups: problems of measuring outcomes. *Small Group Behavior* 1978; 9:221–241.
15. Levy L. Issues in research and evaluation. In Gartner A, Riessman F (eds). The Self-Help Revolution, New York, Human Sciences Press, 1984.

16. Piran N, Kaplan A. A Day Hospital Group Treatment Program for Anorexia Nervosa and Bulimia Nervosa. New York, Brunner/Mazel, 1990.
17. Giannini AJ. Anorexia nervosa: a retrospective view. *Int J Psych Med* 1981; 11:199–202.
18. Vandereycken W, Vanderlinden J, Van Werde D. Directive group therapy for patients with anorexia nervosa or bulimia. In Larocca FEF (ed): Eating Disorders: Effective Care and Treatment. St. Louis, Ishiyaku EuroAmerica Inc, 1986.
19. Goldsmith M. Proliferating "self-help" groups offer wide range of support, seek physician rapport. *J Am Med Assoc* 1989; 261:2474–75.
20. Antze P. Role of ideologies in peer psychotherapy groups. In Lieberman MA, Borman LD (eds): Self-Help Groups for Coping With Crisis. San Francisco, Jossey-Bass Publishers, 1979.
21. Gartner A, Riessman F (eds). The Self-Help Revolution. New York, Human Sciences Press, 1984.

Bibliography

Collins AH, Pancoast DL, Natural Helping Networks: a Strategy for Prevention. Washtington, DC, National Association of Social Workers, 1976.

Gartner A, Riessman F. Self-Help in the Human Services. San Francisco, Jossey-Bass, 1977.

Larocca FEF (ed). Eating Disorders: Effective Care and Treatment. St. Louis, Ishiyaku EuroAmerica Inc, 1986.

Larocca FEF (ed). The Psychiatric Clinics of North America, Vol. 7, No. 2. Philadelphia, WB Saunders Co, 1984.

Richow WC, Training of lay helpers. In Abrams JC (ed): Supervision, Consultation and Staff Training in the Helping Professions. New York, Jossey-Bass, 1977.

16 The Hospital Treatment of Eating Disorders

Michael M. Newman

Introduction

Patients admitted to the hospital with anorexia nervosa or bulimia nervosa often present with a complex constellation of behavioral symptoms, psychological disturbances, and medical complications. Many of the eating disorder patients also have diagnoses of affective disorders, psychoactive substance abuse, and severe personality disorders. While this suggests that the clinician treating these patients may be faced with the challenge of treating an individual who has become quite dysfunctional, the clinician is also faced with shortened lengths of stay and a relatively brief time period to treat the individual in a hospital setting. The role of the hospital in the treatment of all psychiatric patients, including those with eating disorders, has changed considerably over the last several years. Associated with this change is a need to reevaluate treatment programs and, in particular, the goals of hospital treatment.

Indications for Hospitalization

The obvious first decision to be made regarding treatment is whether or not hospitalization is indicated. A combination of behavioral, psychological, and medical factors contribute to deciding whether a patient needs to be hospitalized. In addition, the adequacy of the patient's previous treatment must be carefully evaluated.

Behavioral

The therapist evaluates the severity of the symptoms—frequency of binging and purging, time spent involved in excessive exercise, degree of food restriction, and preoccupation with food and body weight—and determines to what extent the patient's level of functioning has been compromised. Patients may complain they have been unable to function in school or have missed a considerable amount of time at work because of the frequency of their bulimic symptoms. If a patient presents with a significant and persistent deterioration in level of function, hospitalization should be considered.

Psychological

The patient must be assessed for the presence and severity of an associated affective disturbance and hospitalization is indicated for any patient who presents with severe depression. Previous suicide attempts are not uncommon among eating disorder patients[1,2] and patients must be specifically questioned as to whether they have any such history. Clearly, any patient who is considered a risk to suicide or to hurt themselves must be hospitalized.

Medical

Patients with eating disorders may have multiple medical complications.[3,4] For the most part, the medical disturbances may be managed conservatively and do not require an acute medical intervention. Rather, with nutritional rehabilitation and stabilization of eating disorder symptoms, the abnormal findings are reversed. Conversely, the clinician should be alert for several conditions for which hospitalization is indicated.

An abnormally low level of potassium may be present secondary to purging and may place the patient at risk for developing a life-threatening cardiac arrhythmia. Hypernatremia secondary to water loading may result in seizures and should be corrected under close medical supervision. The presence of a cardiac arrhythmia or marked sinus bradycardia (less than 50 beats per minute) warrants hospitalization. The use of ipecac to induce purging may be cardiotoxic and patients who engage in this behavior on a regular basis should be considered for hospitalization.

Some patients may acknowledge profound weakness and fatigue, feeling lightheaded, and having experienced blackouts. Acute medical stabilization of these patients is indicated. Lastly, patients who are severely emaciated require close medical supervision during the early stages of refeeding and weight gain and hospitalization is indicated for patients who are more than 20 to 25 percent below ideal body weight.

Outpatient Treatment Failure

There are some patients who do not meet any of the previously mentioned criteria but for whom hospitalization is indicated. Typically, these patients have had an adequate trial of both psychotherapy and pharmacotherapy and have demonstrated little or no progress in their treatment. Despite antidepressant medication and months to years of individual and/or group therapy, some patients may require hospitalization to interrupt their cycle of binging and purging or to begin to reduce the severity of their food restriction and correct their low body weight.

Developing a Treatment Plan

Initial considerations in developing a treatment plan for a patient with an eating disorder must include interventions targeted to the signs and symptoms of the eating disorder for which the patient was hospitalized. That is, binging and purging, food restriction, excessive exercise, and laxative abuse all must be interrupted. It is difficult to justify hospitalization if one cannot clearly outline the therapeutic measures being taken to manage and help the patient gain control of the symptoms.

Second, the question of comorbidity must be addressed. Affective illness is not uncommon in eating disorder patients[5,6,7] and treatment of a clinical depression may be necessary. Psychoactive substance abuse may be present in one-quarter to one-third[8] of bulimic patients. As such, some eating disorder patients may require withdrawal precautions and drug or alcohol detoxification. Furthermore, substance abuse treatment groups need to be an integral component of any eating disorders program.

Recently, there has been considerable research into the comorbidity of personality disorders and eating disorders. Some but not all research has indicated that borderline personality disorder may be present in a significant number of eating disorder patients.[9,10,11] To better anticipate problems that may arise during the course of hospitalization, patients should be carefully assessed for the presence of prominent disturbances in personality.

While not clearly in the realm of comorbidity, a history of sexual abuse may be found in a significant number of women with eating disorders.[12,13] Interpersonal mistrust, as well as unresolved feelings of anger, guilt, and shame associated with the abuse may complicate the treatment process. The hospital may provide a patient with the first "safe" setting she has experienced in which she can begin to discuss the effect the abuse has had on her life.

All patients should have an educational or a vocational assessment. It is not unusual for patients with eating disorders to place unrealistic expectations on themselves either academically or at their job. Patients may have selected schools or careers more to please family members than to pursue their own interests or strengths. The vocational counselor can assist the patient to better identify her own interests and to learn how to best pursue those interests.

In summary, the individual needs of patients in an eating disorders treatment program may vary considerably. A program must be structured to care for the group as a whole as well as be comprehensive enough to address differences among individuals.

Treatment Interventions

Psychotherapy

By definition, the psychotherapy that takes place during the inpatient phase of treatment is short-term therapy. It is therefore most appropriate to focus on the present and to keep in mind that the immediate goal of treatment is the resolution of the eating disorders symptoms. That does not mean that underlying issues and conflicts should not be identified but, for the most part, the goal of the hospitalization cannot be to resolve these issues and conflicts. It is helpful, if not necessary, for a patient to understand that anorexia nervosa is not simply about body weight and wanting to be thin. Rather, the therapist can help the patient identify how issues such as feelings of inadequacy, poor self-esteem, struggles with independence and autonomy, and family problems may have contributed to the development and perpetuation of the eating disorder. It is generally through long-term treatment that these issues are resolved. During short-term therapy, the patient can learn how these issues trigger the symptoms of her eating disorder.

Cognitive behavioral therapy may be a particularly useful form of psychotherapy for eating disorder patients.[14,15] Working in this way, patients learn how maladaptive thoughts lead to uncomfortable feeling states resulting in behaviors or symptoms of the eating disorder. Typically, patients with eating disorders demonstrate cognitive distortions of dichotomous thinking, magnification, personalization, overgeneralization, and magical thinking.[15]

Dichotomous thinking is when the individual employs "all or none" reasoning. For the bulimic trying to control her weight, eating one cookie may be the same as eating one box of cookies. As such, she may reason how she may binge on a box of cookies after having eaten only one or two cookies. Magnification is generally coupled with catastrofication. The individual overestimates the significance of an event and, in doing so, assumes a terrible consequence will occur. Overgeneralization is making unwarranted conclusions from a single event and magical thinking leads to believing in unrealistic cause and effect relationships.

Patients generally begin treatment believing their symptoms "just happen." While it is true that the symptoms become habits, it is also true that events and thoughts about events trigger the symptoms of an eating disorder. By learning what it is that triggers the symptoms, the patient can begin to learn how to control and avoid the symptoms.

Behavioral Contracts

A form of behavioral therapy is practiced on virtually every inpatient unit. That is, as hospitalized patients respond to treatment, they are generally given more responsibility and more privileges to participate in activities that are less supervised. The latter often includes passes both on and then off hospital grounds. Increased privileges may be helpful in reinforcing the anorectic's weight gain process and a contract for $1\frac{1}{2}$ pounds per week is not unreasonable. Positive reinforcements should not be contingent on behaviors that cannot be clearly and objectively observed or measured. Thus weight gain rather than completion of a meal is a better contingency as staff will otherwise be debating among themselves (and with the patient) whether or not the patient has earned added privileges. Patients and staff should work together to identify weekly goals such as being more assertive in group, contacting a school counselor or job supervisor, making an appointment for aftercare, and no episodes of self-injurious behavior. The meeting of the weekly goals should also be reinforced with additional privileges.

When patients fail to meet the terms of their contracts, they often accuse staff of punishing them by withholding privileges such as passes. It is important that the staff be both consistent and supportive of one another. Decisions made by the treatment team should be presented as staff decisions and not as the decision of one member of the team.

Nutritional Counseling

Eating disorders are not caused by a lack of knowledge about proper nutrition. In fact, many patients know more about nutrition than many of the staff. What patients do not know is how to apply proper nutrition to themselves. Nutritional counseling should assist patients in devising an individualized comprehensive food plan. Rather than obsessing about calories, the patient learns to plan meals with proper balance of food groups.

Caloric requirements of anorectic patients may be quite high[16] and the use of liquid nutritional supplements may be necessary. Otherwise, the patient will face large amounts of food that she will most likely reject. The patient can be reassured that the supplements contain the proper amount of nutrients and are to assist the weight gain process. The staff does not want the patient to "overeat" and without the supplements, she would have to do so. Once a healthy weight is achieved, the supplements can be gradually reduced and discontinued leaving the patient to continue on the meal plan already being following.

Specialized Groups

The category of specialized groups is to highlight the needs of subgroups of patients as well as the need for focused group therapies. In particular, substance abuse meetings and survivor groups are an essential component of any treatment program for eating disorder patients. When first admitted to the hospital, patients should attend psychoeducational substance abuse groups held on the treatment unit. As the patient progresses, she may attend Alcoholics Anonymous and Narcotics Anonymous meetings held in the hospital and then off grounds. Should they be available, many patients benefit from attending groups for family members of substance abuse.

As large, heterogeneous groups are not experienced as "safe," patients with a history of sexual abuse often need a specialized group to begin to openly discuss issues related to their abuse. Depending on the size of the treatment program, a survivors group may also include women who are hospitalized for reasons other than an eating disorder.

Other group therapies include: eating awareness group, which focuses on how thoughts and emotions influence eating; assertiveness training group; leisure planning group; exercise group; relationships group; behavior awareness group, which focuses on how an individual's behavior is interpreted by other patients; problem solving group; psychodrama; and adult children of alcoholics.

Vocational Counseling

Vocational counseling should be an integral part of the treatment plan. Patients with eating disorders not unusually experience difficulties at the workplace. They may take or keep jobs to "prove something" to their family (or boss) rather than pursue their own interests. Alternatively, they may be particularly sensitive to any criticism and this may lead them to frequently be changing jobs.

While in the hospital, patients should be tested for their vocational interests. Patients who are out of work can be helped to look for a job and this would include beginning to have job interviews. Before discharge, patients who do have jobs should visit their workplace to reduce the stress associated with seeing their co-workers and returning to work.

Medication

Patients who are hospitalized with an eating disorder are generally quite symptomatic and have not responded to outpatient treatment. In terms of severity of illness, these patients would therefore represent the more severe end of the spectrum and it is more than likely that a medication trial will be indicated.

The efficacy of antidepressant medications for the treatment of bulimia nervosa has been well documented.[17,18,19] It is not uncommon, however, for eating disorder patients to initially resist the recommendation of medication. Their resistance is often based on misconceptions about medication. Patients frequently ask "If I get better on medication, how will I know if it's me or the medication." Some patients believe antidepressant medications are addicting and other patients are fearful that once they begin medication, they will have to take medication for the rest of their lives.

Patients must be educated regarding the use of medication and they should be counseled that medication is but one component of their treatment. The indications and side effects should be carefully reviewed and the patient should understand why the particular medication was selected. As lengths of stay in the hospital become shorter, patients need to be advised that their response to medication is not fully determined prior to their discharge. Rather, medication is started in the hospital setting and the patient is closely monitored for the development of any side effects. Response to treatment will be determined after the patient returns home.

The use of medication for the treatment of anorexia nervosa is less clear-cut and, as a group, anorectic patients tend to be more resistant than bulimic patients to taking medication. One indication for medication is the presence of a major depression—especially if it can be determined that the depression predated the eating disorder and was not simply a consequence of starvation. Before beginning an antidepressant, patients must be medically stabilized. It is generally advisable to begin the weight gain process before starting medication. This may not only lead to the amelioration of some depressive symptomatology but also help the patient to better tolerate the medication. Otherwise, the patient may begin an antidepressant trial only to shortly thereafter refuse to continue the medication because of distressing side effects that might have been averted.

For many years, clinicians have been aware of the resemblance of anorexia nervosa to obsessive compulsive disorder. Anorectics obsess about their weight and fear of weight gain and often have compulsive behaviors including excessive exercise. Fluoxetine, an antidepressant that has been demonstrated to be effective for obsessive compulsive disorder,[20] may prove to be a useful adjunct to the treatment of anorectic patients.

Treatment Planning

In planning treatment, it may be helpful to divide the treatment program into three phases. This may help to more clearly identify weekly goals and the interventions necessary to meet these goals.

Phase I

The principal goal of the first phase of treatment is to interrupt the cycle of symptoms associated with the eating disorder. Simply, the bulimic patient will stop binging and purging, and the anorectic patient will stop losing weight and begin the weight gain process. An additional goal for the first phase of treatment is to establish a working alliance with the patient and the patient's family.

To interrupt the symptoms of an eating disorder, behavioral interventions and contracts with the patient are generally helpful. The patients should be told they will be closely supervised to reduce the opportunity for them to be symptomatic. Generally, this involves supervising meals and use of bathroom and limiting the time a patient may be alone in her room.

During this phase, patients work closely with the nutritionist to plan their meals from the hospital menu. It is better to emphasize food groups and portion size rather than calories as calories can quickly become another number for the patient to obsess about.

To assist the weight gain process, patients should be prescribed, in addition to their regular meals, a liquid supplement. The purpose of the supplement is twofold. First, it can be emphasized that the patient is medically compromised and the supplement should be considered a medication. Second, patients can be reassured that they will not be expected to "overeat" but that they will learn to eat "a normal amount of food." The supplement takes care of the weight gain and once patients achieve and maintain a healthy weight, they can continue with the portion size they have been eating.

While daily weighing may not be necessary, patients should be weighed at least several times per week. Anorectic patients should be given a goal of gaining no less than $1\frac{1}{2}$ pounds per week and behavioral contracts with positive reinforcement should be drawn to facilitate the weight gain process. To minimize the patient's obsessing about her weight, she should only be told her weight one day per week.

Psychotherapy in the first phase of treatment may be both educational and supportive. It is helpful for the patient to understand that the goals of treatment are to control the symptoms and to begin to identify underlying psychological conflicts that may have contributed to the development of the eating disorder. Family work should likewise focus on educating family members about eating disorders. The family should be reassured that the goal is not to find blame but to better understand what has contributed to the development and maintenance of the eating disorder. This of course includes examining the effect the eating disorder has had on other family members. They should further be reassured that anger and frustration are commonplace in family members of patients with eating disorders.

Medication as indicated should be a component of the first phase of treatment. This is particularly the case for a patient who also presents with significant depression.

Phase II

The second phase of treatment focuses on helping the patient identify the thoughts and feelings that trigger the symptoms of the eating disorder.

Behaviorally, the patient works on developing alternative coping mechanisms to their eating disorder symptoms. The goals of the second phase of treatment include: correction of cognitive distortions, correction of maladaptive family interactions, and stabilization of eating behavior within the hospital.

During this phase of treatment, the patient begins to have therapeutic assignments that include some time spent with family outside of the hospital. Initially it is helpful to exclude meals as they increase the level of stress experienced by both the patient and her family. Once the patient's eating behavior has been observed to be more stable in the hospital and she has spent some time with her family on pass, the patient is then directed to plan passes that include meals.

Behavioral restrictions and the close supervision required in the first phase of treatment may begin to be eased as the patient begins to assume more responsibility for herself. Anorectic patients should have a contract for a minimal amount of weight gain ($1\frac{1}{2}$ to 2 pounds) each week for additional privileges. Bulimic patients who maintain their weight within an agreed upon range may begin, with staff supervision, limited exercise.

It is during the second phase of treatment that a patient also begins to identify some of the underlying issues that may have contributed to the onset of their eating disorder. This work tends to progress most in the individual sessions but group therapy sessions, and in particular, survivors group for women with sexual abuse, also facilitate this process.

Phase III

The third phase of treatment focuses on adequately preparing the patient for discharge and represents a transition to aftercare. It is one thing for the patient to control her symptoms in the supervised setting of the hospital and it is quite another for the patient to begin to handle stressful situations outside of the hospital. Therapeutic assignments now include six hour weekend visits home during which time the patient and her family will have a meal together. To minimize the stress and anxiety of returning to work (and facing co-workers) patients are directed to schedule a visit, prior to discharge, to the jobsite and to plan to meet with her supervisor, representative from her employee assistance program and co-workers. Typically, patients resist this recommendation but are almost always relieved after completing such a visit. Their sense of being ashamed about their hospitalization is diminished as they experience support from their colleagues. Also, by talking with their supervisor, they may be able to modify certin stressful work situations or responsibilities.

A similar visit should be planned by patients returning to school. That is, they should plan a meeting with their guidance counselor or advisor who can help the patient organize meetings with teachers. This enables the patient to let her teachers know what course work she has been able to keep up with while she was in the hospital and allows the teachers to assist the patient with her transition back to school. A meeting at school also helps the patient begin to cope with the anxieties of seeing her classmates.

An essential part of discharge planning is a referral for continued outpatient treatment. Again, it is recommended that prior to discharge the patient have a pass to meet one or two times with her outpatient therapist. This is particularly important if the patient will be beginning with a new therapist as it enables the patient to leave the hospital with a greater sense of support.

Conclusion

The most important aspect of treatment planning for any patient is the setting of realistic treatment goals. To determine the goals of treatment for a patient in the hospital, the clinician must not only consider the strengths and weaknesses of the patient but also the anticipated length of stay. As has been the case in all of medicine, patients' lengths of hospitalization for the treatment of anorexia nervosa and bulimia have become significantly reduced. It is helpful for the clinician to remember that the hospitalization is but one phase in the overall treatment of a patient with an eating disorder.

References

1. Garfinkel PE, Moldofsky H, Garner DM. The heterogeneity of anorexia nervosa: Bulimia as a distinct subgroup. *Arch Gen Psychiatry* 1980; 1036–1040.
2. Mitchell JE, Hatsukami D, et al. Characteristics of 275 patients with bulimia. *Am J Psychiatry* 1985; 482–485.
3. Hall RCW, Beresford TP. Medical complications of anorexia and bulimia. *Psychiatric Medicine* 1989; 165–191.
4. Brotman AW, Herzog DB. Medical complications of eating disorders: Outpatient evaluation and management. *Comprehensive Psychiatry* 1985; 258–272.
5. Hudson JI, Pope HG, Jonas JM, et al. Phenomenologic relationships of eating disorders to major affective disorder. *Psychiatry Research* 1983; 345–354.
6. Walsh BT, Roose SP, Glassman AH, et al. Bulimia and depression. *Psychosomatic Medicine* 1985; 123–131.
7. Lee NF, Rush AJ, Mitchell JE. Bulimia and depression. *J Affective Disorders* 1985; 231–238.
8. Hatsukami D, Eckert E, Mitchell JE, Pyle R. Affective disorders and substance abuse in women with bulimia. *Psychological Medicine* 1984; 701–704.
9. Pope HG, Hudson JI. Are eating disorders associated with borderline personality disorder? A critical review. *Int J Eating Disord* 1989; 1–4.
10. Yates WR, Sieleni B, Reich J, Brass C. Comorbidity of bulimia nervosa and eating disorders. *J Clin Psychiatry* 1989; 57–59.

11. Gartner AF, Marcus RN, Halmi K, Loranger AW. DSM III R personality disorders in patients with eating disorders. *Am J Psychiatry* 1989; 1585–1596.
12. Hall RCW, Tice L, Beresford TP, et al. Sexual abuse in patients with anorexia nervosa and bulimia. *Psychosomatics* 1989; 73–79.
13. Oppenheimer R, Howell K, Palmer RL. Adverse sexual experiences in childhood and clinical eating disorders. A preliminary description. *J Psychiatric Research* 1988; 357–361.
14. Fairburn CG. A cognitive behavioral approach to the management of bulimia. *Psychological Medicine* 1981; 707–711.
15. Garner DM, Bemis KM. A cognitive-behavioral approach to anorexia nervosa. *Cognitive Therapy and Research* 1982; 123–150.
16. Newman MM, Halmi, Marchi P. Relationship of clinical factors to caloric requirements in subtypes of eating disorders. *Biol Psychiatry* 1987; 1253–1263.
17. Pope HG, Hudson JI, Jonas JM, et al. Bulimia treated with imipramine: A placebo controlled double blind study. *Am J Psychiatry* 1983; 554–558.
18. Walsh BT, Stewart JW, Roose SP, et al. Treatment of bulimia with phenelzine. *Arch Gen Psychiatry* 1984; 1105–1109.
19. Hughes PC, Wells LA, et al. Treating bulimia with desipramine: A placebo controlled study. *Arch Gen Psychiatry* 1986; 182–186.
20. Weltzin T, Kaye WH, Hsu LKG, Sebkiewicz T. Fluoxetine improves outcome in anorexia nervosa. NR 497. New Research Program and Abstracts. American Psychiatric Association, 1990.

17
The Treatment of Obesity

PHILLIP M. SINAIKIN

In a 1983 article Susan C. Wooley asked the challenging question, "Should obesity be treated at all?"[1] The source of her question was the growing recognition that all treatments for obesity were generally ineffective over the long run and that biological, not behavioral forces were primarily responsible for body weight regulation. She felt that millions of people with mild to moderate obesity were needlessly suffering through depriving dieting experiences with little or no long-term benefit to health and well being. In fact, the dieting experience was probably doing more harm than good through its negative impact on self-esteem, body image, and self-worth. Physicians and other health professionals were cited as contributing to, not alleviating the problem, by feeding the national obsession for thinness.

At about the same time, the set point theory of body weight regulation was gaining popularity as a comprehensive explanation for the overall biological forces that resist successful long-term weight loss.[2] Also emerging was very strong and compelling evidence for the role of genetic factors in body weight regulation.[3,4] A vocal minority of health professionals were clearly calling for a reexamination of the scientific community's generally supportive stance toward the national obsession for weight loss.

On the other side of the issue, however, was the ongoing concern about the relationship of body weight to health. Evidence continued to mount for both the general and specific health risks of excess body weight. While a few dissenting voices questioned the interpretation of data from large studies such as the Framingham study,[5,6] the consensus remained that excess body weight is an independent or contributing risk factor in a number of serious health problems.[7,8] In light of this, the effort to lose excess body weight was felt to be a worthwhile medical goal.

The informed professional was and still is caught in the dynamic tension between these concerns about the health risks of obesity and the apparent futility of efforts for long-term weight loss. Adding to the pressure in deciding how best to treat overweight patients are tremendous marketing forces that feed a 30 billion dollar a year dieting industry. This business is heavily invested in promoting strong expectations that thinness leads to happiness.[9] The American public has literally been brainwashed into unquestionably accepting the psychological value of weight loss. The vast majority of dieters report that their motivation to lose weight is aesthetic and emotional, not medical.

The point is that the previously mentioned conflict, though felt by the informed professional, is probably doomed to have little impact on the determined dieter. If the health professional tries to convince a mild to moderately obese individual that attempts to lose weight and keep it off will probably fail, chances are that the person will graciously thank the professional for the advice and then march down the street to the nearest weight loss center to enroll. Weight loss is and will remain a passionate goal for millions of people. What the health professional must do then is learn how best to help those who are determined to lose weight for aesthetic reasons as well as those who should lose weight for health reasons. To that end, this chapter examines what we do know about weight control and what does and what does not work. The most popular weight control programs are evaluated in terms of how they meet the current scientific criteria for rational weight loss. And finally, future directions and ideas are explored.

Defining Obesity

In order to assess the health risks presented by excess weight it is necessary to define the term obesity. This is not as clear-cut as might be expected. The terms overweight and obese have often been used interchangeably and imprecisely. The most common definition derives from the Metropolitan Life Insurance Company Table of Ideal Body Weights. This table defines a range of weight in relation to height, frame size, and sex as being ideal. Ten to 20 percent above the midpoint ideal weight is considered overweight. Greater than 20 percent above the ideal is termed obese. Twenty to 40 percent over is mild obesity, 40 to 100 percent over ideal is called moderate obesity while greater than 100 percent over is termed morbid obesity. Morbid obesity is often also defined as 100 or more pounds above ideal body weight.[10]

This most common method of assessing weight suffers from a number of problems. There are now two tables, the first from 1959 and the second from 1983. The second table allows for higher weights but both tables are still commonly used. There is also significant controversy about the validity of defining ideal weights from actuarial life insurance data.[11] Finally, and most importantly, it is now widely accepted that body weight in relation to height is the least precise method of assessing health risks because health risks are not associated with body weight but the percentage and distribution of body weight that is made up of fat.[12]

A more precise measure is the Body Mass Index (BMI). The BMI is calculated by dividing weight in kilograms by height in meters squared. The resulting number is more closely reflective of body fat percentage and a normogram can then be used to assess general health risks.[12] Overweight is defined as a BMI between 25 and 30 and obese as a BMI greater than 30.

A more recent finding is that health risk is closely associated with the ratio of waist to hip measurement. This reflects the understanding that the android distribution of body fat (central or male pattern obesity) represents a much higher risk for heart disease, hypertension, stroke, and diabetes than gynoid (lower body or female) obesity. The Waist Hip Ratio (WHR) then becomes an easily calculated assessment of relative risk, with a ratio of greater than 1 in the male and greater than 0.8 in the female being associated with higher risk.[13]

More sophisticated methods to measure percentage of body fat exist but these are often cumbersome, expensive, or imprecise.[12] That, of course, has not stopped enterprising entrepreneurs from promoting procedures such as electrical impedance as more precise guidelines for measuring body fat . . . for a fee. For the health professional, utilizing the BMI and WHR should offer sufficient data to made a reasonably intelligent assessment of body weight loss needs. Of course, individual data derived from lab testing and medical history should also be considered in setting weight loss goals.

Weight Loss

It is generally recognized that rational weight loss and long-term weight control involve three chief components: diet, exercise, and behavior modification.

The Diet

The principles of thermodynamics still define the basic weight loss equation. In essence, change in body weight is determined by the equation: Energy ingested minus energy expended equals change in body weight. Dieting concerns the energy ingested side of the equation. The goal in dieting is to reduce the amount of energy ingested relative to energy expended so weight can be lost. This can be accomplished by fasting (zero calories ingested), very low-calorie diets (up to 800 calories a day), or low-calorie diets (more than 800 calories a day).

Fasting

Treating obesity with a program of little or no caloric intake has been attempted in the past. While it certainly was an effective way to reduce weight, the medical complications were numerous and often severe. This method of weight control has all but disappeared except for research purposes.[14]

The most troublesome problem with fasting is the negative nitrogen balance created through the excessive loss of lean body tissue. Recognition of this problem lead to the development of the Protein Sparing Modified Fast (PSMF), in which high quality protein, usually in the from of fish or chicken, was added to the diet to "spare" the body the need to ingest its own protein for necessary internal chemical processes.[15] In this form, the diet remained essentially in the province of medical centers and was used for the treatment of a few severely obese patients, until the marketing machinery seized upon the idea of modified fasting and the liquid diet boom was born.

Very Low-Calorie Diets (VLCD)

In the 1970s the eager and characteristically desperate dieting public was introduced to this radical form of weight loss in the aptly titled book *The Last Chance Diet*. This book advocated the use of the Pro-Lin formula, a hydrolyzed collagen protein source liquid diet available over the counter in drugstores and supermarkets, to promote rapid weight loss. It rapidly gained wide popularity, until people started to die.

Deaths related to the use of this liquid diet began to be reported to the FDA soon after its introduction. Investigations of 58 reported deaths lead to the conclusion that 17 deaths were attributable solely to the use of the diet, although are exact etiology was not clear.[16] During the heyday of the Pro-Lin diet the Cambridge diet, another liquid protein diet, gained even greater popularity. After a few highly publicized deaths associated with its use the VLCD business took a significant downturn, until Oprah Winfrey nearly single-handedly revitalized the industry.

In November of 1988 the highly popular obese talk show hostess Oprah Winfrey had a big surprise for her millions of fans. Lugging a wagon filled with 67 pounds of beef fat behind her, Oprah proudly informed an admiring public that she had indeed lost 67 pounds and reached her dream of a size 10 body. Vowing never to be fat again, Oprah let the country in on the secret of her success, Optifast, a very low calorie liquid diet.

Following the Pro-Lin disaster, researchers had begun to investigate the problem with the liquid diet formula and found that the quality and bioavailability of the protein (the early formulas had used proteins derived from collagen and other connective tissues) was crucial, as was careful monitoring and replacement of electrolytes and minerals. New formulations using protein from egg whites and milk were developed to be utilized in hospital-based, medically supervised programs. Clinical data proved this type of supplemented fasting to be both safe and effective. This "new and improved" liquid fasting industry of the 1980s moved slowly forward until Oprah helped catapult it to a 5 billion dollar a year industry.[17]

The liquid diet fad is supported primarily by three products: Optifast, HMR, and Medifast. The first two are available only in hospital-based programs while Medifast is prescribed by private practitioners. All three programs, when done properly, involve close medical monitoring throughout the weight loss phase. All three also advocate untritional education, an exercise program, and behavior modification. There have been no reported deaths associated with these high quality protein, balanced nutrition liquid diets.[18]

The VLCD is an effective diet with reported average weight losses of 4.5 pounds per week in men and 3.1 pounds per week in women.[19] There are a number of reported side effects and complications. The less serious ones include headache, hypotension, nausea, vomiting, diarrhea, constipation, fatigue, cold intolerance, and hair loss. More severe complications include gall bladder disease, kidney stones, and gout.[20]

VLCDs are recommended for people who are at least 30 percent overweight and have been most thoroughly studied in people at least 50 percent overweight. The diet should be administered by a professional experienced in its use.[21] Both of these safety standards are routinely violated because, once again, obesity is big business. There have been reports of weight loss programs offering VLCDs to people as little as 15 percent overweight,[22] and since liquid diets are widely marketed to all physicians as a good way to supplement their income, many inexperienced physicians have begun their own part-time office based liquid diet practices.[21]

A final concern about VLCDs has to do with long-term results. All of America has witnessed the tragic picture of Oprah Winfrey, the former champion of the liquid fast, slowly at first and then rapidly regain all of her lost weight within two years. Sadly to say, this is the likely outcome for most dieters on supplemented fasts.[21] In this regard, very low-calorie diets differ little from the longer lived, better known low calorie diets.

Low-Calorie Diets

The backbone of the dieting industry has always been the low-calorie diet. Ranging from 800 to 1800 calories, these planned menus of daily intake have come out in literally thousands of forms over the years but actually fall into only a few distinct categories.

Balanced Nutrient Diets

This is the type of diet most familiar to physicians in which all three basic nutrients—carbohydrates, protein, and fat—are incorporated. The American Diabetic Association concept of the exchange diet is the most widely used, balanced nutrient diet. Caloric intake can be tailored to the needs of the individual by adjusting the number of exchanges per day. The advantage of this type of diet is that it most closely mimics real world eating and can help the dieter begin to learn new eating habits and skills to help maintain the weight loss after the diet. There is also minimal health risk in a balanced nutrient diet. The chief disadvantage of this form of diet is its complexity (it is often difficult to figure out the exchange allowances for many foods), and the variety of foods in the diet, which can present too many choices to the dieter and diminish compliance.[22]

Unbalanced Nutrient Diets

A very popular technique in generating new diet rages has been to reduce or eliminate one class of nutrients in favor of another. All possible combinations have been popular at one time or another. The high protein-low carbohydrate diet in particular had a long and profitable life in American culture.

It's not surprising that the high protein diet was popular; weight losses early in the diet are particularly dramatic. When carbohydrate is reduced or eliminated from the diet a profound diuresis occurs that results in many pounds being lost.[23] This is the way people are able to lose 10 or more pounds the first week on a diet. Physiologically it is impossible to lose 10 or more pounds of fat in a week. This would require creating a calorie deficit of 35,000 calories (one pound of fat is equivalent to 3500 calories of stored energy). Even with an extremely high daily caloric maintenance need of 3000 calories, which in itself would be quite unusual, total starvation would create a weekly deficit of only 21,000 calories, far short of the deficit needed to lose 10 pounds. In addition, this diuresis is only temporary. As soon as carbohydrate is reintroduced to the daily food intake, the pre-diet water equilibrium is rapidly restored, and the hapless dieter faces a totally demoralizing weight gain of all of the water pounds lost in the first week or two of the diet.

The allure of protein has also been reinforced by the widely held false assumption that carbohydrates are "fattening." For years dieters have made the fundamental mistake of forgoing the bun for the hamburger, when just the opposite would be the more rational decision.

Current scientific thinking is that carbohydrates are the cornerstone of healthy lifetime weight control, especially the so-called complex carbohydrates. Carbohydrates are polymers of glucose molecules. The complex carbohydrates are long chain polymers frequently complexed with nondigestible fibers and other nutrients. Their digestion, absorption, and breakdown into essential nutrients is slow. This lends a healthy sense of satiety to the ingestion of these foods and leads to a slow, steady rise in plasma insulin, helping to maintain a steady state rather than a widely fluctuating plasma glucose level.

Fruits, vegetables, and whole grains are among the class of foods called complex carbohydrates. These foods should be an intergral part of any weight loss diet and lifetime eating plan as well. There is no justification for eliminating or reducing these foods in favor of protein in a weight reduction plan.

Another supposed advantage of a high protein diet was the alleged "specific dynamic action" of proteins. The theory was that it took more calories to digest protein so the caloric "cost" of eating protein was less, almost a free food. These theoreticians had the right idea, but the wrong food. This digestive cost issue is relevant to another class of food, the one getting the most attention in terms of both weight control and health—fat.

Recent research has supported a new conceptualization of fat as being more efficiently absorbed during digestion and more readily stored as body fat. The theory is that while up to 25 percent of the caloric content of carbohydrate or protein foods is used up in the digestion and fuel storage process, only 3 percent of the calories in fat is needed for digestion, leaving up to 97 percent available for storage.[24] Of course the amount of fat stored is also dependent on the energy needs of the body and whether the current caloric intake exceeds demand. Exceeding the energy requirements of the body is also more likely with fat due to the fact that fat has twice the caloric density of protein or carbohydrates.

Protein and carbohydrates (including sugar) are each 4.5 calories per gram while fat is 9 calories per gram. So each bite of fat is at least twice as "fattening" as protein or carbohydrates without even factoring in the differences in efficiency of digestion. Add to this the well-known negative impact on health of a high fat diet and it is clear that the chief culprit in weight control and health is dietary fat.

Fortunately the dieting industry is finally catching onto this reality and "low fat" is the newest marketing buzzword. This is really only a recent phenomenon. Even the so-called frozen dietary dinners that have been so popular for years used to contain a high percentage of their calories from fat. Recently, however, in response to public demand, these and many other foods have lowered their fat content to keep in line with the well-known American Heart Association requirement of less than 30 percent of daily caloric intake from fat. This is a very healthy trend and the informed professional should always prescribe a low fat diet for weight loss and lifetime health.

Fad Diets

Fortunately, this topic requires a lot less attention than in the past. There was a time, not too long ago, when each year saw the emergence of a new batch of fad diets in the local book store. The cornerstone of the fad diet industry was some magical combination or elimination of certain foods that would result in rapid, painless weight loss. Sometimes the recommended diet was simply ludicrous, at other times there was a modicum of truth, often a recent scientific discovery taken out of context, to justify the recommendations. The goal was always the same, to sell a lot of diet books, and sell they did. It was not unusual to find that the majority of best-selling nonfiction books for the year were diet books. Each program would garner its share of die-hard fans, only to fade into relative obscurity within a year or two.

The current diet business does not seem to involve fad diets or best-selling diet books. Programs and products are the new mainstays of the diet business. These are explored more fully below. However, the diet business is fickle and the fad diet might someday reemerge. The informed clinician therefore should have some idea how fad diets work to be prepared to answer questions and concerns from clients and patients.

The efficacy of fad diets derives from two primary factors: novelty and monotony. The novelty factor can be very powerful, especially for the typical cyclic dieter, always searching for a magic solution that will work once and for all. A novel diet then evokes an initial enthusiasm that enhances compliance. Since most fad diets are low calorie, adherence to the diet will lead, of course, to weight loss. And since many fad diets are imbalanced, often low carbohydrate, the initial weight loss is often rapid and dramatic, reinforcing the dieter's faith that this is indeed a magic weight loss plan.

The second success factor often seen in fad diets is monotony. Fad diets frequently recommend the overconsumption of a single food or class of foods and the total elimination of other foods. Early in the diet this monotony can enhance compliance by eliminating food choices and thus temptation to "cheat." This same monotony, however, can lead to significant difficulties following the diet for an appreciable length of time. An unnatural diet does little to teach the dieter about nutrition or the long-term changes in eating behaviors that will be needed to maintain the weight loss.

There is a promising trend in our society away from fad dieting and towards low-fat, balanced nutrition. As long as this lasts the clinician will probably not be confronted by questions about outlandish diets. That will free up time to concentrate on a much more important concern in long-term weight control, exercise.

Exercise and Obesity

The previously discussed thermodynamic equation tells us that energy ingestion is not the only variable involved in body weight regulation; equally important is energy expenditure. In human beings energy expenditure has three components: resting metabolic rate (RMR), physical activity, and thermogenesis (increase in energy expenditure following a meal or other sympathetic stimulation such as caffeine or cold weather).

A lot of research has been done to answer the question of whether a diminished RMR is the primary etiology of obesity. The findings are surprising to say the least. Although not without some controversy, the general consensus is that the RMR is generally increased in obese versus lean individuals.[25] Why this is so is not that mysterious. RMR tends to be related to the absolute level of lean body tissue, which is much more metabolically active than fat tissue. While obese people have a greater absolute amount and percentage of body fat, they also tend to have a greater absolute amount of lean body tissue when compared to lean individuals.

The energy cost of physical activity also tends to be greater in the obese since they are moving around a larger mass. However, obese individuals tend to be less physically active and burn off fewer calories in volitional physical activity.[26]

A final consideration in energy expenditure in weight loss is the well-demonstrated impact of caloric restriction on metabolic rate. During a diet, the reduction in caloric intake is accompanied by a drop in metabolic rate as the body responds physiologically to what it interprets as a famine.

Turning back to the thermodynamic equation, it is clear that on the energy expenditure side of the ledger, it is imperative to compensate for the dietary induced drop in metabolic rate and to also increase physical activity to obtain optimal results. This can be accomplished through a program of regular physical exercise.

Aerobic Exercise

There are two types of exercise, aerobic and anaerobic. Aerobic exercise utilizes oxygen and is the type of sustained exercise associated with cardiovascular fitness and improved health. This is the type of exercise most frequently recommended to aid in weight loss and lifetime weight control. Anaerobic exercise is resistance training and oxygen is not utilized to fuel this activity. Anaerobic exercise is used to strengthen and enlarge muscle tissue and was not generally recommended as an adjunct to weight loss. Recent evidence, however, suggests that anaerobic exercise may indeed be an important part of a successful weight control program.

Since metabolic rate is increased by increasing the amount of metabolically active muscle tissue, the first question to be answered is whether aerobic exercise increases muscle mass. Common sense would seem to dictate that a program of regular aerobic exercise should improve the lean-to-fat ratio. Research on this topic, however, is far from conclusive. Most studies demonstrate mixed results or only modest improvements in muscle mass except at very high levels of exertion on a daily basis.[27]

Another supposed advantage of aerobic exercise is the notion that a session of exercise can raise the metabolic rate for hours. Early research suggested that this positive effect could last as long as 48 hours.[28] Careful recent research, however, has shown that this effect is extremely modest at best and that the extra amount of calories expended is trivial compared to the overall energy deficit needed for weight loss.[29]

Does aerobic exercise have any place then in the treatment of obesity? The answer is still a definite yes. First, aerobic exercise directly burns calories. It is perfectly reasonable to suggest that nearly anyone can work their way up to an eventual goal of directly burning 1500 to 2000 calories a week in an aerobic exercise program. This obviously speeds weight loss but, even more importantly, builds in a safety margin during weight loss maintenance that will allow for the occasional indulgences that inevitably follow a diet. Also, the health benefits of aerobic exercise are well documented. Regular physical exercise clearly reduces morbidity and mortality from cardiovascular related diseases.[30] Finally, exercise has proven psychological benefits. A program of regular aerobic exercise enhances self-image and raises self-esteem. It is associated with improved job performance and an increased daily energy level. In this sense, exercise is clearly not only for obese or postobese individuals, but for everyone.

Anaerobic Exercise

Turning back to the question of anaerobic exercise and its place in the treatment of obesity, recent research suggests that resistance training is an important exercise activity for weight loss and even more so for weight loss maintenance. The reason anaerobic exercise was not traditionally included in weight loss programs was the low direct energy cost of this type of activity. Lifting weights, for example, does not typically raise the pulse above 60 percent of maximum, the lowest rate that is recommended in aerobic exercise programs. In one study, obese women lifting weights for 42 minutes burned an average of only 132 calories.[31] This rate of caloric expenditure would hardly allow these women to reach a goal of burning 1500 to 2000 calories per week. But if a program of modest weight training is added to an aerobic training program, the gain in muscle mass would help elevate the overall RMR, thus augmenting the weight loss and helping to insure a successful program of weight loss maintenance.

Behavior Therapy

The final component of a rational weight control program is behavior therapy. Exactly what form that therapy should take, however, is not fully clear because there is still a lot of controversy about the exact nature of the behaviors that cause a person to gain weight, resist weight loss, or regain lost weight.

A common sense notion that guided early behavioral thinking about obesity was that there must be a set of eating and activity behaviors that distinguish obese from lean individuals. The obvious goal was to identify these behaviors and then, through behavior therapy, reshape the obese person's behavior into the behavior of a lean person.

Among the early behavioral theories were the concepts that: 1) obese people are more sensitive to food cues and overeat in response to them; 2) there is a particular eating style that leads to obesity; and 3) obesity is basically the result of learned maladaptive behavior, not biological forces.

In response to these ideas, elaborate behavioral programs were developed to be used alone or combined with a dietary program. The concept that the obese are more sensitive to food cues led to recommendations for stimulus control such as keeping all forbidden foods out of sight, avoiding dangerous situations such as buffets, and limiting all eating activities to one designated eating spot in the home. The notion of a distinct obese eating style (basically "wolfing" down food in large rapid bites) led to recommendations to chew slowly, put the fork down between bites, chew each mouthful a specified number of times, and to cut up food into small bite-size pieces. Finally, the concept that obesity is the result of early learned behavior led to a great number of recommendations to recondition new behaviors in place of the learned maladaptive behaviors. For example, the obese individual was instructed to develop new rewards to substitute for maladaptively learning to use food as a reward as a child.[32]

There was an initial enthusiasm for the behavioral approach to obesity, sparked by reports of remarkable success rates. When long-term follow-up data became available, however, the initial enthusiasm began to wane. Follow-up studies showed a nearly invariant pattern of weight regain in patients treated with behavior therapy.[33] In part this was due to the typical pattern of failure in compliance so common to all of medicine. But the failure of behavioral treatment was also due to the fact that the foundational theories were flawed.

Empirical investigation has demonstrated that the behavioral variables distinguishing obese from lean individuals are not nearly as clear-cut as originally thought. Careful studies have shown that obese people do not as a rule eat more than thin people; they do not characteristically wolf down their food nor are they more responsive to food cues or the enticing properties of tasty foods.[34]

This is not to say that behavioral therapy no longer has a place in the treatment of obesity. After all, obesity is at least, in part, a reflection of past behavior and losing weight and keeping it off definitely requires long-term changes in behavior. The question that needs to be asked is not what behaviors need to be changed in all obese people, but what particular behaviors need to be changed in the particular person in treatment. In other words, an individual behavioral analysis needs to be done and a specific program designed for each individual. Often, the best first step is a food diary.

It is important for the obese individual to gain an awareness of the thoughts, feelings, and stimuli that precede and accompany eating, especially the inappropriate and often mindless type of eating that causes weight gain. With the help of the food diary, the patient and therapist can begin to identify the behavioral patterns that are causing problems. Then the behavior can be modified through behavioral techniques or alternately, the antecedent thoughts and feelings that lead to self-destructive eating can become the focus of therapy.

Psychotherapy in general and cognitive therapy in particular are becoming important weapons in the fight against obesity. The particular value of cognitive therapy is its effectiveness in helping to reverse the cognitive distortions that come from being obese. One of the most important growths in understanding the plight of the obese individual has been the recognition that obesity, while not characteristically caused by psychological conflict, more often than not results in significant psychological distress.

Being obese in a society that so highly values thinness can and often does do significant damage to the sense of self-worth of the obese individual. This damage often manifests itself as frequent, desperate attempts to diet and lose the hated fat. If the diet fails to produce the desired results, the self-esteem sinks even lower. This is hardly the state of mind that supports long-term and often difficult positive changes in behavior. That is why it is so crucial to support changes in the sense of self-worth and personal effectiveness at the same time that the weight problem is being treated. Cognitive therapy is particularly well suited to help the obese patient identify and then modify irrational beliefs about the self and the world that come about through the experience of being obese in modern society.

Another approach to the behavioral treatment of obesity borrows from the field of addiction treatment. Here, minor deviations from dietary guidelines are conceptualized as a "slip." Falling back into a pattern of overeating and then gaining back lost weight is called a relapse. The goal in this form of therapy is to help the patient identify high risk situations and anticipate that there may be a problem with dietary adherence. Forewarned, the patient can then prevent a slip from turning into a full-blown relapse.[35]

The application of an addiction model to weight control is relatively new. While Overeaters Anonymous, a lay organization, has directly translated the 12-step model into terminology applicable to overeating, a more rigorous and refined model of the relationship of addictive behavior to obesity has yet to emerge. It is this author's opinion that this model, when developed, will be of significant value to a weight control program because I believe that the addict and the obese person face a nearly identical challenge. They both need to make long-term changes in behavior and attitude that will be supported by a radically different reward system. Clearly, a lot that has been learned in the treatment of addiction can be applied to the treatment of obesity. But I do not believe that this can be the direct translation that has been attempted by Overeaters Anonymous. The psychological damage from drug addiction is spiritual and requires a 12 step spiritual program to repair but the damage from obesity is to the self-esteem and requires an addiction-model program geared toward enhancing self-esteem.

A multifactorial, multidetermined, and highly prevalent problem such as obesity will obviously not yield to a single explanatory model. The informed therapist should be familiar with a number of behavioral and psychological strategies that can be geared to the needs of the individual. A final area that the therapist should be familiar with is what the popular weight loss programs offer in terms of their recommendations for diet, exercise, and behavior therapy.

Weight Loss Programs and Products

As mentioned before, the fad diet craze has now yielded to the commercial weight loss programs and products. It behooves the health professional to gain an understanding of what these programs and products offer because the vast majority of people seeking help to lose weight turn to them. The currently popular programs and products fit into a few basic categories: 1) medically supervised liquid diets; 2) over-the-counter liquid diet products; 3) prepackaged meal programs; and 4) exchange diet programs.

Medically Supervised Liquid Diets

The medically supervised liquid diets include Optifast, Medifast, HMR, and United Weight Control. These programs are generally comprehensive and include nutritional counseling, recommendations for exercise, and behavior therapy. For example, the Medifast Patient's guide is a 210 page spiral bound workbook that covers topics ranging from food shopping guides to cognitive therapy for self-esteem. There is a chapter on exercise that recommends five 30 to 60 minute aerobic exercise sessions per week. Optifast, HMR, and United Weight Control also offer comprehensive weight loss and weight loss maintenance programs.

The primary problems with medically supervised liquid fast programs are cost and compliance. Requiring active physician participation, these programs tend to be costly, often running into the thousands of dollars. The compliance problem starts right from the beginning. Giving up all solid food is simply too difficult for a substantial portion of the dieters and they drop out. For those who complete the programs, willingness to continue to attend the recommended one year of follow-up counseling and/or group sessions is often low. In summary, medically supervised liquid fasting programs are well-designed, comprehensive programs that are indicated for people with substantial amounts of weight to lose and who can tolerate completely giving up solid food. If they participate in and comply with follow-up programs all of the elements necessary for weight loss maintenance will be made available to them.

Over-the-Counter Liquid Diets

The over-the-counter liquid diet products are often mistakenly confused with medically supervised liquid diets but they are, in fact, quite different. Medically supervised liquid diets are very low-calorie diets, 450 to 800 calories a day. The over-the-counter liquid diets (such as Ultra Slim Fast, Dyna Trim, and Dick Gregory's Bahamian Diet) are liquid meal replacement low-calorie diets of at least 1000 calories per day. The diet products are balanced nutrition, vitamin, and mineral supplemented powders that are mixed with milk, fruit juices, or water. They generally supply around 200 calories per drink. Two or three drinks per day are recommended along with low-calorie meals and snacks.

The theory behind these products is simplification. Two meals a day are drinks, simple to prepare and monotonous enough to help curb the appetite. Food choices are then made at only one meal a day. The novelty fractor is also at work here, helping the dieter maintain compliance.

A major disadvantage with these products is that the only help the dieter receives aside from the product is a package insert that recommends appropriate food choices, exercise, and behavior changes. There is little detail and, of course, no face-to-face evaluation or treatment by a professional. A major advantage is cost. Unlike the medically supervised liquid diets, costs for these programs is only the price of the product, which is usually less expensive than the meals being replaced.

The medical risks of these liquid diets should be no different than any other balanced low-calorie diet. The consumer is cautioned not to use the drinks as the sole source of nutrition and not to consume less than 1000 calories per day.

Prepackaged Meal Programs

Another type of meal replacement concept are the prepackaged meal programs represented by the well-known Nutri System and Jenny Craig weight loss programs. In these programs the dieter purchases all the foods they will eat from the program itself. The meals are nutritionally balanced with the calorie total geared to the needs of the individual. The dieter is exposed therefore to a wide range of real foods without needing to make choices. Other services include counseling, group education, and therapy as well as recommendations for exercise. A criticism of these programs involves concerns about the qualifications of the counselors and nutritionists.

Exchange Diet Programs

The final type of program is also the oldest, the exchange diet program. The best known commercial representative of this type of program is Weight Watchers. Another is the Richard Simmons Deal A Meal program. Health professionals are generally familiar with the exchange concept. Dieters choose their own foods with the help of exchange lists, but initially in Weight Watchers, certain foods are forbidden (although the degree of freedom to choose seems to change each year to serve marketing needs). Weight Watchers' main claim to fame, however, is the group support they offer. Groups are often lead by former successful dieters so the level of expertise can be questionable. But Weight Watchers does keep up with the times and recommendations for exercise and behavior therapy are now integral parts of the program.

In all, today's commercial diet products and programs are reasonable. Each offers certain advantages that might make it better for a specific individual. None are specifically geared toward weight loss maintenance since weight loss is the product that sells. The health professional needs to recognize this and perhaps lend expertise in the areas of compliance, motivation, and long-term behavior change as an addition to what these programs have to offer.

Conclusion

This chapter opened with the question of whether obesity should be treated at all. We have seen that whether or not it *should* be treated, it most decidedly *will* be treated by a 30 billion dollar a year industry. We have also seen that scientific knowledge about weight control continues to grow and, fortunately, seems to be filtering down to the commercial weight control businesses. We are hopefully witnessing the demise of the outlandish and sometimes dangerous fad diet. What has not as yet changed, and perhaps never will, are the unrealistic expectations that anyone can be thin and that being thin will automatically improve the quality of life.

The most important role of the health professional in weight control could be to help modulate these unrealistic expectations. We need to continue to carry to the dieting public the message that while weight loss is generally a healthy goal, it must not become an all-consuming obsession and that the quality of life and overall health can be improved in many other ways that do not require a scale for verification.

References

1. Wooley SC, Wooley OW. Should obesity be treated at all? *Psychiatric Annals* 1983; 13:11–18.
2. Bennett W, Gurin J. The Dieter's Dilemma. New York, Basic Books, 1982.
3. Stunkard AJ, Sorensen TIA, Harris C, et al. Adoption study of human obesity. *N Engl J Med* 1986; 314:193–198.
4. Price RA, Cadoret RJ, Stunkard AJ, et al. Genetic contributions to human fatness: An adoption study. *Am J Psychiatry* 1987; 144:1003–1008.
5. Knapp TR. A methodological critique of the ideal weight concept. *JAMA* 1983; 250:506–510.
6. Sorlie P, Gordon T, Kannel WB. Body build and mortality: The Framingham study. *JAMA* 1980; 243:1828–1831.
7. Van Itallie TB. Health implications of overweight and obesity in the United States. *Ann Intern Med* 1985; 103:983–988.
8. Bray GA. Complications of obesity. *Ann Intern Med* 1985; 103:1052–1062.
9. Hall A, Stewart R. Obesity: Time for sanity and humanity. *New Zealand Med J* 1989; 102:134–136.
10. Lerman RH, Cave DR. Medical and surgical management of obesity. *Adv Intern Med* 1989; 34:127–164.
11. Seltzer CC. Limitations to height-weight standards. *N Engl J Med* 1965; 272:1132.
12. Bray GA. Classification and evaluation of the obesities. *Med Clinics NA* 1989; 73:161–185.
13. Bjorntrop P. Regional patterns of fat distribution. *Ann Intern Med* 1985; 103:994–995.
14. Bray GA. Obesity: Basic Considerations and Clinical Approaches. Chicago, Yearbook Medical Publishers, 1989.
15. Linder PG, Blackburn GL. Multidisciplinary approach to obesity utilizing fasting modified by protein sparing therapy. *Obesity Bariatric Med* 1976; 5:198–216.
16. Sours HE, Frattali VP, Brand CD, et al. Sudden death associated with very low calorie weight reduction regimens. *Am J Clin Nutrition* 1981; 34:453–461.
17. Stoffel J. "What's new in weight control"? NY Times, Nov 2, 1989.
18. Howard AN. The historical development of very low calorie diets. *Int J Obesity*. 1989; 13(Suppl 2):1–9.
19. Kirshner MA, Schneider G, Ertel NH, et al. An eight-year experience with a very low calorie formula diet for the control of major obesity. *Int J Obesity* 1988; 12:69–80.

20. Atkinson RL. Low and very low calorie diets. *Med Clinics NA* 1989; 73:203–215.
21. Wadden TA, Van Italie TB, Blackburn GL. Responsible and irresponsible use of very low calorie diets in the treatment of obesity. *JAMA* 1990; 263:83–85.
22. Pope T, Watkins T. Opting to take it off fast is one thing. . . . *Med Tribune* 1989; 1:9–10.
23. DeHaven I, Sherwin R, Hendler R, et al. Nitrogen and sodium balance and sympathetic nervous system activity in obese subjects treated with low-calorie protein or mixed diet. *N Engl J Med* 1982; 302:477–482.
24. Jecquier E, Acheson K, Schutz Y. Assessment of energy expenditure and fuel utilization in man. *Ann Rev Nutr* 1987; 7:187–208.
25. James WPT, Bailes K, Davies HL, et al. Elevated metabolic rates in obesity. *Lancet* 1978; 1:1122–1125.
26. Thompson JK, Jarvie GJ, Lahey BB. Exercise and obesity: Etiology, physiology and intervention. *Psych Bull* 1982; 91:55–79
27. Wilmore JH. Body composition in sports and exercise: Directions for future research. *Med Sci Sports Exercise* 1983; 15:21–31.
28. deVries HA, Gray DE. After-effects of exercise on resting metabolic rate. *Res Quarterly* 1963; 34:314–321.
29. Segal KR, Gutin B, Albu J, et al. Thermic effects of food and exercise in lean and obese men of similar lean body weight. *Am J Physiol* 1987; 252:E110–E117.
30. Paffenbarger RS, Hyde RT, Wing AL, et al. A natural history of athleticism and cardiovascular health. *JAMA* 1984; 252:491–495.
31. Ballor DL, Katch VL, Becque MD, et al. Resistance weight training during caloric restriction enhances lean body weight maintenance. *Am J Clin Nutrition* 1988; 47:19–25.
32. Wooley SC, Wooley OW, Dyenforth SR. Theoretical, practical and social issues in the behavioral treatment of obesity. *J Applied Behavior Analysis* 1979; 12:3–25.
33. Kramer FM, Jeffery RW, Forster JL, et al. Long term follow-up of behavioral treatment for obesity: Patterns of weight ragain among men and women. *Int J Obesity* 1989; 13:123–136.
34. Rodin J, Shank D, Streigel-Moore R. Psychological features of obesity. *Med Clin NA* 1989; 73:47–65.
35. Schlundt DG, Sorocco T, Bell C. Identification of high-risk situations in a behavioral weight loss program: Application of the relapse prevention model. *Int J Obesity* 1989; 13:223–234.

18
Eating Disorders and Drug and Alcohol Dependency

NORMAN S. MILLER

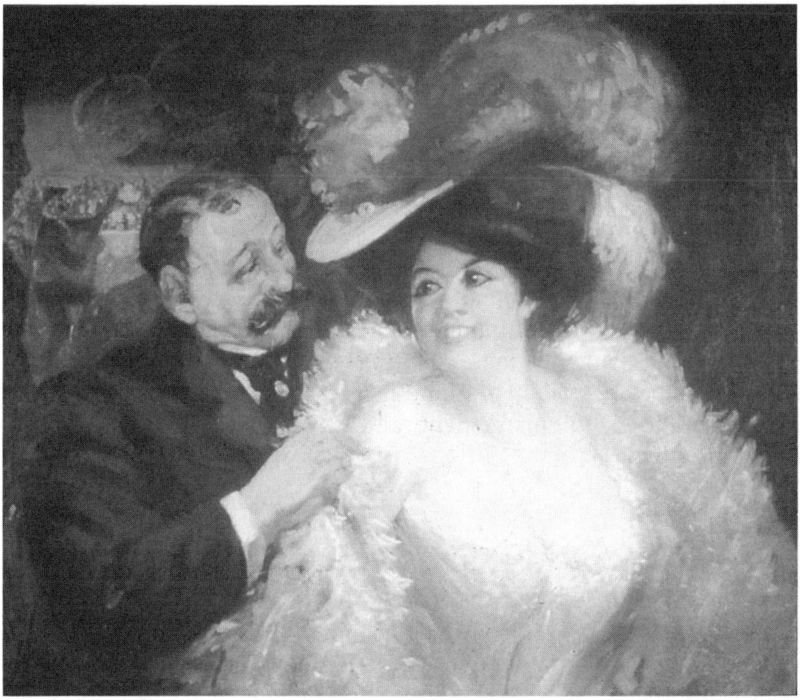

Luks, George—*Cafe Francis*—(Butler Institute of American Art, Youngstown, Ohio)

Definitions and General Characteristics of the Disorders

Anorexia Nervosa and Bulimia Nervosa

The essential features of anorexia nervosa according to DSM-III-R criteria are a refusal to maintain body weight over a minimal normal weight for age and height; intense fear of gaining weight or becoming fat, even though underweight; a distorted body image; and amenorrhea (in females).[1]

Age of onset of anorexia nervosa is usually early to late adolescence, occurs predominately in females (95%), and may have an unremitting, episodic course, or consist of a single episode. The disorder is more common among female family members of those with the disorder than among the general population. The mortality rates in follow-up studies range from 5 to 18 percent.[1,2]

The essential features of bulimia nervosa according to DSM-III-R criteria are recurrent episodes of binge eating (rapid consumption of a large amount of food in a discrete period of time); a feeling of lack of control over eating behavior during the eating binges; self-induced vomiting, use of laxatives or diuretics, strict dieting or fasting, or vigorous exercise in order to prevent weight gain; and persistent overconcern with body shape and weight.[1,2]

The age of onset of bulimia nervosa is usually in adolescence, and has a chronic and intermittent course over years. No clear family history of bulimia has been found but bulimics tend to have parents who are obese. Morbidity from binge eating, vomiting, and use of laxatives include electrolyte imbalance, dehydration, megacolon, esophageal tears, esophogitis, paratid gland enlargement, and occasionally sudden death from cardiac arrhythmias.[1,2]

Alcohol and Drug Dependence

The essential features according to DSM-III-R criteria can be reduced to a preoccupation with acquiring alcohol and drugs, compulsive use (use despite adverse consequences), a pattern of relapse to alcohol and drug use over time, and tolerance and dependence to alcohol and drugs.[1]

The age of onset is usually in adolescence and early adulthood, and 50 percent or greater of the family members report a history of alcohol dependence in probands who are alcoholic. The rate of familial drug dependence among drug dependents is less, and reports are in the 15 to 23 percent range. Reports also indicate that 50 percent or greater of family members of drug dependents report a history of alcohol dependence.[36]

Prevalence of the Disorders

The Prevalence Rates for Bulimia Nervosa and Anorexia Nervosa

In the general population, eating disorders are common in middle class females. These disorders also are seen almost exclusively in industrialized societies where there is an abundance of food and where slimness is highly deemed. Whereas in societies where thinness is not highly valued, the prevalence of these disorders is rare.[2,4,5]

In the Epidemiologic Catchment Area Study (ECA), the rate of anorexia nervosa was found to be 0.1 percent in the general population, and rarely among blacks. Rates of bulimia nervosa were not reported. Many of the studies concentrate on young females, and find that the prevalence rate for bulimia ranges from 1 to 8 percent, whereas the rate for anorexia was just under 1 percent of young females.[6]

A recent study college freshmen found that 4.5 percent of females and 0.4 percent of males had a history of bulimia.[7] The prevalence of anorexia nervosa has been reported in a range from 1 in 800 to as many as 1 in 100 females between the ages of 12 and 18. As can be seen both categories of disorders, alcohol and drug dependence and bulimia and anorexia nervosa, are relatively common in the general population. The rates for the eating disorders are less well characterized but are certain to be higher than in the general population.[1]

The Prevalence of Drug and Alchohol Dependence

The prevalence of a lifetime diagnosis of alcohol dependence in the general population is 16 percent, 5 percent for females and 24 percent for males. The rates for clinic and hospital populations are considerably higher as 25 to 50 percent of a general medical practice consists of alcoholics and drug addicts, and 50 to 75 percent of psychiatric patients are alcoholic and drug addict.[3]

The age of onset of alcohol dependence is young as with eating disorders. The mean age of onset for alcohol dependence in females is 25 years old whereas for males it is 22 years old according to the ECA study. In the same study, the majority of the alcoholics experienced their first alcoholic symptom between the ages of 15 and 19 years, and the vast majority of those interviewed at any age had an onset of alcoholism in their twenties.[3]

The Co-occurrence of Alcohol and Drug Dependence and Eating Disorders

Prevalence of Alcohol and Drug Dependence in Eating Disorders

The co-occurrence of alcohol and drug disorders and eating disorders is substantially high. When the focus of the population studied is eating disorders, the rates for alcohol and drug disorders in eating disorders appear to increase with age, ranging from 13 to 22 percent for high school students and college freshman to 31 to 50 percent in studies of ages in the thirties and forties.[2]

The rates for a lifetime diagnosis of alcohol and drug dependence in those with anorexia nervosa range from 0 to 19 percent depending on the methods employed in the studies. Of interest is that the rates tend to be higher among those anorectics who are also bulimic than without. The studies are not numerous, and are performed by those whose primary interest is in eating disorders, Table 18-1.[8,9,10]

The rates for a lifetime diagnosis of alcohol and drug dependence in bulimia nervosa have been studied in larger numbers of populations than for anorectics. Both controlled (studies done only in bulimia nervosa populations) and uncontrolled studies (comparisons between bulimic and non-bulimic populations) have been performed, and while high rates are found in both, rates tend to be consistently higher in uncontrolled studies. Also greater numbers of uncontrolled studies have been done. The rates range from 13 to 50 percent in older bulimics, Table 18-2.[8,11,12,13,14,15,16,17,18,19]

Prevalence of Eating Disorders in Alcohol and Drug Dependence

When the focus of the population studied is alcohol and drug patients, the rates are still substantial but not as striking as in primary eating disorder populations. Also, fewer studies have been done in alcohol and drug populations. The rates have ranged from 2 to 30 percent depending on

TABLE 18-1. Drug and alcohol dependence in anorexia nervosa.

Study	Year	N	Age	Results
Eckert et al.	1979	105	27.3	6.7% lifetime DSM-III diagnosis of alcohol abuse
Hudson et al.	1983	16	25	19% lifetime DSM-III diagnosis of substance abuse disorder (DIS)
Viesselman	1985	13	22.1	0% had diagnosis of alcohol or drug abuse (Feighner criteria)

TABLE 18-2. Drug and alcohol dependence in bulimia nervosa.

Uncontrolled Studies Study	Year	N	Age	Results
Pyle et al.	1981	34	24	High rate of drug/alcohol problems; 24% treated for CD
Hudson et al.	1983	49	17–49	31% lifetime prevalence of substance use disorder (DIS)
Mitchell et al.	1985	275	24.8	34% history of drug/alcohol problems; 18% history of CD treatment
Beary et al.	1986	112	24.9	Alcohol abuse and excess usage increased with age; to 50% by age 35
Hudson et al.	1987	70	18–45	49% lifetime prevalence of substance use disorder (DIS)
Mitchell et al.	1987	22 22	<20 >25	More substance abuse and affective disorder in the later age onset group (36% vs. 5%)

Controlled Studies Study	Year	N	Age	Results
Pyle et al.	1983	1355	college freshman	More alcohol and drug abuse in bulimics than nonbulimics
Bulik et al.	1987	35 bulimics 35 healthy controls	30 31	More alcohol/drug abuse in bulimics (48%) than in age and sex matched healthy controls (8.6%)
Hudson et al.	1987	70 bulimics 28 bulimics controls	26 31	More total substance abuse disorders in bulimics (49%) vs. controls (3%)
Killen et al.	1987	1728	tenth graders	More drunkenness and drinking in female purgers (22%) than nonpurgers (6%)

the methods used, and whether specific types of eating disorders were studied or only eating disorders in general, Table 18-3.[2,12,20]

A study was performed by Jonas et al. in 1987 using a structured clinical interview to diagnose eating disorders in 259 consecutive callers to

TABLE 18-3. Eating disorders in drug and alcohol populations.

Study*	Year	N	Results
Katzman & Strauss	1982	34 women	9% DMS-III-R diagnosis of bulimia nervosa and 12% diagnosis of anorexia nervosa
		46 men	2% DSM-III-R diagnosis of bulimia nervosa
Beary et al.	1986	20 women	30% had diagnosis of eating disorder (BN = 4; AN = 2)
Hoffman	1989	243 men	3% had an eating disorder
		2,519	18% had an eating disorder
		6,680	5% had an eating disorder
Hudson et al.	in press	143 women	15% had an eating disorder (AN = 5; BN = 11; AN/BN = 6)

the National Cocaine Hotline who met DSM-III-R criteria for cocaine abuse. Thirty-two percent of this sample met criteria for an eating disorder. Of these, 22 percent met DSM-III-R criteria for bulimia, 7 percent met criteria for anorexia nervosa and bulimia, and 2 percent met criteria for anorexia nervosa only. Interestingly, 44 percent of the callers who met criteria for bulimia nervosa were males.[21] Lacey et al. in 1986 studied 27 consecutive alcoholic women between ages 15 and 45 where eleven were bulimic and 16 were nonbulimic. The bulimics tended to be younger, to have an earlier onset of problem drinking, to weigh more, and to have a lower prevalence of alcoholism in their fathers.[22] In an earlier study by Lacey in 1983 in a treatment study of 30 severely bulimic outpatient women, ages 17 to 45, a history of alcohol abuse and bulimia was associated with a poor outcome.[22]

Familial Rates in the Disorders

There have been studies of family history of drug and alcohol dependence in relatives of patients with anorexia nervosa and bulimia nervosa. The studies have found higher rates of drug and alcohol diagnoses in family members of bulimics and anorectics than in the general population and in controls. The explanation for the increased association is unclear but supports the findings of the co-occurrence of drug and alcohol disorders with eating disorders.

Theander in 1970 reported that 6.4 percent of the fathers and none of the mothers of 94 women with anorexia nervosa had a drug or alcohol diagnosis.[23] Two controlled studies in relatives of bulimia nervosa patients have been reported. Bulik in 1987 found in a comparison of 35 bulimics and 35 controls that 49 percent of the bulimics and 20 percent of the controls met criteria for a drug or an alcohol diagnosis.[24] Hudson et al. in 1987 reported in a comparison of 69 bulimics and 28 nonpsychiatric controls that 19 percent of bulimics and 6.5 percent of controls had relatives with a drug or an alcohol diagnosis.[20]

Claydon in 1987 identified a group of college students who were children of alcoholics, and found that they were more than twice as likely to report an eating disorder than in controls, particularly in male subjects.[25] Pyle et al. in 1983 reported that 50 percent of their bulimic population indicated alcoholism in at least one first degree relative, and that 21 percent reported that their fathers were alcoholic.[26] Others studies substantiate an increased prevalence of drug and alcohol dependence in families of those probands with bulimia nervosa or anorexia nervosa.[1]

Common Interactions Between the Disorders

Onset of the Disorders

The studies and clinical experience tend to demonstrate that the onset of eating disorders precedes that of alcohol and drug disorders. Further studies need to be performed to further confirm the sequence of the onset of the disorders, as the respective disorders appear to interact throughout their courses. Some patients tend to binge-eat when intoxicated while others tend to substitute binge-eating for drugs and alcohol addiction. A common finding is an escalation of bulimic or anorectic behaviors following abstinence from drugs and alcohol.[2]

Hatsukami et al. in 1986 reported in a study of 46 bulimics without drug and alcohol addiction and 39 bulimics with drug and alcohol addiction that those with both disorders were likely to be older at the time of evaluation, were significantly more likely to report unprescribed use of diuretics for weight control, and reported significantly more financial, social, and work problems. They were more likely to report a history of suicide attempts, stealing behavior (both before and since the onset of the eating disorder), and prior inpatient and outpatient treatment.[27]

Addictive Behaviors

Many of the behavioral patterns and psychological states of bulimia and anorexia nervosa are similar to the well-established behavioral and psychological characteristics of drug and alcohol addiction. The cardinal manifestation of "loss of control" over drugs and alcohol is clearly present in the use or lack of use of food in eating disorders, and in the subjective feeling of loss of control over food as in the binging. As with drug and alcohol addiction, bulimics and anorectics are preoccupied with acquiring food, using it compulsively despite adverse consequences, and demonstrating a pattern of relapse over time. Bulimics clearly show this behavior in bulimic binges, that is, accumulating food, consuming large amounts and purging despite psychological and medical complications, and doing it repetitively. The sense of loss of control, fear, and apprehension of being out of control are overwhelming but reexperienced seemingly endlessly in both bulimics and anorectics.

The adverse psychological consequences in bulimia—anxiety, depression, shame, guilt, and remorse—can be severe. Also, bulimic behavior and mood states can interfere significantly with interpersonal relationships in similar ways to drug addicts and alcoholic. The denial is not only of the abnormal use of drugs and alcoholics. As with many psychiatric disorders, the subject state of the individual is not well characterized but clinical self-reports indicate extreme demoralization and destruction to the sufferer's self-esteem and confidence.

In anorectics who are also bulimic, the aforementioned psychological profile and behavioral patterns apply. However, anorectics have additional symptoms that are similar to those seen in the drug addict and alcoholic. The self-delusional "fatness" in the face of starvation and cachexia in the anorectic is akin to the self-destructive delusion of denial in the drug addict and alcoholic. The denial is not only of the abnormal use of drugs and alcohol but also of the consequences of addictive use of drugs and alcohol. This denial is also in the face of extraordinary evidence of deterioration in personality and interpersonal relationships, and high psychiatric and medical morbidity and mortality for the drug and alcohol addiction.

Common Biological Mechanism

The limbic system serves as a neurosubstate for alcohol and drug addiction as well as for eating disorders, particularly bulimia nervosa and anorexia nervosa. The limbic system houses primitive and instinctual drive states that are essential to the survival of the individual. These drive states pertain to eating (hunger), drinking (thirst), sex (reproduction), and emotions (moods). These instincts are ordinarily regulated by complex neurological and psychological modulators in the brain that are only partially understood.[28]

The limbic system is phylogenetically old, and is relatively constant from species to species, and over evolution. The limbic system is composed of the hypothalamus that contains the substrate for appetite and thirst, the septal areas for mood and sex, and the hippocampi for immediate memory encoding for longer storage. The neurotransmitters that are messengers for functioning in these areas are also affected by alcohol and drugs. These neurotransmitters are norepinephrine, dopamine, and serotonin, and are increased, decreased, or otherwise stimulated or depressed by many drugs of addiction including alcohol.[28]

What can be appreciated is that drive states produce behaviors that are similar to those seen in addictive disorders, for both drug and alcohol and eating disorders. Drive states are spontaneous, stereotypic, and autonomous, and are accompanied by an increased tension state that requires reduction to the normal states. The object of the drive state is often what is needed to reduce the tension and satisfy the source of the drive, namely food for hunger, liquid for thirst, and ejaculation or orgasm for sex. Under normal conditions the drive states are under control of higher cortical centers, particularly the frontal lobe that contains inhibitory input to the limbic system. The function of the frontal lobe includes ethics, judgment, planning, and foresight among others. The frontal lobe is responsible for modulating the drive states by regulating their expression through inhibitory influences.[28]

What appears to occur in addictive behavior in the case of drugs and alcohol, and bulimia and anorexia nervosa, is an alteration of these drive states. The drive states become relatively autonomous and spontaneously arise in pursuit of drugs, alcohol, and food, and less regulated by the normal mechanisms. The drugs, alcohol, and food appear to entrain the drive states to set up aberrant drives that are manifested by a loss of control, and unresponsive to regulation of the use of drugs and alcohol. In short, addiction to drugs, alcohol, and food appear to be drives that have gone awry.[28]

Treatment

General Principles

The overall approach to eating disorders and drug and alcohol disorders is similar. The therapies tend to be behavioral and cognitive, and are aimed at stopping the behaviors of addiction as the first priority. For drug and alcohol patients, this would mean requiring abstinence from all drugs and alcohol except for those prescribed. For the bulimic and anorectic patient, this means abstaining from bulimic behaviors and other pathological eating patterns such as starvation and poorly nutritious foods in hazardous schedules. The emphasis is on modifying under supervision the essential pathological eating behaviors that would then allow progression to other phases of treatment. The initial target is not on attitudes or feeling state, as these tend to change in response to behavioral alterations.[29,30]

Concurrently, a thorough medical and psychiatric evaluation for comorbid diagnoses should be undertaken. The prevalence of concomitant medical and psychiatric problems is significant in this population, and their identification may require careful assessment.[2]

The current approaches to treatment typically employ a major and minor focus on either the drug/alcohol disorder or the eating disorder. It is not only unusual but it remains to be proven possible to hold simultaneous foci in one particular treatment setting. Attempts have been made to employ dual tracts for the psychiatric disorders on the one hand and drug and alcohol addiction on the other. No clear documentation has been presented for the simultaneous, successful treatment of eating disorders and drug/alcohol disorders. In actual clinical practice it is too distracting for the patient and often confusing for the staff to concentrate on both categories of disorders at the same time.[29,30]

The model that is generally used in clinical practice in many treatment programs is a combination in sequence of both approaches. While not ignoring any disorder, a major focus of drug and alcohol addiction may be attended to first. Strong clinical experience and evidence confirm that until the drug and alcohol use is eliminated, little else can be accomplished in the treatment of concomitant eating, psychiatric, or medical disorders. A minor focus for the treatment of eating disorders can be instituted during the treatment of the major disorder either for those cases of eating disorders that are clearly out of control or routinely in a prescribed program. Specialized groups for treatment of eating disorders and attendance at meetings of Overeaters Anonymous (OA) can be mandatory during the treatment of the drug and alcohol disorder. It is important to note that skill should be employed to avoid making the eating disorder a focus to the exclusion of adequate treatment of the drug and alcohol disorder. This is a prevailing risk in the treatment of many addictive disorders.[29,30]

A subsequent referral to either an inpatient or outpatient treatment program for eating disorders can be made for those patients who are diagnosed as having bulimia or anorexia in the drug/alcohol treatment population. It is clinically well known but not well documented in studies that bulimic and anorectic behaviors tend to escalate in abstinent alcoholics and drug addicts. These eating symptoms can be severely incapacitating as to require psychiatric and medical intervention in an outpatient or inpatient setting. Abstinent alcoholics and drug addicts with bulimia can experience significant depression and anxiety that qualify for DSM-III-R diagnoses of major depression and anxiety disorders. For these patients, adequate treatment of the eating disorder often results in an amelioration of these psychiatric symptoms.

For those patients with an eating disorder who have a drug and an alcohol disorder as well, treatment of the eating disorder first as a major focus in the sequence may be indicated, particularly in the case of severely anorectic patients or bulimics who are severely out of control with binging and purging. The treatment of the drug and alcohol disorder as a minor focus can occur in the setting of the eating disorder treatment program. Specialized groups for treatment of drug and alcohol disorders and attendance at meetings of Alcoholics Anonymous can be mandatory during treatment of the eating disorder in either an inpatient or outpatient setting.

Treatment Process

The general principles of the abstinence based programs of 12 step programs can be applied to both categories of eating disorders and drug/alcohol disorders. The abstinence in drug/alcohol disorders is from drugs and alcohol whereas in eating disorders abstinence is avoiding addictive behaviors such as binging and purging, compulsive exercise designed to reduce weight, and obsession with "fatness" and pathological eating patterns, particularly starvation in anorectics. While in a technical sense abstinence from food is not possible, eliminating aberrant eating behaviors, and eventually attitudes that are fundamental to pathological eating, are possible.[32,33,34]

Because eating disorders do follow the model clinically for addictive disorders and share a common theoretical basis with drug and alcohol disorders, similar treatment strategies have been developed and employed successfully. Eating disorders do respond to behavioral and cognitive techniques similar to those that are used for drug and alcohol addiction. The desired changes in attitudes in behavior, cognition, and moods are similar for eating disorders as for drug/alcohol disorders. An acceptance of the disease concept and an establishment of a commitment to recovery are the initial treatment goals for both categories of disorders. An open and honest attitude, and a willingness to participate in the steps in the treatment process are the early and essential enduring features that are required for successful treatment of both categories of disorders.[35]

Family programs directed at treatment of family members are often necessary for the successful treatment of the patients with either category of disorders. The enabling behaviors of families and significant others are similar in eating disorders as with drug and alcohol disorders. The parallel processes of coaddiction including denial, minimization, and rationalization occur in the family as well as in the addicted whether addiction is to food, drugs, or alcohol. Family members may be suffering from psychological and psychiatric symptoms as well, and can include anxiety, depression, and psychosomatic and medical complications. A complete evaluation of the family is therefore indicated. Specific therapy aimed at the coaddictive behaviors is required for all family members who have been and will be involved with the patients.[29,30,31]

Long-Term Follow-Up

The long-term treatment of addictive disorders, especially eating disorders and drug and alcohol disorders, is indicated because of the relapsing nature of the addictive process. Also, treatment of comorbid psychiatric and medical conditions may be necessary. The minimum and core standard of long-term treatment currently is regular attendance at Overeaters Anonymous (OA), Alcoholics Anonymous (AA), or Narcotics Anonymous (NA). These are essential parts of treatment plans for relapse prevention for these addictive disorders. Although each "self-help" organization uses the same 12 steps, it is often necessary for the patient with a concomitant eating disorder and drug and alcohol disorder to attend both OA and AA or NA. While there is clear overlap of addictive behaviors and attitudes, clinical empirical experience at this point recommends the simultaneous treatment of both categories of disorders in the initial months and years. No studies have been performed that have substantiated that continued treatment of either disorder may not be necessary.[29,30,31]

Future Research

Considerably more research is needed to determine the natural history of eating disorders, particularly the co-occurrence of eating disorders with drug and alcohol disorders. While substantial overlap occurs, the interactions between the categories of disorders is poorly understood. Although the fundamental similarities of the behavioral and cognitive states can be derived from common mechanisms, the pathophysiology of either category is not well understood. Both categories of disorders appear to be psychiatric and neurological in origin but the specific neuroanatomy and neurochemistry have only been minimally elucidated. Moreover, the concurrent and long-term treatment of both disorders in the same individuals is in critical need of further research.

References

1. Diagnostic and Statistical Manual of Mental Disorders (third edition revised, DSM-III-R). Washington, DC, American Psychiatry Association, 1987.
2. Mitchell JB, Pyle RL, Echert ED, Specker S. Eating disorders and drug and alcohol addiction. In Miller N (ed): Comprehensive Handbook of Drug and Alcohol Addiction. New York, Marcel Dekker Inc, 1991; 193–202.
3. Helzer JE, Burnam A, McEvoy LT. Alcohol abuse and dependence, Chapter 5. In Robins LN, Regier DA (eds): Psychiatric Disorders in America. New York, The Free Press, Macmillan, Inc, 1991.
4. Anderson AB, Hay A. Racial and socioeconomic influences in anorexia nervosa and bulimia. *Int J Eating Disord* 1985; 4:479–487.
5. Mitchell JE, Eckert ED. Scope and significance of eating disorders. *J Counselling and Clin Psychol* 1987; 55:628–634.
6. Robins LN, Helzer JR, Weissman MM, Orvaschel H, Gruenberg E, Burke JD, Regier DA. Lifetime prevalence of specific disorders in three sites. *Arch Gen Psychiatry* 1984; 41:949–958.
7. Hesse-Biber S. Eating patterns and disorders in a college population: Are college women's eating problems a new phenomenon? *Sex Roles* 1989; 20:73–89
8. Hudson JI, Pope HG, Jonas JM, et al. Family history study of anorexia nervosa and bulimia. *Br J Psychiatry* 1983; 142:133–138.
9. Eckert ED, Goldberg SC, Halmi KA, et al. Alcoholism in anorexia nervosa. In Pickens RW, Heston LL (eds): Psychiatric Factors in Drug Abuse. New York, Grune & Stratton, 1979.
10. Viesselman JO, Roig M. Depression and suicidality in eating disorders. *J Clin Psychiatry* 1985; 46:118–124.
11. Mitchell JE, Eckert ED. Scope and significance of eating disorders. *J Consult Clin Psychol* 1987; 55:628–634.
12. Beary MD, Lacey JH, Merry J. Alcoholism and eating disorder in women of fertile age. *Br J Addict* 1986; 81:685–689.
13. Hudson JI, Pope HG, Yurgelun-Todd, et al. Psychiatric disorders in bulimic outpatients. *Am J Psychiatry* 1987; 144:1283–1287.

14. Mitchell JE, Hatsukami D, Eckert ED, et al. Characteristics of 275 patients with bulimia. *Am J Psychiatry* 1985; 142:482–485.
15. Mitchell JE, Hatsukami D, Pyle RL, et al. Late onset bulimia. *Comp Psychiatry* 1987; 28:323–328.
16. Pyle RL, Mitchell JE, Ecket ED, Halvorson PA, Neuman PA, Goff GM. The incidence of bulimia in freshman students. *Int J Eating Disord* 1983; 2:75–85.
17. Hudson JI, Pope HG, Jonas JM, et al. A controlled family history study of bulimia. *Psychological Medicine* 1987; 17:883–890.
18. Bulik CM. Alcohol use and depression in women with bulimia. *Am J Drug Alcohol Abuse* 1987; 13(3):343–355.
19. Killen JD, Taylor CB, Telch MJ, et al. Evidence for an alcohol-stress link among normal weight adolescents reporting purging behavior. *Int J Eating Disord* 1987; 6:349–356.
20. Giannini AJ. Drug abuse and depression possible models for gerintric anorexia. *Neurobiol Aging* 1988; 9(1):26–27.
21. Jonas JM, Gold MS, Sweeney D, et al. Eating disorders and cocaine abuse: A survey of 259 cocaine abusers. *J Clin Psychiatry* 1987; 48:47–50.
22. Lacey JH, Moureli E. Bulimic alcoholics: Some features of a clinical subgroup. *Br J Addict* 1986; 81:389–393.
23. Theander S. Anorexia nervosa—a psychiatric investigation of 94 female patients. *Acta Psychiatrica Scandinavia Suppl* 1970; 46:1–194.
24. Bulik CM. Drug and alcohol abuse by bulimic women and their families. *Am J Psych* 1987; 144(12):1604–1606.
25. Claydon P. Self-reported alcohol, drug, and eating-disorder problems among male and female collegiate children of alcoholics. *J Am Coll Health* 1987; 36:111–116.
26. Pyle RL, Mitchell JE, Eckert ED, et al. The incidence of bulimia in freshman college students. *Int J Eating Disord* 1983; 2:75–85.
27. Hatsukami D, Mitchell JE, Eckert ED, et al. Characteristics of patients with bulimia only, bulimia with affective disorder, and bulimia with substance abuse problems. *Addict Behav* 1986; 11:399–406.
28. Miller NS, Gold MS. A neuroanatomical and neurochemical approach to drug and alcohol addiction. In Miller N (ed): Comprehensive Handbook of Drug and Alcohol Addiction. New York, Marcel Dekker Inc, 1991.
29. Hoffman L, Halmi K. Hospital treatment of eating disorders with drug and alcohol addiction. In Miller N (ed): Comprehensive Handbook of Drug and Alcohol Addiction. New York, Marcel Dekker Inc, 1991.
30. Cocores J. Outpatient treatment of drug and alcohol addiction. In Miller N (ed): Comprehensive Handbook of Drug and Alcohol Addiction. New York, Marcel Dekker Inc, 1991.
31. Harrison PA, Hoffman NG, Sneed SG. Drug and alcohol addiction treatment outcome. In Miller N (ed): Comprehensive Handbook of Drug and Alcohol Addiction. New York, Marcel Dekker Inc, 1991.
32. Zweben JE. Eating disorders and substance abuse. *J Psychoactive Drugs* 1987; 19:181–192.
33. Scott DW. Alcohol and food abuse: Some comparisons. *Br J Addict* 1983; 78:339–349.

34. Brisnan J, Siegel M. Bulimia and alcoholism: Two sides of the same coin? *J Substance Abuse Treatment* 1984; 1:113–118.
35. Garner DM, Bemis KM. Cognitive therapy for anorexia nervosa. In Garner DM, Garfintel PE (eds): Handbook of Psychotherapy for Anorexia Nervosa and Bulimia. New York, Guilford Press, 1984; 107–146.
36. Miller NS, Gold MS, Belkin BM, Klahr AL. Family history at diagnosis of alcohol dependence in cocaine dependence. *Psych Res* 1989; 29:113–121.

19
Occupational Therapy Treatment of Anorexia Nervosa

DAVID J. FOLTS, KENT TIGGES, and GARY JACKSON

Anorexia nervosa affects the biological, social, and emotional competence of the patient. This eating disorder which affects young women is multi-faceted and requires a global approach to treatment intervention. The occupational behavior model proposed by Reiley is such an intervention.[1] It is based on Adolph Meyer's continuum of the balance between work, rest, play, and sleep.[2] Occupation means not only employment but also includes all other activities that occupy a person's time. In anorexia nervosa there is an unhealthy imbalance of time directed towards weight loss, exercise, and food related issues. This chapter uses the occupational behavior paradigm as a foundation for exploring occupational deficits and discusses treatment interventions for anorexia nervosa.

Occupational Behavior: A Model of Practice

In occupational behavior, the starting point is to examine fundamental assumptions about people, occupation, principles about patients, occupational therapy, and how these relate to anorexia nervosa.

People

People have a need to master their environment, to alter and improve it.[3] The inherent drive towards mastery is a prerequisite for attaining competence and influencing one's world. Personal effectiveness results from many different situations where competency is achieved.

People with anorexia nervosa do not feel mastery. Their obsessional desire to master their bodies through weight control is repeatedly thwarted through ongoing dissatisfaction with body weight.

Despite mastery in other areas of their lives, competencies do not impact on the anorectic's feelings of mastery and do not alter perceptions of incompetence. Anorectics feel helpless against forces outside their control such as family and other social spheres.

There is a relationship between levels of aspiration and expectancy established in prior socialization and current patterns of success or failure.[4] The ways in which people have learned to succeed or fail in the past is directly related to how they will adapt to the present and future.

Anorectics doom themselves to failure by establishing unrealistic performance standards that have been referred to as "cycles of inflationary self-evaluation."[5] Their view that they must perform without error prevents anorectics from acknowledging performance that is viewed by others as adequate. As with any self-fulfilling prophesy, their expectation of failure is reinforced by maintaining unachievable standards.

Food restriction and exercise become attempts to achieve success. Rather than being a failure, they become a paragon of thinness. Their proclivity to rely on others' opinions and their lack of trust in themselves continues to feed their feelings of failure.

Anorectics' distorted expectancy patterns are related to difficulties observed in anorectic families including: 1) family emeshment that undermines achievement and success related experiences; 2) overprotective parents who shelter the anorectic from risk-taking experiences that would allow them to achieve success, or rescue the anorectic from any experience that may be remotely connected to failure; 3) families that avoid direct confrontation which does not allow for successful negotiation and compromise in the interpersonal sphere; and 4) rigidness and strict limit setting which discourages individuality and personal freedom.[6] In attempting new things, anorectics learn to turn to their bodies for success experiences.

Anorexia nervosa appears most often in middle and upper socioeconomic status levels.[7] In these families, high achievement and exceptional performance become the norm. Rigidly following high standards results in numerous perceived failures that reinforce the anorectic's belief that they are failures. The lack of preparation by their families, the multitude of options available to the adolescent anorectic, and the need for a perfect score results in inevitable feelings of failure.

People have a vital need for occupation.[3] Purpose and meaning are developed through the productive engagement in activity.

Despite excellent performance in activity, anorectics report that they do not feel productive or derive meaning from activities that are not food related.[8] Instead, they find successful completion of activity as meaningless, so that competency and skills do not impact on feelings of well being.

While anorectics are often high achievers with a wide range of skills and abilities, internally they do not perceive themselves as competent.[9]

Occupation

Achievement has a developmental nature.[4] Early successful performance lays the foundation for future success experiences. Unfortunately, psychosomatic families preclude many achievement experiences. The anorectic's family organization develops and maintains the lack of self-perceived achievement because of the inability to adapt itself to changing circumstances, which is a necessary prerequisite for success. Any attempt by the anorectic to make a positive change is viewed by other family members as a violation of established codes of behavior.

Developmental changes of the adolescent such as increasingly independent behavior are perceived as threats to the family. It becomes virtually impossible for the anorectic to achieve success in expected developmental tasks. In addition, the anorectic has a childlike dependency on the family which makes it difficult for the anorectic to progress. Instead of obtaining competency through achievement experiences, the young female regresses into anorectic behavior.

Roles are learned through the process of socialization.[10] The roles taken by people are influenced by the social system they are in and result in certain occupational behaviors. Roles influence the skills that are developed by the person which in turn influences socialization patterns.

Socialization for the anorectic begins in her family relationships. Anorectic families are characterized by few boundaries. There is a lack of delineation in tasks and roles between parents and children. In these families, the children can assume the parenting role with parents and siblings.

This stems from family expectations that others will know their wants and desires without expressing them. Triangulations occur when two family members are interrupted by the third resulting in confusion and role blurring.

Occupational Therapy

Occupational therapy focus lies in the area of creativity.[3] Creativity is an action producing a result that is useful. It is effective, solves a problem, helps, and stimulates. It enriches and changes a person's life. In creativity, a change in direction is required. However, the rigid and compulsive behaviors of anorexia dampens creative ability.

Certain features of the creative process are diametrically opposed to the anorectic's life style. These include the lack of guideposts to direct them which may explain academic success but difficulty when choosing a vocation.[11] In order to be creative, anorectics must first allow themselves to be open to new ideas—a difficult task when control is central to their lives. Because of their rigid behavioral style, they have difficulty changing directions which is a prerequisite for finding a new solution.

The task of occupational therapy is to prevent and reduce the incapacities resulting from illness.[4] The job of occupational therapy is to activate the residual adaptation forces within the patient.[4]

Because of their denial systems, anorectics are frequently admitted to the hospital in an acute medical crisis lacking the ability to identify their adaptive forces. When asked what their assets, are, they may be unable to identify them. Even though anorectics deny their abilities, they often possess a wide range of capacities that can be used to remediate dysfunction.

Occupational therapy should be directed towards achievement.[4] Achievement orientation is directly opposite the anorectic's upbringing as a child. Bruch[12] describes the anorectic's situation as "seemingly well functioning homes where parents raise children who mistrust their ability to face the future and shy away from adult living. On one level, child care appears to be excellent, everything is provided for materially, psychologically and culturally. However, little attention is paid to the child's expression of wants, needs or feelings." Even though anorectics learn to build skills, they do not possess feelings of achievement due to the inelasticity of their environment.

Principles About patients

1. Patients are to be considered at high risk.
2. Patients are the pivotal initiative in assessment and treatment.

Anorexia nervosa is a life-threatening disease with the highest incidence of death among psychiatric patients (2%–8%).[13] Patients are encouraged to work towards cessation of their illness by establishing specific treatment goals.

Anorectic patients are asked to assume responsibility for their behavior. They are free from constant supervision so as to become their own therapeutic agent. Responsibility implies choice of action. To recover from anorexia nervosa, the patient needs to freely choose not to engage in eating-disordered behavior. By assuming responsibility, anorectics are forced to examine their motives for continuing to engage in eating-disordered behavior.

Concepts: Occupational Behavior

A fundamental concept in occupational behavior is that of intrinsic motivation. Intrinsic motivation is the force that propels a person towards achievement. Intrinsic motivation can be divided into a behavioral continuum of "pawn" and "origin" behaviors. Depending on their pawn or origin position, people attempt to control and master the environment.[14] An origin orientation refers to the perception of events as being a consequence of one's behavior and under personal control. Pawn orientation refers to the opposite whereby events are viewed as unrelated to one's behavior due to lack or future and thereby out of personal control. This concept is similar to Bruch's sense of ineffectiveness.[5]

Pawn or origin behaviors have been correlated with health behaviors. Strickland[16] concluded that origin-oriented individuals faced with health problems engaged in more adaptive behavior.

A major component of pawn or origin behavior is that of self-esteem. Self-esteem determines how anorectics face their illness. When recovering, they need to adjust to how significant others value them when they are free of eating-disordered behavior. This new perception makes up the foundation of their recovery.

Treatment Strategies, Assessment, and Treatment Intervention

As theory must integrate with practice, Table 19-1 refers to occupational role performance components and Table 19-2 refers to biomedical performance elements.

Assessment

Work History

While anorectics do not display dysfunction in the student role, obsessiveness represents a block to performance satisfaction. Even though anorectics are competent in academia, they have difficulty making the transition to the adult worker role. Starvation becomes the mechanism to settle the conflict over wanting to remain emeshed in the family while understanding the need for vocational preparation.

TABLE 19-1. Elements of medicosocial performance.

Performance area	Elements
1. Medical	A. Bodily Interpretation
	B. Sensory Adaptation
	C. Motor Competence
2. Personal	A. Cognitive Skills
	B. Coping Skills
	C. Interpersonal Skills
	D. Self Concepts
	E. Self Identity
3. Social	A. Assimilation of Cultural Norms
	B. Dyadic Interpretation
	C. Familial Identification
	D. Subcultural Identification/Resection

* Adapted from DJ Folts. Occupational therapy in treatment of substance abuse disorder. In AJ Giannini and AE Slaby (eds) *Drugs of Abuse*, Oradell, NJ, Medical Economics, 1989.
Standard Terminology for Reporting Occupational Therapy Services. American Occupational Therapy Association, 1979.

TABLE 19-2. Elements of role performance.

Performance area	Elements
1. Leisure	A. Amusement
	B. Creative Expression
	C. Relaxation
	D. Exercise
2. Personal Maintenance	A. Dressing
	B. Eating
	C. Hygiene
	D. Mobility
3. Work	A. Child care
	B. Home management
	C. Vocational preparation

* Adapted from DJ Folts. Occupational therapy in treatment of substance abuse disorder. In AJ Giannini and AE Slaby (eds) *Drugs of Abuse*, Oradell, NJ, Medical Economics, 1989.
Standard Terminology for Reporting Occupational Therapy Services. American Occupational Therapy Association, 1979.

Deficits in vocational functioning occur when work habit structure deteriorates as a result of severe malnutrition. Extreme anorexia can cause impairment in concentration, attention to task, decision making, ability to follow directions, problem solving, and frustration tolerance.

In terms of occupational choice, certain vocations place females at risk for developing anorexia nervosa. Occupations where physique is important such as modeling and ballet display a greater frequency of anorexia nervosa.[17]

Home management is a critical assessment area and includes skill and performance in meal planning, shopping, meal preparation, eating, meal cleanup, household chores, and money management.

To assess performance in home management, a functional Eating Evaluation is completed.[18] Since anorectics have high performance anxiety, it is explained that the evaluation is not passed or failed. Rather, her performance will be used to plan treatment.

The Functional Eating Evaluation, Table 19-3, is a series of semistructured tasks involving a kitchen and grocery store.

Specific instructions are given prior to beginning each task. The anorectics are scored on such factors as choice of appropriate foods, flexibility, number of minutes food is consumed, compulsive behavior regarding cleanup, frustration tolerance, anxiety level, communication, and cooperation. Difficulties experienced during completion of the evaluation are processed and the patients are encouraged to consider their reactions as they relate to eating-disordered behavior. Table 19-3 is the Functional Eating Disorders Evaluation used with anorectic patients.

Family History

Anorectics are questioned about their relationship with significant others to determine dysfunctional family patterns. Key issues explored include the level of: 1) emeshment defined as very close relationships between family members without any boundaries being available for each individual in the family: 2) rigidity, or the inability of the family to adapt itself to different situations: 3) overprotectiveness which is characterized by overconcern and overreaction of family members to each other's distress: and 4) conflict avoidance or inability to negotiate conflictual situations in the family.

Other dysfunctional patterns assessed include pseudomutuality[19] in which family members agree that there are no difficulties except those medical problems associated with anorexia. Pseudohostility is assessed to determine if family members exert pressure on the patient to eat. Since anorectics will lead family members into a trap over eating, power struggle intensity

TABLE 19-3. Functional eating evaluation.

Planning
(uses shopping list appropriately, accurate estimation of money spent, estimates food required accurately, uses balance of four food groups)
4- no problem in any area
3- problem in one area
2- problem in two areas
1- problem in three areas
0- problem in four areas

Shopping
(chooses appropriate foods, chooses appropriate qualities of food, avoids diet foods, maintains appropriate pace)
4- no problem in any area
3- problem in one area
2- problem in two areas
1- problem in three areas
0- problem in four areas

Preparation
(does not eat food drug preparation, estimates correct size to eat food, flexability in choosing food quantity)
4- no problems in any areas
3- problem in one area
2- problem in two areas
1- problem in three areas
0- refuses to participate

Eating
(completes meal within 30 minutes, absence of negative statements regarding food, portions appropriate, quantity of food without measuring)
4- no problem in any area
3- problem in one area
2- problem in two areas
1- problem in three areas
0- refuses to participate

Meal Cleanup
(remains seated while others finish, makes adequate decisions regarding remaining food, cleans without excessive rabbling and shinning)
4- no problem in any area
3- problem in one area
2- problem in two areas
1- problem in three areas
0- refuses to participate

Anxiety Level
4- no signs of anxiety
3- anxious, no effect on results
2- anxious, minor effect on results
1- anxious, major effect on results
0- unable to work on tasks

is measured. This includes the severity of arguments, yelling, threatening, punishments, and other adversive experiences.

In order to assess the roles played by the anorectic in the family, the Role Performance Scale is utilized.[20] An interview is performed with a format that includes twelve roles yielding a view of past performance in that role and performance using time intervals prior to completion of the interview. Changes in role performance are noted with factors that precipitated changes and their relationship to stress and performance.

Temporal Adaptation

How people spend their time has been associated with competency and achievement.[21] Anorectics live restricted lives. As a group, anorectics work effectively but have low rates of interpersonal relationships.[22] The role of friend is virtually nonexistent.[22] Former anorectics have low rates of marriage and sexual satisfaction. Many continue to live at home and remain dependent on their parents, economically and socially.

Anorectics complete the Life Attitude Profile[23] which gives data relevant to the purpose and meaning in the anorectic's routine and the anorectic's future orientation.

To assess specific time use, the Occupational Questionnaire is used.[24] It consists of an activity configuration that investigate specific information on use of time and competence felt when engaged in an activity. Information is gleaned on time rigidity, habits, and reactions to time use. Rigidity and habits are of particular importance in view of the anorectic's compulsive behavioral style.

Leisure

Although anorectics do not lack leisure interests, they possess minimal awareness of their own needs and values.[25] In order to gain an understanding of the anorectic's use of leisure, a Leisure Satisfaction Questionnaire is utilized to view their motivations for engaging in leisure.[26] This includes whether the leisure activity is solitary or social; motivation for beginning, terminating, or resuming an activity; and how much enjoyment is derived from reaction.

The next assessment is biomedical-(see Table 19-2) which examines the sensorimotor, personal/emotional, and social factors that have restricted the biosocial elements.

Sensorimotor Performance

While chronic starvation does not result in impaired task performance in dressing, transfers, or personal hygiene, sensation is evaluated to determine sensory loss as a result of peripheral neuropathies. In addition, the anorectic is assessed for peroneal nerve palsy which can be a result of chronic malnutrition. Anorectics with peripheral neuropathies are at increased risk for developing localized compression neuropathies secondary to subcutaneous tissue loss.[27]

As a result of starvation and excessive exercising, muscle strength and endurance are reduced. Symptoms of anorexia also include mitral valve prolapse, blood pressure irregularity, seizure activity, and electrolyte imbalance.

A task evaluation is conducted to assess cognitive functioning. Since anorectics have obsessive performance standards, they are informed that it is not a test that can be passed or failed. The task evaluation is a highly structured activity. Four instructions are given and the anorectic is asked to complete the task. Factors assessed include short-term memory, distractibility, dexterity, problem solving, and the ability to generalize.

The disturbed body image in anorexia nervosa is an essential diagnostic characteristic. To assess body image distortion, the Askevold method is used.[28] It consists of patients self-recording certain body parts chosen for measuring. A piece of wrapping paper is taped to the wall. To determine the accuracy of anorectics' measuring dimensions, the patient works on a vertical and horizontal line the length of two equal dimensions. Patients visualize themselves standing in front of a mirror. The occupational therapist stands behind the anorectic and touches the body parts selected for marking. The anorectic then makes a mark on the paper where she perceives the points in the mirror.

Personal/Emotional

During the evaluation process, the anorectic is assessed for the presence of defense mechanisms. Most observable is denial and presents as denial of an eating disorder, denial of the need for treatment, and denial of medical problems associated with anorexia nervosa. Defense mechanisms also include rationalization, minimization, and intellectualization. Rationalization legitimizes anorexia through the anorectic's perception of societal expectations of a lean body type. Minimization is used to explain medical problems associated with malnutrition and excessive exercising and occurs when the patient distorts the quantity of food consumed and the frequency and intensity of exercise performed. Interllectualization hides the anorectic's feelings about the eating disorder through focusing on matters not directly related to her eating problem.

Lack of mastery in life tasks,[29] low personal competence,[30] and powerless feelings[31] are associated with an increase in eating-disordered behavior. Since there is a strong correlation between feelings of powerlessness and anorectic behavior, several assessments are used to measure internal versus external orientation. The first is the I.E. Scale (Generalized Expectancies for Internal Control) which measures the degree one feels controlled by forces beyond one's control versus one's feeling in control of one's destiny.[32] The Reid Ware-Factor Internal External Scale[33] supplements the I.E. assessment. This instrument yields three scores which measure: 1) a belief in self-control; 2) a belief in control by social systems; and 3) the degree of fatalism.

Social Functioning

An evaluation of social functioning is completed to determine anorectics relational skills. Despite high level verbal and cognitive functions, anorectics display reduced intellectual skills.[22] It is interesting to note that several researchers have found anorectics to be deficient in nonverbal reception[34] and transmission.[35]

Treatment Planning and Implementation

Following are seven steps used in treatment planning and implementation for the anorectic patient.

Step 1. Assessment Review

Through the use of previous assessment tools, an identification is made of those skills that will allow the anorectic to not engage in eating-disordered behavior.

Step 2. Establish Intrinsic Motivation

The anorectic patient is given a pawn origin rating based on the results of the I.E. Scale and Reid Ware assessment. By determining intrinsic/extrinsic motivation, early identification is made of anorectics at higher risk of relapse and difficulty during treatment.

Step 3. Identify Patient's Self-Esteem

Anorectics may be best described as obsessive compulsive with contricted affect perfectionism, and having a strong achievement orientation. However, this does not lead to feelings of adequate self-esteem. Rather, it results in dysfunctional self-concept, insecurity in social relationships, and a general sense of inadequacy.

Step 4. Review Assumptions of Occupational Behavior

Intrinsic motivation, achievement, competency, and temporal adaptation are reviewed to determine if the anorectic is building skills that promote a life style without eating-disordered behavior.

Step 5. Develop and Prioritize Goals

The anorectics are asked to identify three goals they would like to achieve. When discussing eating-disordered behavior, the patient may experience extreme difficulty finding goals which may require assistance. The patient is then guided in exploring possibilities in areas such as leisure and stress management by providing them with cues to an achievable goal. When the patient successfully chooses a goal developed with the occupational therapist, there is an increased possibility that other goals will be identified.

Goals are established and agreed to in how they will be accomplished. No goal in itself is therapeutic. For a goal to become therapeutic, it is important for the patient and occupational therapist to be committed to designing goals that will assist the patient in change. The occupational therapist listens to determine if the patient is willing to accept alternatives to goal achievement.

Step 6. Review Goals in Acquisition of Life Skills

Areas of performance include:

1. Abstinence from eating-disordered behavior
2. Treatment participation
3. Competency in demonstration of life skills
4. Treatment follow-through

Step 7. Modify Goals and Treatment Methods Based on Performance

Treatment goals and methods are graded according to the needs and changing status of the patient. If the patient is not able to abstain from eating-disordered behaviors goals are graded accordingly.

Treatment

Since recovery from anorexia nervosa is a dynamic process, patients receive consistent reinforcement on maintaining an active role in treatment. The principles of transfer of training are applied so that skills learned in treatment can be implemented upon discharge.

Research has demonstrated a significant relationship between anorexia nervosa and type A behavioral patterns.[36] Since anorectics are high achievers who are more reactive to stressors, stress management focuses on the patient developing adaptive coping skills. Anorectics are asked to identify the psychological symptoms of stress. Emphasis is placed on the patient's stress response regarding food. In order to minimize the stress response, anorectic patients participate in progressive/autogenic relaxation, visual imagery, and biofeedback.

In stress management group, clients are provided with support and guidance as they undertake a change in their eating behavior. The anxiety produced by not starving themselves can overwhelm them; regaining control through renewed starvation can be a destructive form of stress abatement.

Since changing eating behaviors is stressful, patients keep an eating record which they discuss in stress management group. The daily record includes time that eating occurs, quantity eaten, hunger level, and stress before and after eating.

Discussion of the eating record focuses on the stress involved in the patient moving away from dieting towards normal eating, the ingesting of larger quantities of food, and the relationship of food intake to stress.

In goal setting group, patients begin to establish priorities. They are asked to categorize and follow goals as follows: 1) long-range goals are those concerned with the overall life style that they want, whether or not they wish to be married, the kind of family they want, and the general situation they wish to live in.

Although they are asked to develop on overall idea of what they want, they are not expected to plan long-range goals in detail, due to the many changes that will occur. It is emphasized that they need a plan but they should keep it flexible; 2) medium-range goals are goals covering the anorectic's next five years; these goals are concerned with the kind of training or education that they will be seeking. It is stressed that they have more control over these goals and that they can determine whether they are going to be successful and modify their efforts accordingly; 3) short-range goals cover from one month to one year. These include postdischarge goals in which concerns can be set quite realistically. Patients are encouraged not to set impossible goals for themselves but to stretch themselves in terms of risk taking; 4) mini goals are goals covering from one day to one month and include those things that the anorectic had control over during hospitalization. Anorectics learn that they can plan a program for the next week and that their chances of successfully carrying it out (assuming their plans are reasonable) are good. If they planned too ambitiously, they can modify it after a period. By learning to think in abbreviated lengths of time, they learn greater control over each portion; 5) micro goals are goals covering the next 15 to 60 minutes. Realistically, these are the only goals over which they have direct control. Because of direct control, these goals can be extremely important in the anorectic's life. It is through micro goals that the anorectic is able to achieve longer term goals related to abstaining from eating-disordered behavior.

Since anorectics are often above average in intelligence, they appear to have no social skill deficits. However, unlike their peers, anorectics have few social connections and friendships that they develop are short lived.[22]

The communication skills group includes basic concepts of control in relationships related to women with anorexia nervosa. Anorectics experience a narrow range of emotional reactions and often feel that their emotions do not count.[31] Thus, a group priority is the identification and expression of appropriate feelings in relationships. The occupational therapist assists the anorectics in identifying a range of feelings in themselves and others. Patients examine how their passive and aggressive behaviors intensify negative feelings in significant others and lead to continued eating-disordered behavior. Since anorectics need to develop peer relationships, communication skills focus on the establishment of new relationships and prerequisite skills such as initiating, continuing, and terminating a conversation. Table 19-4 lists those skills taught in the communication group.

TABLE 19-4. Social skills for anorexia nervosa.

1. Initiating a conversation. Speaking to another person about a specific topic.
2. Continuing a conversation. Beginning the main topic of discussion, expounding on it, and resonding to the other person's points of discussion.
3. Terminating a conversation. Allowing the other person to know through verbal and nonverbal cues that he or she has been attended to and then ending the conversation appropriately.
4. Making a request. Describing to a person how they can fulfill desire.
5. Requesting assistance. Asking another person for help in a specific situation.
6. Following directions. Completing instructions as informed to do so and requesting any additional clarification.
7. Active listening. Focusing on the speaker and responding to the speaker's message through verbal and nonverbal cues.
8. Giving directions. Clearly explaining in specific steps how a task should be completed.
9. Giving compliments. Telling another person that something that they did was liked.
10. Empathic assertion. Acknowledging an understanding of another person's feelings, beliefs, or wants while clearly stating one's own position.
11. Criticizing. Objecting to another person's behavior while offering a suggestion for change.
12. Expressing anger. Telling a person about a justifiable annoyance that he or she has caused without humiliating that person.
13. Expressing feelings. Being able to define an emotion that is being experienced and communicating that feeling to another person.
14. Admitting a mistake. Disclosing to a person that an error was made which affected that person.
15. Accepting criticism. Using a firm tone of voice and direct eye contact in explaining what will be done about the mistake.
16. Reacting to another's anger. Acknowledging that the other person's angry feelings have been heard and calming the person so that the issue can be discussed.
17. Responding to nonverbal communication. Being able to identify aspects of nonverbal communication that can help to interpret a person's feelings.
18. Dealing with mixed messages. Identification of contradictory and sometimes confusing messages that occur when a person states something but acts in the opposite manner.
19. Bargaining. Being able to compromise so that each person's needs are met.
20. Assertiveness. Standing up for one's feelings, thoughts, and actions in nonthreatening fashion.
21. Problem-solving. Being able to define alternatives to solving a problem and then choosing the correct one.
22. Decision-making. Deciding on a specific course of action that will be in one's best interest.

The anorectic's disdain for eating and inappropriate behavior regarding food is a central theme. The patient's obsession with caloric content prevents the ability to produce a well-balanced meal. In the cooking group, meals include nonanorectic foods and do not involve food fads.[38]

During treatment, patients are taken shopping. If they do not possess the skills, patients are taught to prepare a shopping list, estimate quantities of food to purchase, cook a nutritionally balanced meal, and to store unused food appropriately. Initially in the cooking group, patients prepare their own meals beginning with precise amounts of ingredients for themselves. Subsequently, they will plan a meal, shop, and cook. As patients progress, there is the expectation that they will cook a group meal without using measuring devices to determine exact amounts.

Since food has become associated with anxiety, substitution responses are practiced. This involves social reinforcement for appropriate eating behavior. Researchers have shown that eating is facilitated by involvement in a group.[39] Eating with others provides modeling, encouragement, and support. Eating out is scheduled on a weekly basis and later in treatment families are encouraged to take the anorectic dining.

Since excessive exercising is a hallmark of anorexia, patients learn how to moderate their activity level. Patients participate in weight lifting to tone/strengthen muscles and for cardiac conditioning. They learn to self-monitor body cues that indicate adequate exercise.[40] The patient also learns to adjust food intake to maintain a constant weight. During exercise, cardiac performance is monitored and is most relevant to those with metabolic abnormalities such as hypokalemia.

Summary

Anorexia nervosa is a very complex and multifaceted illness that effects young women in personal, biological, family, and community dimensions. As such, it would appear logical that a model of intervention founded on organismic, humanistic, biosocial, and developmental assumptions and concepts would have particular usefulness in treating the person with anorexia. Therefore the occupational behavior model of practice was employed within the realm of general systems theory to describe the complexities of this illness and to discuss assessment and treatment intervention.

References

1. Reilly M. A psychiatric occupational therapy program as a teaching model. *Am J Occup Ther* 1966; 20:61–67.
2. Meyer A. Philosophy of occupational therapy. *Arch Occup Ther* 1922; 1:6.
3. Reilly M. Occupational therapy can be one of the greatest ideas of 20th century medicine. *Am J Occup Ther* 1962; 16:300–308.

4. Reilly M. The educational process. *Am J Occup Ther* 1969; 23:299–307.
5. Zellner DA, Harner DE, Adler RL. Effects of eating abnormalities and gender on perceptions of desirable body shape. *J Abn Psychol* 1989; 98: 93–96.
6. Humphrey LL. Observed family interactions among subtypes of eating disorders using structural analysis of social behavior. *J Consult Clin Psychol* 1986; 37:206–214.
7. Sykes DK. Preliminary findings of demographic variables in patients suffering from anorexia nervosa and bulimia. *Int J Psychosom* 1986; 33(4):27–30.
8. Rumpling D. Ascetic ideals and anorexia nervosa. *Psychiatric Research* 1985; 19(2–3):89–94.
9. Dura JR, Bornstein RA. Differences between IQ and school achievement in anorexia nervosa. *J Clin Psychol* 1989; 45(3):433–435.
10. Kielhofner G, Burke J. Components and determinants of human occupation. Baltimore, Williams and Wilkins, 1986.
11. Eckert ED. An overview of treatment of anorexia nervosa. *Psychiatric Medicine* 1989; 7(4):293–315.
12. Bruch H. Four decades of eating disorders. In Garner D, Garfinkel D (eds): Handbook of Psychotherapy for Anorexia and Bulimia. New York, Guilford Press, 1985.
13. Herzoy DB, Keller MB, Lavori PW. Outcome in anorexia nervosa and bulimia nervosa. Nerv Ment Dis 1988; 176(3):131–143.
14. Wolman BB. Dictionary of Behavior Science. New York, Von Nostrand Reinhold, 1973.
15. Bruch H. Eating Disorders. New York, Basic Books, 1973.
16. Strickland BR. Internal-external expectancies and health related behavior. *J Consulting and Clin Psychol* 1978; 46:1192–1211.
17. Hamilton LH, Brooks-Gunn J, Warren MP, Hamilton WG. The role of selectivity in the pathogenesis of eating problems in ballet dancers. *Medicine and Science In Sports and Exercise* 1988; 20(6):560–565.
18. Folts D, Giannini J. The Functional Eating Disorder Evaluation (unpublished instrument).
19. Gross M. Aspects of the family with anorexia nervosa or bulimia. *Int J Psychosom* 1986; 33(3):3–8.
20. Good-Ellis M, Fine SB, Spencer JH Jr. The Role of Performance Scale (unpublished instrument).
21. Hultsch D. Personal time perspective in adulthood. A time sequencial study. *Dev Psychol* 1974; 10:835.
22. Jones D. Structural discontinuity and the development of anorexia nervosa. *Sociological Focus* 1981; 3:233–247.
23. Reker GT, Peacock EJ. The life attitude profile: A multidimensional instrument for assessing attitudes towards life. *J Behav Sci* 1981; 13:264–273.
24. Riople NJ. An examination of the occupational behavior and life satisfaction of the elderly. 1982. Unpublished master's project. Virginia Commonwealth University, Richmond, VA.
25. Nowell R. The role of therapeutic recreation with eating disorder patients. *Psychiatric Medicine* 1989; 7(4):285–292.
26. Beard JG, Ragheb MG. Measuring leisure satisfaction *J Leisure Research* 1980; 12:20–33.

27. Mackenzie JR, LaBan MM, Sackegfio AH. The prevalence of peripheral neuropathy in patients with anorexia nervosa. *Arch Phys Med Rehabil* 1989; 70:827–830.
28. Askevold F. Measuring body image. *Psychother Psychosom* 1975; 26:71–77.
29. Hood J, Moore TE, Garner DM. Locus of control as a measure of ineffectiveness in anorexia nervosa. *J Con Clin Psychol* 1982; 50:3–13.
30. Harding TP, Lachenmeyer JR. Family interaction patterns and locus of control as predictions of the presence and severity of anorexia nervosa. *J Clin Psychol* 1986; 42(3):440–447.
31. King M. Locus of control in women with eating pathology. *Psychol Medicine* 1989; 19:183–187.
32. Rotter J. Generalized expectancies for internal versus external control of reinforcement. *Psychol Monogr* 1966; 80:1–28.
33. Reid DW, Ware EE. Multidimensionality of internal versus external control. Can *J Behav Sci* 1973; 5:264–271.
34. Giannini AJ, Folts DJ. Impaired reception of nonverbal cues in anorexia. *J Abn Psychol* (submitted).
35. Bolzani R, Matinelli P, Falmigni C. Gaze and eye contact with anorexia adolescents. *J Med Psychol* 1989; 62:365–369.
36. Brunner RL, Maloney MJ, Daniel S, et al. A controlled study of Type A behavior and psychophysiologic responses to stress in anorexia nervosa. *Psych Research* 1989; 30:223–230.
37. Swift WJ, Bushell MS, Hanson D, et al. Self concept in adolescent anorexics. *Am Acad Child Psychiatry* 1986; 12:826–834.
38. Garner DM, Garfinkle PE, Bemis KM. A multidimensional psychotherapy for anorexia nervosa. *Int J Eating Disord* 1982; 1(2):1–15.
39. Jenkins ME. An outcome study of anorexia nervosa in an adolescent unit. *J Adolesc* 1987; 10(1):71–81.
40. Collins ME. Education for healthy body weight: Helping anorexics exercise. *J Sch Health* 1988; 58(6):227–231.

20
Occupational Therapy Treatment of Bulimia Nervosa

DAVID J. FOLTS and A. JAMES GIANNINI

The mission of occupational therapy in treating bulimia nervosa is teaching increased competency and achievement through participation in meaningful activity. As reliance on binging, purging, laxative abuse, and exercise increases, functional behavior decreases. It is important for those with bulimia nervosa to learn how their eating disorders affect habits, skills, and values.

Occupational therapy is in a unique position to treat bulimia nervosa. Therapies that treat psychological problems without providing concrete assistance in remediating eating disorders display minimal efficacy.[1] In this chapter, a treatment model for bulimia nervosa is proposed utilizing the occupational behavior paradigm. This treatment model is used to illustrate occupational therapy interventions.

Bulimia Nervosa

By age eighteen, 80 percent of females in the United States have begun dieting.[2] Young women feel pressured to conform to the unrealistic standard for a lean body. Self-worth, happiness, and beauty have become equated with thinness and success. Over the past ten years, Miss America contestants and Playboy centerfolds have become thinner while the average woman's weight has increased.[3] The growing disparity between actual and ideal weight standards is shown by the 70 percent increase in dieting articles by women's magazines during the past ten years.[4]

An increasing number of young women are attempting to push themselves below their biological weight.[5,6,7] Research on the effects of semistarvation reveal that the onset of binge eating is an inevitable response.[8,9]

Symptomatology and Etiology

Although the majority of bulimic women weigh close to their normal body weight,[10] they possess an extreme desire for thinness.[11,12] According to the DSM-III-R,[13] bulimia nervosa is an eating disorder that has three central features. First, there are various behaviors designed to control shape and form. These include excessive exercising, extreme dieting, self-induced vomiting, and use of laxatives or diuretics. Second, there are repeated instances of overeating referred to as binges. Third, there is heightened concern over weight and shape.

Bulimic women present in their middle twenties and have older mothers when born.[14] In terms of family composition and social class, there are no significant differences in social class, family size, birth position, and sibling sex ratio than similar comparison groups.[15]

Frequently, bulimia nervosa is diagnosed with other psychiatric disorders. These include personality disorders, the most common being borderline, avoidant, and self-defeating.[16] High life time rates of major affective disorders have been noted.[17] It has also been reported that there is a higher incidence of sexual abuse among bulimics.[18] Researchers have also shown a high frequency of psychiatric disorders among first degree relatives of bulimics including eating disorders, alcoholism, and major affective disorders.[19]

It has been hypothesized that family dynamics play an important role in the etiology of bulimia. Several studies have indicated that bulimics are less cohesive than those of nonproblematic comparison groups.[20,21] There is also a relationship between disengaged family cohesion and compulsive eating.[22]

Fear of fatness and dissatisfaction with body size envelopes the bulimic's thought processes. Denial of the eating disorder is observed and is accompanied by overestimation of body size.

A Theoretical Model in Treatment of Bulimia Nervosa: Occupational Behavior

When treating bulimia nervosa, methodological concerns require a theoretical model that provides the organizing principles for treatment. Following are the major concepts of occupational behavior relevant to treatment.

Intrinsic Motivation

This arises from the satisfaction of performing or completing a task.[23] Intrinsic motivation is divided into a behavior continuum of pawn and origin behaviors.[24] Pawn orientation consists of: 1) feelings of being controlled by uncontrollable forces; 2) not behaving responsibly; 3) nonresponsiveness to environmental feedback; 4) perception of few options; 5) minimal risk taking; 6) disbelief in skills influencing the environment; 7) minimal motivation to acquire skills; and 8) external orientation resulting in the belief that fate and luck dictate success.

An origin orientation consists of: 1) feelings of being in control of one's destiny; 2) assuming responsibility for one's behavior; 3) improving performance through attention to feedback; 4) many options observed; 5) moderate risk-taking behavior; 6) belief in efficacy of skill; and 7) internal orientation resulting from expectancy of success or failure being skill based.

No person is totally pawn or origin since specific situations influence these behaviors. However, there is an unhealthy dominance of pawn behaviors in the bulimic population.

Control is a central issue for bulimics. Binging and purging is paradoxical in terms of control. Binging is an extreme example of control loss while purging allows the bulimic the regaining of control. Johnson[25] has shown a pawn orientation in bulimic women related to sex role behavior. Even though female bulimics did not differ from their counterparts in sex role attitudes, their sex role behaviors displayed the viewpoint that women are not in control of their lives.

Bulimics have little belief in their skills being able to influence the environment. College women engaging in eating-disordered behavior have stated feeling unable to match their high performance standards.[26]

Those with bulimic nervosa are resistive to treatment. This is until their physical condition necessitates medical attention. Eating-disordered patients conceal their condition with the typical patient reporting symptoms of bulimia three to five years before seeking treatment.[10] However, since there are oversocialized and hypersensitive to external demands, their hospitalization often results in an overt show of responsibility.

In terms of choices, bulimics display uncertainty regarding vocation. They also show conflict between feminine occupational values and changing societal expectation.[27] In addition, social and leisure interests are restricted with bulimics engaging in fewer leisure pursuits than their peers.[28] Kaufman[29] has reported that they view their leisure participation and satisfaction decrease due to time spent coping with the effects of illness.

Because of rigid and compulsive behaviors, bulimics are not responsive to feedback from their environment. Contributors include familial patterns associated with psychosomatic families. These characteristics consist of emeshment, rigidity, overprotectiveness, and lack of conflict resolution skills. Their external control becomes reinforced by an overdependency on significant others. Because of tight boundaries, risk-taking behavior is not encouraged and the environment is not explored.

Competency Motive

Competency relates to the bulimics' attempts to master their environment.[30] When interacting with the environment, the competency motive determines adjustment and success. Bulimics spend inordinate time and energy in obsessional thinking, and compulsive and ritualistic behavior.[31]

Examples of these behaviors include overexercising, binging/purging food, and eating rituals. Minimal time remains for mastering the environment.

While bulimics have assumed the worker role, their performance is dysfunctional with work-related stress being a major concern.[32,33] When experiencing an increase in vocational stress, they also display greater severity of binge eating.

Achievement Motive

This is based on problem solving tasks and involves meeting performance standards for task completion.[23] Bulimics place considerable importance on others' approval and tend to denigrate themselves when not meeting performance standards. Their self-imposed pressures create chronic tension. Several studies have found bulimics have high expectations, demand for approval, low self-esteem, and feelings of failure.[34,35] Since the performance standards established are unrealistic, they feel trapped between what they perceive as socially unacceptable behavior (binging and purging) and the overwhelming desire for acceptance and approval.

Despite self-reported feelings of inadequacy and lack of success, bulimics are accomplished.[36,37] Irrational and unrealistic performance standards do not allow them a sense of adequacy. In addition, attainment of performance standards becomes nearly impossible.

The social environment sends contradictory messages to the bulimic regarding achievement. One category is that of feminine beauty and physical attractiveness while another is accomplishment and achievement. Ambivalence is created regarding recognition versus physical attractiveness. The competency motive is weakened due to the importance of compulsiveness and rituals in the bulimic's daily life. As they become more dependent on habit and routine, competency becomes extinguished.

Problem Solving

Solving problems is the manner in which persons discover the correct sequence leading to a goal.[38] Bulimics perceive their shape as a problem and weight reduction as the goal. Except for exercise used as a weight control device, their ability to see cause and effect is faulty. Ironically, the cognitive effects of binging and purging prevent them from successful problem solving.

When making decisions concerning food, bulimics experience difficulties. When hospitalized, they often require training in choosing the appropriate food groups. Even after choosing the correct items, they experience indecision regarding the quantity of food required for an individual meal.[39]

Assessment

When utilizing the occupational behavior paradigm, the primary evaluation tool is the occupational history. The occupational history assesses the bulimic's past and current work, leisure, temporal functioning, and family history.

Work History

Although bulimics have assumed a vocational role, their performance is frequently impaired.[25] Deficits in vocational functioning are a result of the habit structure. Compulsive behavior in eating transfers to the work situation creating dysfunctional patterns. Binging, purging, and excessive exercising results in impaired concentration, lassitude, sleep disturbances, and inner tension bringing about a disintegration in work habits.[40]

In terms of vocational dysfunction, there is a striking incidence of bulimia among ballet dancers and professional models. This suggests that chronic dieting behaviors followed by these professions may be important in the pathogenesis of bulimia nervosa.[41,42]

Management of the home is assessed and consists of meal planning, meal preparation, laundry, chores, shopping, and money management. Planning a meal is difficult because they do not know what portions to use or how to balance the basic food groups.

Food preparation habits are assessed to determine if the bulimic patient eats food while preparing it and whether the person uses reasonable portions for food consumption. Patients are timed to assess how rapidly they eat, their ability to eat with others, and their ability to control their impulses to binge with remaining food left on the table.

During the cleanup phase of the meal, the bulimic is monitored for compulsive behaviors including excessive rubbing and shining and if they can store excess food without consuming it.

Money management is assessed and is a deficit area since bulimics spend a significant portion of their money on binge foods and laxatives. Impulsive spending is also a problem. Research has shown that impulsivity is a hallmark among those diagnosed with bulimia nervosa.[43]

Since there is a codependency relationship between the bulimic and one or both parents, it is determined if either parent is acting in the role of the enabler. If the enabler has assumed responsibility for completion of performance area, skill deficits will be noted.

Family History

Dysfunctional familial patterns are assessed through questions about significant others. The circumplex model of family functioning is utilized since it is a system model compatible with occupational behavior.[44] Two dimensions of the model are emphasized, that of family adaptation and cohesiveness.

Three central areas of family functioning are identified: cohesion, adaptability, and communication. Family cohesion contains four levels ranging from disengaged to emeshed. Included within family adaptability are four levels ranging from extremely low (chaotic) to extremely high (rigid). Three types of family functioning result: balance, midrange, and extreme.

Since families of bulimics show a higher incidence of eating disorders, alcoholism, and drug abuse,[45] patients are questioned to identify the level of codependency with significant others. Because there is a high incidence of sexual abuse in bulimia nervosa,[46,47] patients are gently questioned about this area.

Temporal Adaptation

How persons use their time is directly related to feelings of competency and achievement. Due to bulimics' impairment in perceiving cause and effect, they have difficulty planning for the future, developing short-term objectives, and establishing long-term goals. Obsessive thoughts and compulsive behaviors reduce confidence in their ability to impact on the present and to control their future.

Patients are asked to compose a typical day and to highlight times engaged in eating-disordered behavior. It becomes evident that significant time is spent on eating-disordered behavior with binging and purging most in the evening.[25] As a result of the surreptitious nature of the disorder, temporal functioning is isolated with peer relationships less common than the norm.

Leisure

Hospitalized bulimics are likely to display the adverse effects of prolonged binging and purging, laxative abuse, and excessive exercising.[48] As a result, their participation in recreational activities is diminished. Bulimics display an inability to relieve stress or feel pleasure.[28] Kaufman[29] has reported that bulimics' participation and satisfaction from leisure is reduced because of the time expended in coping with their eating disorder.

The feelings of satisfaction that the bulimic derives from exercising is distorted. Many joggers participate in jogging as a stress management tool or for its pure enjoyment. However, for the bulimic jogging is compulsive. Several authors have suggested a similarity between exercise dependence and bulimia nervosa. Katz[49] has reported on patients who developed characteristics of bulimia following a drastic increase in exercise. Other researchers have hypothesized a relationship between obligatory running and bulimia nervosa.[50,51]

As part of the leisure assessment, patients complete a leisure survey. Those with bulimia nervosa engage in fewer recreational pursuits than their peer group. In terms of leisure adjustment, it has been shown that bulimics displayed a significant impairment being most similar to alcoholic females serving as a comparison group.[52]

Sensorimotor Performance

When assessing bulimics, they rarely have difficulty with dressing, personal hygiene, or object manipulation. However, they do have perceptual difficulties. In the revised third edition of the *Diagnostic and Statistical Manual of Mental Disorders*,[13] there is one change in the criteria for bulimia nervosa, that is, a preoccupation with weight and shape of the person's body. Several researchers have shown bulimics to have body shape distortion.[53,54]

Personal/Emotional

Perceived lack of mastery in life tasks,[55] low personal competence,[56] and powerless feelings[57] are associated with an increase in eating-disordered behaviors. Since feelings of low personal competence and powerlessness are associated with an increase in bulimic behavior, a Multidimensional Locus of Control Scale is utilized.

The Multidimensional Locus of Control Scale[58] has been revised to fit bulimia nervosa.[59] It measures the degree that bulimics feel controlled by outside forces (pawn orientation) versus feeling in control of their destiny (origin orientation). Their score is based on the cumulative total of their internal and external choices. Those with higher pawn scores show a higher rate of relapse.

Social Functioning

Social Functioning is assessed to determine social skills. Previous studies have noted that social functioning of the bulimic is extremely impaired.[25] Deficiency in the social realm is caused by food obsessions and food related activities that lead to reduced concern in previous interest areas.

Treatment

Treatment is based on building occupational behaviors such as achievement and competency which will decrease the bulimic's reliance on eating-disordered behavior.

Stressful life changes are associated with relapse into eating-disordered behavior.[60] Since binging, purging, laxative abuse, and excessive exercising are utilized to minimize tension, stress management teaches coping skills that can be used to substitute for eating-disordered behavior. The patient is encouraged to identify sources of stress and the physiological and psychological symptoms of their reaction to life changes.

As an adjunct to stress management, the patients participate in a relaxation group. Since not engaging in bulimic behavior leads to increased anxiety, relaxation is used as a therapeutic substitute. The treatment goal becomes practicing relaxation skills for future control of their anxiety state.

The hour long session is divided into two parts. The first half of the session is devoted to teaching a variety of relaxation techniques. These include slow stretching exercises, yoga positions, diaphragmatic breathing, self-massage, meditation, concentration, and visualization techniques. The last half of the session includes discussion and a variety of progressive relaxation exercises.

Since temporal dysfunction exists, patients participate in a time management group. Bulimic patients are asked to complete a retroactive time log based on the week proceding their admission. After discussing the temporal imbalance created by bulimic behavior, patients write a time log based on their expectations of time use post discharge. A comparison is made between the two time logs and discussion relates to the importance of structuring meaningful activity that can be used to substitute for dysfunctional behavior.

While obsessive compulsiveness is destructive when paired with an eating disorder, it can be refocused. In goal setting, bulimics establish short- and long-term goals related to changing their eating-disordered behavior. Their short-term goals consist of: 1) feeling that their dysfunctional eating patterns are under control; 2) being able to eat at normal time with no binging or purging; and 3) reducing the binging and purging to manageable limits. When setting long-term goals, patients are reminded that their goal is not to "cure" themselves but to work towards marked improvement. Additionally, if relapses do occur, the patient needs to plan a strategy for coping with them.

Bulimics are socially isolated due to the time spent engaging in and recovering from the effects of their disorder. Thus, assertiveness training focuses on conversational skills and the establishment of new relationships. Assertiveness training also assists patients in identifying feelings in themselves and others. Bulimics are asked to identify how their nonassertive behaviors contribute to friction with significant others. To increase intimacy, patients learn basic assertiveness skills such as making a request, accepting criticism, and reacting to another person's anger.

Mediums used to promote transfer of training after hospitalization include videotaping, audio cassettes, handouts, and role playing. The bulimic patients are encouraged to practice their assertive skills with staff members on the unit and with significant others on therapeutic home leaves.

Leisure planning is used to provide the patient with understanding about recreation. The negative effects of their eating disorder on their leisure life style are identified. Community resource information is provided and encouragement is given for patients to take an active role in planning their recreation.

Motivation for engaging in leisure activities and satisfaction derived from them are explored. Emphasis is placed on the degree to which the recreation is social or solitary, reasons for beginning or terminating activities, playfulness versus routinization, and the level of mastery felt when having fun.

Since cognitive distortion is a central feature of bulimia nervosa,[34] a rational ideas group is used to discuss fundamental premises and beliefs about thinness and weight. The main thrust of the group is to examine the patient's cognitions regarding eating and food. In the rational ideas group, the therapeutic techniques used help identify, test, and remediate distorted cognitions. Patients learn to self-monitor negative automatic thoughts to overcome them through cognitive override and to recognize how thinking and behavior are interconnected. Patients are encouraged to view the rationality of their thoughts and are taught to substitute beliefs that lead to healthy adaptive behavior.

Because body image disturbance is a significant issue patients participate in a body image group. The primary goals of the group are 1) clarification of present body image versus normative standards; 2) identification of roadblocks impeding perception; 3) disregarding of negative beliefs associated with media and peer/family pressures; and 4) acceptance of present body shape. Methods to achieve group goals consist of image recording, caliper measurement, didactic presentation, guided imagery, handouts, written assignments, and group discussions.

Summary

The occupational behavior model provides a framework for treatment of patients with bulimia nervosa. The occupational therapist shares responsibility with the physician for problem identification and determination of treatment goals. The ultimate focus of the occupational therapist is to assist the bulimic patient in building competence and intrinsic motivation through meaningful involvement in purposeful activity.

References

1. Lacey JH. An outpatient treatment program for bulimia nervosa. *Int J Eating Disord* 1983; 2:209–214.

2. Mintz LB, Benz NE. Prevalence and correlates of eating disordered behavior among undergraduate women. *J Counseling Psychol* 1988; 35:463–471.
3. Garner DM, Garfinkel PE, Schwartz D. Cultural expectations of thinness in women. *Psychol Reports* 1980; 47:483–491.
4. Berzins L. Starving in an affluent society (unpublished).
5. Gross J, Rosen JC. Bulimia in adolescents: Prevalence and psychosocial correlates. *Int J Eating Disord* 1988; 7:51–61.
6. Greenfield D, Quinlan DM, Hurding P, et al. Eating behavior in an adolescent population. *Int J Eating Disord* 1987; 6:99–111.
7. Crowther JH, Post G, Zaynor L. The prevalence of bulimia and binge eating in adolescent girls. *Int J Eating Disord* 1985; 4:29–42.
8. Rossiter EM, Wilson GT, Goldstein L. Bulimia nervosa and dietary restraint. *Behav Res Ther* 1989; 27(4):465–468.
9. Charnock DJ. A comment on the role of dietary restraint in the development of bulimia nervosa. *Br J Clin Psychol* Nov 28, 1989; 329–340.
10. Drewnowski A, Hopkins SA, Kessler RC. The prevalence of bulimia nervosa in the U.S. student population. *Am J Public Health* 1988; 78(10):1322–1325.
11. Baba KA. Body image of patients with eating disorders. *Seishin, Shinkeiggka, Zasshi* 1989; 61(6):682–689.
12. Hall RC. Bulimia nervosa: Diagnostic criteria, clinical features and discrete clinical sub syndromes. *Psychiatric Medicine* 1986; 7(3):13–15.
13. Diagnostic and Statistical Manual of Mental Disorders (third edition revised). Washington, DC, American Psychiatric Association, 1987.
14. Giannini AJ, Newman M, Gold MS. Anorexia and bulimia. *Am Family Physician* 1990; 41(4):1169–1176.
15. Dolan BM, Evans C, Lacey H. Family composition and social class in bulimia. *Ab J Psychol* 1989; 77(5):267–272.
16. Gartner AF, Marcus RN, Halmi K, et al. DSM-III-R personality disorders in patients with eating disorders. *Am J Psychiatry* 1989; 146(12):1585–1591.
17. Hudson JI, Pope HG, Todd-Yurgelan D, et al. A controlled study of the lifetime prevalence of affective and other psychiatric disorders in bulimic outpatients. *Am J Psychiatry* 1987; 144(10):1283–1286.
18. Bulik CM, Sullivan PF, Rorty M. Sexual abuse in women with bulimia. *J Clin Psychiatry* 1986; 50(12):460–464.
19. Kassett JA, Gershon ES, Maxwell E, et al. Psychiatric disorders in the first degree relatives of probands with bulimia nervosa. *Am J Psychiatry* 1989; 146(11):1468–1471.
20. Coburn J, Ganony L. Bulimic and non bulimic college females' perceptions of family adaptability and family cohesion. *J Adv Nurs* 1989; 14:27–33.
21. Humprey L. Observed family interaction among subtypes of eating disorders using structural analysis of social behavior. *J Consult Clin Psychol* 1989; 57(2):206–214.
22. Kagan DM, Squires RL. Family cohesion, family adaptability and eating disorders among college students. *Int J Eating Disord* 1986; 4(3):267–279.
23. Florey L. Intrinsic motivation: The dynamic of occupational therapy theory. *Am J Occupat Ther* 1969; 23:319–322.
24. DeCharms R. Personal Cauzation. New York, Academic Press, 1968.
25. Johnson C, Lewis C, Hagman J. The syndrome of bulimia: Review and synthesis. *Psychiatric Clin NA* 1984; 7:247–273.

26. Goebel M, Spalthoff G, Schulze G, et al. Dysfunctional cognitions, attributional style and depression in bulimia. *Psychosom Res* 1989; 33(6):747–752.
27. Stein A, Fairburn CG. Children of mothers with bulimia nervosa. *Br Med J* 1989; 99(6700):777–778.
28. Nowell R. The role of therapeutic recreation with eating disorder patients. *Psychol Medicine* 1989; 7(4):285–292.
29. Kaufmann JE, McBride LG, Hultsman JT, et al. Perception of leisure and an eating disorder: An exploratory study of bulimia. *Therap Rec J* 1988 (first quarter); 55–63.
30. Wolman B. Dictionary of Behavior Science. New York, Van Nostrand, 1973.
31. Hart K, Ollendick T. Prevalence of bulimia in working and university women. *Am J Psychiatry* 1985; 142:851–854.
32. Cattanach L, Malley R, Rodin J. Psychologic and physiologic stressors in eating disordered individuals. *Psychosom Medicine* 1988; 50:591–599.
33. Lacy JH, Coker S, Birtchnell SA. Bulimia: Factors associated with its etiology and maintenance. *Int J Eat Disord* 1986; 5:475–487.
34. Carter BS, Hamilton SA, O'Neil PM, et al. Depression and bulimia: The link between depression and bulimic cognitions. *J Abn Psychol* 1989; 98(3): 322–325.
35. Butterfield PS, Leclair S. Cognitive characteristics of bulimia and drug abusing women. *Addiction Behav* 1988; 13:131–138.
36. Schlesier-Stropp B. Bulimia: A review of the literature. *Psychol Bull* 1984; 95:247–257.
37. Strober M. Locus of control, psychopathology and weight control in bulimia nervosa. *J Abn Child Psychopathology* 1982; 10:97–106.
38. English H, English A. A Comprehensive Dictionary of Psychological and Psychoanalytic Terms. New York, McKay, 1958.
39. Shimp SL. Short-term treatment for eating disorder patients with a high level of functioning. *Mental Health: Special Interest Section Newsletter* 1989; 12(3):1–3.
40. McSherry J, Ashman G. Bulimia and sleep disturbance. *J Fam Prac* 1990; 30(1):102–103.
41. Hamilton LH, Brooks-Gunn J, Warren MP, et al. The role of selectivity in the pathogenesis of eating problems in ballet dancers. *Med Sci in Sports and Exercise* 1988; 20(5):560–565.
42. Garner DM, Garfinkel PE, Rockert W, et al. A perspective study of eating disorders in the ballet. *Psychother Psychosom* 1987; 48:170–175.
43. Sohlbery S, Norring C, Holmgren S, et al. Impulsivity and long term prognosis of psychiatric patients with anorexia nervosa/bulimia nervosa. *J Nervous Mental Disease* 1989; 177(5):249–257.
44. Kagan DM, Squires RL. Family cohesion, family adaptability and eating disorders among college students. *Int J Eating Disord* 1986; 4(3):267–279.
45. Bulik C. Drug and alcohol abuse by bulimic women and their families. *Am J Psychiatry* 1987; 144:1604–1607.
46. Bulik CM, Sullivan PF, Rarty M. Childhood sexual abuse in women with bulimia. *J Clin Psychiatry* 1989; 50(12):460–464.
47. Hull RC, Tice L, Beresford TP, et al. Sexual abuse in patients with anorexia and bulimia. *Psychosomatics* 1989; 30(1):73–74.

48. Sedlet KL, Berger M. Energy expenditure and the abnormal eating pattern of the bulimic: A case report. *J Am Diet Assoc* 1989; 89(1):74–77.
49. Katz JL. Long distance running, anorexia and bulimia. A report of two cases. *Comprehensive Psychiatry* 1986; 27:74–78.
50. Lyons HA, Cromey R. Compulsive jogging: Exercise dependence and associated disorders of eating. *The Ulster Medical J* 1989; 58(1):100–102.
51. Chalmers J, Catalan J, Deg A, et al. Bulimia nervosa presenting as morbid exercising. *Lancet* 1985; 1:286–287.
52. Johnson C, Berndt DJ. Preliminary investigation of bulimic and life adjustment. *Am J Psychiatry* 1983; 140:774–777.
53. Williamson DA, Davis CJ, Goreczny AJ, et al. Body image disturbance in bulimia nervosa: Influences of actual body size. *J Abn Psychol* 1989; 98(1):97–99.
54. Powers PS, Schulman RG, Gleghorn AA. Perceptual and cognitive abnormalities in bulimia. *Am J Psychiatry* 1987; 144(11):1456–1460.
55. Schneider JA, O'Leary A, Stewart WA. The role of perceived self-efficacy in recovery from bulimia: A preliminary examination. *Behav Res Ther* 1987; 25(5):429–432.
56. Rost W, Neghous M, Florin I. Bulimia nervosa: Sex role attitude, sex role behavior and sex role related locus of control in bulimorexic women. *J Psychosom Research* 1982; 26(4):403–408.
57. King M. Locus of control in women with eating pathology. *Psychosom Medicine* 1989; 19:183–187.
58. Herzog D, Keller M, Lavori P. Outcome in anorexia and bulimia nervosa. *J Nervous Mental Disease* 1988; 176(3):131–143.
59. Folts D, Giannini J (unpublished manuscript).
60. Cattanach L, Phil M, Malley R. Psychology and physiological reactivity to stressors in eating disordered individuals. *Psychosomatic Medicine* 1988; 50:591–599.

21 Dietary Management of Eating Disorders

JUNE VENTIMIGLIA

Dietetics is the science or art of applying the principles of nutrition to feeding. Webster's dictionary defines a dietitian as "a specialist in dietetics."[1] As a specialist in applying the principles of nutrition to feeding, the dietitian is a valuable member of the team working with patients with eating disorders. The dietitian possesses many qualifications to assess the patient with an eating disorder. The dietitian is knowledgeable of the process of nutrition; is highly skilled in communication; is devoted to conceptual thinking; and is oriented to research. The main quality the dietitian possesses is being the only professionally educated person whose primary concern is the application of nutritional science to the health care of people. Through the use of nutritional assessment, development of a nutritional care plan, nutrition management, and education the dietitian can provide for the needs of the patient with an eating disorder.

Nutrition Assessment

Several definitions of nutrition assessment exist. For some it is defined as a dynamic process, everchanging and evolving. For others it means simply the identification of current nutritional status and requirements. Still for others it has evolved into a comprehensive process of identifying individuals and populations at nutritional risk and involves planning, implementing, and evaluating a course of action. Another definition is the systemic method of gathering data on individual patients, classifying the degree of malnutrition, and instituting appropriate treatment and intervention. Nutrition assessment involves looking at the total person, taking into account individual variables, and then planning for the nutritional well being of that person based on the information obtained. Nutritional assessment involves evaluating:

- anthropometric data
- biochemical data

- dietary history data
- clinical data, and
- psychosocial data

The anthropometric data used by the dietitian includes weight, height, skinfold thickness, and the mid-upper arm circumference. Accurate and consistent measurements of weight and height over time provide valuable information. Changes in weight reflect current nutritional status, while changes in height reflect chronic nutrition or undernutrition.[2] Weight in infants and children is a good indicator of growth and changes in weight indicate nutritional inadequacy. In adults, regular weight measurements are especially important in chronic illness. The inability to meet nutritional requirements can be verified by documenting weight loss in children and adults. How to properly measure weights and heights in children and adults is outlined in a number of nutrition textbooks.

In infants and children, weight and height are plotted on the appropriate growth charts. In adults, heights and weights are compared to the Metropolitan Life Insurance tables. The tables offer age related weight ranges with three frame sizes in one inch increments of height. Weight measurements can be used to determine the percent of weight change:

$$\frac{\text{usual weight} - \text{present weight}}{\text{usual weight}} \times 100$$

Weight change can be reflective of the patient's ability to meet nutritional needs. Table 21-1 shows weight change over time and the severity of malnutrition.

Skinfold thickness is a measurement of subcutaneous fat and is used to assess body fatness and muscle protein reserves. Measurements include the triceps, biceps, below the scapula, or above the iliac crest. The triceps and subscapular area measurements are easiest to compare to standard tables. Age and sex appropriate charts should be used for individual evaluations of data. Mid-upper arm circumference and tricep skinfold measurements can give a better assessment of protein and energy. These numbers can be used to determine muscle area and fat area. Arm muscle area is an indicator of lean body mass and skeletal protein reserve.

Biochemical data obtained from analysis of blood and urine can add to the evaluation of a patient. Essential nutrients can be low in the body due

TABLE 21-1. Assessment of weight loss over time.

Time	Significant (%)	Severe (%)
1 week	1–2	>2
1 month	5	>5
6 months	10	>10

Adapted from Walker[8]

to a dietary deficiency, poor absorption, impaired transport, abnormal utilization, or any combination of these. When used in conjunction with the dietary history, the medical history, and the clinical data, biochemical data can help to assess the status of a patient more thoroughly. Laboratory tests used to evaluate nutritional status usually measure:

- nutrient levels in the blood
- urinary excretion rate of the nutrient
- urinary metabolites
- abnormal metabolic products in the blood
- changes in blood components or enzyme activities that can be related to intakes of the nutrient, and
- response to a load, saturation, and isotopic test[3]

Laboratory tests of value in nutritional assessment include: zinc, magnesium, alkaline phosphorus, calcium, phosphorus, Vitamin K, Vitamin E, Vitamin D, Vitamin A, water soluble vitamins, B_{12} and folate, iron, albumin, total protein, cholesterol, triglycerides, and glucose.

The dietary history gives a picture of the patient's intake. Several methods can be used to accurately question what has been consumed. A 24 hour recall asks the patient to recall what food and liquids have been consumed in the past 24 hour period of time. The food frequency asks how often a food is eaten. The diet history includes questions regarding food allergies, physical activity, appetite, oral health, medications, food dislikes, meal patterns, snack consumption, and recurrent weight loss. In the food diary or record the patient records intake over a period of time. Often the dietitian must decide which method will give the most accurate and useful information. Evaluation of information obtained can be done using food groups or nutritional composition. Many computer programs are currently available to provide detailed information regarding the nutritional intake of patients.

The clinical data includes information obtained by a physical examination as well as visual examination by a dietitian. Is the hair glossy or dull? Are the eyes bright and clear? What does the skin look like? What does the patient's teeth, lips, and gums look like? All of these observations add to the total picture of the nutritional health of the patient.

Psychosocial data important to the overall nutritional assessment include who cooks in the household, who does the patient live with, the number of people in the household, where they shop, outside activities the patient is involved in, who does the patient eat with, bowel habits, and is the patient involved in any food programs. These and other questions deemed necessary by the dietitian can help to complete the nutritional picture of the patient.

After the nutritional assessment is completed by the dietitian, information obtained and evaluated is used to plan for the nutritional care of the patient. The nutritional care plan involves developing goals for the patient and suggestions for meeting those goals. A specific time frame should be established for meeting the goals and carrying out the nutritional care plan. It is the dietitian's job to not only develop the care plan, establish goals, and establish the time frame to meet the goals, but also to manage the care plan. Management of the nutritional care plan involves the implementation of the plan and also the evaluation and continual monitoring of the plan. Education of the patient/family and other health professionals is part of the dietitian's responsibility. The dietitian is the professional knowledgeable of the patient's nutritional needs and how the patient's nutritional status can be improved to benefit the patient.

Eating Disorders

The dietitian's role in eating disorders is to apply knowledge of nutrition, use the skills of nutritional assessment develop and monitor the nutritional care plan, and educate the patient regarding the nutritional needs of the body. In working with eating-disordered patients, the dietitian must avoid certain attitudes and/or situations that can cause problems. Some things the dietitian should avoid are listed in Table 21-2.

Anorexia Nervosa

In dealing with patients with anorexia nervosa, the dietitian assesses the nutritional needs of the patient, plans the nutritional care, manages the plan, and educates. If available, several records of height and weight help, when plotted on a growth chart, to provide a picture of normal growth and then weight loss. The height begins to level off also if under-nutrition has been chronic. Biochemical values add to the nutritional picture. The diet history becomes a very important tool. The dietitian must use the diet history to obtain information regarding the current diet

TABLE 21-2. What the dietitian should avoid.

1. Counseling patients who lack psychiatric or medical backup (anorectic and bulimic patients)
2. Conflicts with the patient
3. One-time visits
4. Expectations of uninterrupted progress
5. Threatening anorectics who refuse to eat
6. Overfeeding at first
7. Catering excessively to the anorectic's whims

Adapted from Dwyer[4]

regime and to determine when the dieting started, why it started and what the dietary intake was prior to dieting. Questions also to be included are

Does the patient exercise—how much and how often?
Are there any food aversions?
Did these food aversions exist before the dieting?
Are there any ritualistic eating behaviors?
Are there any bowel problems—diarrhea or constipation?
Who does the patient eat with, and who cooks?

The answers to these quesions help to evaluate the total picture of anorexia. It is important for the dietitian to develop a trusting relationship with the anorectic patient and to present the questions as patients participate in the treatment plan. Clinically, what does the patient look like? Is there lanugo, is the anorectic cold all the time? Do they layer clothes? Is the hair dull? Are the lips cracked at the corners? Has amenorrhea occurred? These are all observations that can be made during the interview or obtained from the medical history. Again, these add to the assessment of the anorectic patient. Observation of the patient eating can give the dietitian an accurate view of the ritualistic eating behaviors.

After the data is gathered, the dietitian must develop a nutritional care plan for the patient. This occurs if the patient is hospitalized or treated as an outpatient. Treating the patient with anorexia nervosa involves working with the physician, nursing staff, and psychological staff as a team.

Specific nutritional goals should be established by the dietitian. Goals for the patient with anorexia should include

- cessation of weight loss
- improvement of nutritional status
- gradual increase in weight, and
- education regarding normal diet and the body's need for food

The initial diet prescription for the anorectic, whether an inpatient or outpatient, will be low calorie. Most anorectic patients are not able to tolerate a large quantity of food; in fact prescribing a high calorie diet may set up the patient to fail. The initial diet is based on a comparison of usual intake as ascertained by the diet history and a determination of the basal needs based on present weight, height, age, and sex.[5] If the basal calories are 200 to 300 more than the current intake, that figure is used. If there is less than a 200 to 300 calorie difference, then that amount of calories should be added to the basal amount.[5] For some patients, a current estimate of calorie intake may not be attainable; in that case the basal calorie figure is used. In hospitalized patients, weight gain of $\frac{1}{2}$ to 3 pounds a week should be sufficient.[6] Constipation problems frequently seen in patients with anorexia can be alleviated with the use of increased fluids or increased whole grain foods. The initial diet is divided into three meals daily; if the patient is unable to take the full prescribed meal, then a high calorie supplement may be used to replace the meal or part of the meal. Education of the anorectic patient occurs daily during hospitalization. The dietitian stresses the importance of growth, what a normal intake of food consists of, and what foods are needed by the body and why. The dietitian constantly reinforces the idea that the anorectic patient will not become fat. Daily weights are taken, and the calories are constantly reevaluated to provide an appropriate weight gain. Observation of the anorectic actually eating a meal is a valuable experience for the dietitian in the ritualistic behavior of the patient. Taking patients to the cafeteria to allow them to choose their own food can provide the dietitian with another observation of how well patients will do on their own. As calories increase it may become necessary to add snacks to the meal pattern. During hospitalization, the dietitian continues to meet with others members of the team to discuss the progress being made by the anorectic. On discharge of the patient, the dietitian needs to provide the patient with a diet. This information should consist of a meal pattern, food exchange lists, and the dietitian's phone number to call with any problems or questions after discharge. It is important for the patient to continue to record daily intake after discharge and to have this evaluated by the dietitian. Follow-up of the anorectic patient involves working with the therapist, reevaluating calorie needs as the patient approaches goal weight, evaluating the diet diary, providing continued support and education to the patient and/or family, and providing a maintenance diet when appropriate.

The dietitian's input into the therapeutic plan of the outpatient anorectic is similar to the inpatient plan. The dietitian meets with the patient and/or family, determines the initial calorie level, provides a food exchange diet, and of course provides follow-up and readjustment of calories as needed. Again, the dietitian must educate the anorectic about the nutritional needs of the body and how to meet those needs. In dealing with the anorectic patient and their family, the dietitian must be accessible to the patient and the therapist and be able to answer questions and solve problems as needed.

Bulimia

In working with the bulimic patient, the dietitian must complete a thorough nutritional assessment. The diet history plays an important part in revealing the type of meal pattern the patient consumes; the foods that are forbidden; what constitutes a binge for the patient; do they fast; do they use laxatives; is there purging; or a combination of these. Again it is important to develop goals for the bulimic patient. These goals can include breaking the binge-purge cycle, establishing a normal pattern of eating, and changing the bulimic's attitude toward food. Most bulimics are of normal weight or very close to a normal weight for height. The dietitian needs to plan a diet that will maintain the current weight of the patient. Weight loss should not be instituted until the cycle of binging and purging has successfully been eliminated. The diet prescription is based on the current diet or what can be estimated to be the normal diet. The meal pattern is divided into 5 to 6 meals a day to prevent the binging and purging. Education needs to occur regarding the normal needs of the body for food, the role of food in our daily lives, and the fact that food is not harmful to us. The dietitian needs to work with the therapist to help the bulimic patients take control of their food intake. The bulimic patient needs follow-up with the dietitian in regard to intake records, weight maintenance, and diet modification if needed. The diet should include the use of food exchanges and a well-balanced diet pattern.

Obesity

Obesity generally reflects a long-term imbalance in energy intake and energy expenditure. Obesity can be associated with many health risks, among them hypertension, coronary heart disease, diabetes, gall bladder disease, hyperlipidemia, and respiratory disease.[7] Obesity is probably one of the most frustrating problems to face the dietitian.

In children, anthropometric data of height and weight plotted over time can give a good picture of obesity. A child whose height is at the 50 percentile, and with a weight that is continually crossing percentiles up to and beyond the 95 percentile, has a weight problem. In adults using height and weight tables, visual measurements, and tricep skinfold can give a picture of overweight or obesity. With increasing weight, tricep skinfolds may be hard to measure. Laboratory data can help to rule out metabolic causes and any other complicating factors. The diet history data can indicate the types of food eaten, when and with whom, how food is cooked, physical activity, eating and watching television, school lunches or business lunches, what times the food is eaten, etc. A good picture is given if the dietitian has at least 3 to 4 days of records to examine. Psychosocial evaluation involves asking who the patient lives with, are other relatives overweight, and if the patient is a child, with whom they spend free time or summer vacation. All of these questions give a thorough picture of the obese patient and their life style.

The dietitian must develop a trusting relationship with the overweight/obese patient. The dietitian becomes a support system encouraging the patient to reach the goals that have been established by the patient and the dietitian. In the case of children, goals must be established with the parent. Often in the case of small children, the main goal is weight maintenance with continued growth in height. The goals should be short term and long term, so that the patient will be successful. Education must occur in regard to very low-calorie diets, fad diets, the appropriate amount of food needed by the body, and the need for physical activity. The dietitian should help the patient and/or family identify the following:

- habits and activities that lead to obesity
- that no food is a reward
- that regular exercise is important
- how obesity can contribute to health risks, and
- the proper role of food in the nutrition and well being of patients

The dietitian can provide the patient and/or family with an exchange type of diet or a simple menu plan to follow. What is important is individualizing the diet and treatment plan to meet the needs of the patient and/or family and to be supportive of the patient and/or family. In some cases, working with a psychologist may be beneficial to the success of the patient. Depending on the diet restrictions implemented, a vitamin and mineral supplement may be necessary.

Summary

The dietitian's role in eating disorders is one of working as part of the health team and using knowledge of how the body uses and needs food to improve the nutritional health of the patient. The dietitian assesses the patient's nutritional status and uses the data this information provides. The dietitian must develop the nutritional care plan for the patient to meet the needs of the patient. The care plan must be individualized to the patient. The dietitian manages the care plan and continues to evaluate its effectiveness in meeting the goals established for the patient. A good therapeutic relationship must exist between the patient and the dietitian. This enables the care plan to work and meet the nutritional needs of the patient. The dietitian educates the patient and/or family as well as other members of the health care team regarding the care plan for this patient and the importance of nutrition to the overall well being of people. Working with the team, dietitians will be able to provide for the optimal nutritional health of their patients.

References

1. Webster's New Collegiate Dictionary. Springfield, MA, G and C Merriam Company, 1980.
2. Krause MV, Mahan LK. Food, Nutrition, and Diet Therapy (seventh edition). Philadelphia, W.B. Saunders Company, 1984.

3. Simko MD, et al. Nutrition Assessment. Rockville, MD, Aspen Publishers, Inc, 1984.
4. Dwyer JT. Role of the nutritionist in eating disorders. *New Directions for Mental Health Services* 1986; 31:21–8.
5. Huse DM, Lucas AR. Dietary treatment of anorexia nervosa. *J Am Dietetic Assoc* 1983; 83:687–690.
6. Weinsier RL, Krumdieck CL. Death resulting from overzealous total parenteral nutrition: The refeeding syndrome revisited. *Am J Clin Nutrition* 1980; 34:393.
7. Frankle RT, Yang M-U. Obesity and Weight Control. Rockville, MD, Aspen Publishers, Inc, 1988.
8. Walker WA, Hendricks KM. Manual of Pediatric Nutrition. Philadelphia, W.B. Saunders Company, 1985.

22
Administration and Management of Eating Disorder Units

DOMINICK L. FLAREY

Health care executives across the nation are accepting the challenge of the development and management of eating disorder units. The core of this challenge centers on the issues of resource and criteria establishment for the delivery of quality health care. Few, if any, standards or regulations exist, however, to guide executives in the development and maintenance of eating disorder units. This chapter focuses on the issues surrounding their administration and management. An ideal strategic analysis that guides executives in establishing quality standards for care and management is presented.

Health care institutions today exist in a turbulent environment of ever-changing rules and regulations guiding the delivery of care. Unexpectedly, there is a certain lack of such guidelines specific to eating disorder units. At present, the Joint Commission on Accreditation of Health Care Organizations and the American Osteopathic Association have no specific standards or regulations for these units.

Admission Criteria and Procedure

The first and most critical component centers on the appropriateness of admissions to an acute care eating disorder unit. Acute care admissions are costly yet provide for a comprehensive physical and psychosocial model of health care delivery.

Health care executives must guide a sound utilization review program to ensure appropriate admissions and lengths of stay. Criteria can best be established by following the diagnostic outline by the American Psychiatric Association in its Diagnostic and Statistical Manual of Mental Disorders (DSM III).[1]

The DSM III criteria for both anorexia nervosa and bulimia may be summarized as follows:

Anorexia Nervosa. The patient has an intense fear of becoming fat. When weight loss has occurred, this fear does not abate. The patient has a persistent self-image of being overweight. There is a loss of body weight of more than 25 percent and the patient refuses to maintain a normal body weight for age and height.

Bulimia. In this condition, there is a history of repeated binge eating. Other accompanying characteristics include: consumption of high caloric foods during a binge, unassuming binge eating, a fear of uncontrollability of the behavior, and attempted weight loss by restricted dieting, self-induced emesis, or the use of cathartics or diuretics.

Health care executives need to work with third party reimbursers to establish appropriate lengths of stay. Treatment modalities of eating disorders are usually complex as therapies vary according to medical practitioners. Lengths of stay may be quite prolonged when there is extensive emaciation causing multiple system effects.

Length of stay criteria related to Medicare's Diagnostic Related Groups is seldom significant when hospitalization is necessary. The vast majority of patients afflicted with these diseases are well below the age of medicare recipients. Estimates of the incidence according to age groups has shown to be 1 to 50 percent of adolescent women and approximately 10 percent of college age men.[2] Reports of primary eating disorders in the geriatric population are rare.

Health care agencies dedicated to the treatment of eating disorders will establish separate facilities for the development of an eating disorders unit.[2] The unit should be created away from medical and surgical, as well as psychiatric patient care units.[3] This helps to lessen the perception of the illness as being primarily psychiatric. A setting distinct from a medical-surgical nursing unit is necessary due to the highly specialized care involved with eating disorders. The ideal eating disorders unit may mirror a modern day psychiatric unit, but without a locked door policy or seclusion areas.

It is important to provide areas on the unit for group therapy, for private consultation, and for enhancing patient interactions and socialization. Health care executives need to tailor such designs based on the treatment modalities and philosophies of care of the medical staff specialists.

A primary benefit of establishing a dedicated eating disorders unit is the creation of a specialty staff of nurses and ancillary personnel. Maximum patient outcomes will likely be realized when the staff has developed expertise in the care of anorectics and bulimics.[4] The nursing process and plans of care can be developed around the focal nursing and medical problems with which such patients present. Staff who become specialized in the care of these patients develop expertise not only in the biophysiologic approach to treatment, but in the psychosocial components as well.

The health care executive needs to give considerable attention to the necessity for ongoing staff education and skill attainment. Nurse executives should encourage the unit's nursing staff to obtain certification in Psychiatric-Mental Health nursing by the American Nurse's Association. Such certification exemplifies a high level of psychosocial intervention available by the staff and invariably raises the quality of care.

The admission process should encompass a comprehensive psychosocial patient assessment conducted by the admitting nurse. The psychosocial assessment should include the following critical indicators: a history of amenorrhea, use and abuse of laxatives and/or diuretics, any past history or familial history of psychiatric illness, employment and education history, any history of or recent suicide attempts or ideations, a meticulous history of weight loss patterns, effects of the illness on activities of daily living, history of sexual dysfunction and current sexual behaviors, history of drug abuse, binge/purge history, nutritional assessment and food preferences, perception of body image, history of cosmetic surgery, religious affiliation, social relationship patterns, interfamily relations, occupation and effect of illness on job productivity, use and/or abuse of vitamin supplements, coffee consumption, tea consumption, alcohol consumption, any current or past history of financial difficulties, history of weight problems in childhood, history of depression and/or anxiety states, history of psychosis, educational history, history with fad diets, and history of counseling/therapy. While the preceding list is not exhaustive, integration of these components in a psychosocial history will provide the health care team with a more solid basis for diagnosis and planned treatment.

Upon admission of a patient to an eating disorder unit, it is essential that an accurate weight be taken. The patient should be weighed wearing only a patient gown. Shoes or slippers should not be worn and any excessive or heavy jewelry should be removed. It is most ideal if the patient is weighed at approximately the same time each day,[5] again only clothed in a traditional hospital gown. Accurate and daily weights are essential not only as an indicator of treatment response, but weight gain may reap rewards if a behavior modification-reward systems approach is used.

The patient admission process must also include a search for and confiscation of any laxatives or diuretics. This is essential because patients frequently deny such medication use and often try to sneak such drugs onto the unit. A patient search and confiscation should be conducted only after the patient has been thoroughly informed of its necessity and process. Two staff members should conduct the search in the presence of the patient. Ideally, a search of the patient's personal belongings should also be conducted in front of a family member of the patient. It is necessary to adequately document that a search and confiscation has occurred.[6]

Nutritional Assessment and Treatment

Health care executives need to ensure that the eating disorder unit is provided with a full-time registered dietitian, preferably with experience in the assessment and treatment of eating disorders. The role of the dietitian or nutritionist should be integrated on the unit as an essential member of the health care team.

A nutritional assessment is conducted and documented on the medical record within several hours of the patient's admission. This assessment is crucial to the planning of both medical and nursing care. "The nutritionist performs four essential assessment tasks: first, to document exactly what abnormal eating behaviors are present in each case; second, to review food intake data to obtain an estimate of intakes of energy, protein, vitamins, and minerals; third, to take anthropometric measurements; and fourth, to draft a preliminary assessment of nutritional status for review by the physician" (p. 21).[2]

The job design of the dietitian/nutritionist includes a role definition to facilitate involvement in patient care conferences with the staff as well as family conferences and counseling. A quality assurance assessment should be developed to assess the four major functions of the nutritionist as described above. This person is also granted privileges to document continuing assessment and patient progress on a daily basis. He or she works collaboratively with the nursing staff to establish mutual goals for the patient's nutritional treatment and outcomes. The nutritionist also functions in an educational consultant role to both the nursing and physician staff.

Patient Classification

Relatively soon after admission to the eating disorder unit, patients are classified by a primary registered nurse. Patient classification systems are a valid and reliable method of quantifying staff resources to meet identified patient needs. Such systems also assist unit managers and administrators with the development of budgetary systems and productivity analysis for the unit.

In terms of eating disorders, relatively few such classification systems have appeared in the literature. Table 22-1 presents a comprehensive patient classification tool for eating disorders in which reliability and validity have been established. Patients are classified into one of four levels of care based on assessments and identified needs. Five major care areas of assessment are given in Table 22-1 in which to assess patient needs.

Developed patient classification systems may be expanded further to measure actual direct and indirect care time required per level of classification. Such an evaluation may be done using a sophisticated methodology to measure care hours in relation to level of classification.[7]

To adequately plan for staffing needs as well as budgetary requirements, a valid and reliable classification tool must be developed and implemented.

TABLE 22-1. Eating disorders: Patient classification tool.

	Level I Minimal Care	Level II Average Care	Level III Above Average Care	Level IV Maximal Care
ADLs	Unobserved bathroom and shower Sleeps through the night Eats meals without difficulty	Observe bathroom and shower Wakes rarely during the night Locked bathroom Eats meals and snacks with minimal problems	Observe bathroom and shower Sleeps in dayroom; wakes frequently during the night Weights done with difficulty	Requires two people for ADLs Awake most of the night
Eating Disorder Assessment	Observe 1 meal Requires no replacements Requires no dayroom	Takes replacement without problems Requires infrequent (1–2/shift) replacements Dayroom observation without problems such as testing, acting out	Requires frequent (almost every meal and snack) replacement Total dayroom observation Replacement done with difficulty	Requires 1:1 observation 24 hours/day
Teaching and Emotional Support	Attends group support support meetings	Requires only one 1:1 during day and p.m. shift Attends one nursing group during day and p.m. shift	Requires more than one 1:1 per shift High level of anxiety in new admit Requires frequent (more than twice a shift) reminding of rules and program	Extremely high level of anxiety in patient who has been on the unit over 72 hours
Treatments	Routine specimen collection (UA, throat culture, etc.)	Escort to therapies and Outpatient Routine vital signs Return from pass search protocol	Suicide/elopement precautions Tube feeding for meals and replacements rarely required	Extremely uncooperative for tube feedings Restraints
Coordination of Care	Infrequent contact or telephone calls with family, outpatient nurse, dietary for menus, trays, or meal planning	Family meetings weekly 1 call/shift to family, outpatient nurse 1 contact/shift with OT, teacher, social worker	Requires more than 1 contact per shift with other disciplines to prevent splitting and program disruption	Requires several contact hours per shift with doctor or other discipline to manage patient

Olson B, Peterson C. Patient classification on an eating disorders unit. *Nursing Management* 1990; 21(5):68–70.

Such a tool must include the major modalities of assessment, care, and treatment commonly included in eating disorder patients.

Quality Assurance and Control

An essential element of the management and administration of an eating disorder unit is the development of a comprehensive quality assurance (QA) program. The eating disorder unit should be represented on the hospital-wide quality assurance committee. The nurse manager of the unit, along with the physician director should oversee the completion of a unit QA program.

The unit's program should include a written statement of philosophy as well as a written plan outlining the program's primary goals and objectives. The plan and program should include an assessment of the unit's structure (i.e., staffing requirements and modalities, patient-staff ratios, ancillary services, forms, records, the nursing process, medical and nursing documentation). Process is the second component of the program and focuses on policies, guidelines, and protocols for total patient care. The third component is outcome. This provides for direct patient evaluation, assesses outcome of treatment modalities, and provides for evaluation of established patient care goals.

The assessment of patient outcome is the prime focus in today's quality assurance programs. Outcome assessment provides an evaluative means by which to measure patient progress and quality of care services by the health care team. Table 22-2 is a sample outline of criteria from which unit patient care outcomes can be developed and evaluated.[8]

All developed QA audits should be reported to the hospital QA Committee. The unit manager and the unit physician director should share all audit results with the staff. Evaluation of the established audits should guide the revision of policies and protocols to ensure quality patient care.

Unit Standards

Of paramount importance in the development and management of an eating disorder unit is the existence of standards that govern and lead to outcomes of quality care. Few, if any, regulatory standards exist today to provide for adequate guidelines in monitoring the structure, process, and outcomes of a unit.

The following are proposed standards that may be implemented in the management of eating disorder units. The standards are generic and thus health care executives can utilize a wide variety of processes to guide adherence to and provide for institutional specifics to foster compliance.

TABLE 22-2. Anorexia nervosa evaluative criteria for patient care and outcome.[8]

Patient management:
1. Patients are given high carbohydrate, high fat diets.
   a. Diet menus include solid foods.
   b. Liquid food supplements are used if there is a resistance to solid food.
   c. Peripheral or central hyperalimentation therapy is used if there is resistance to oral intake.
2. There is documented implementation of a psychosocial treatment plan.
   a. Routine psychotherapeutic interventions are made with the patient.
   b. There are documented therapy sessions with family members.
   c. Milieu therapy is guided toward the objectives of enhancing the patient's sense of worth and independence and acceptance of weight gain without guilt or depression.
   d. There is observation and charting of failure to gain weight following outside visits.
   e. Suicide ideations are documented and a plan for suicide precautions is implemented.
   f. There is evidence of patient assistance with development requirements, that is, school, recreational activities, and social interaction.
   g. There is documentation of patient progress in the physician's progress notes (at least three times weekly).
   h. There is evidence of periodic reassessment with documentation of any resulting revisions in the treatment plan.

Length of Stay:
1. The patient is hospitalized until she/he has maintained a weight that is at least 90 percent of the ideal for a period of at least two weeks.

Discharge Status and Outcomes:
1. The patient has the following outcomes at discharge:
   a. Weight is at 90 percent of the ideal.
   b. Electrolytes are WNL.
   c. There is no evidence of depression or expressed guilt.
   d. The patient can meet identified development requirements.
   e. There is documentation and an initial schedule for continuing outpatient treatment and therapy.
   f. There is documentation of patient teaching related to diet, ADL, and follow-up treatment and care.

Standards are developed around five core components in which compliance can be identified and measured: 1) facilities, 2) personnel, 3) therapeutics and treatment, 4) documentation, and 5) quality control.

Facilities

1. There shall be a separate, dedicated patient care unit for the comprehensive care and treatment of eating disorders.
2. There is a central nursing station on the unit that includes a medication storage area accessible only to unit staff.
3. A private area is provided for patient consultation and counseling by the professional staff.

4. Patient care rooms are designed semiprivately; there shall be at least one patient room available for private occupation when deemed necessary for therapeutic treatment, in cases of medical isolation, or to enhance patient safety.
5. There shall be a separate kitchen facility accessible to patients. Provisions are made for the safe storage of food for patients and shall be accessible at all times.
6. There shall be provided a common group room or area to facilitate socialization and planned group activities for patients.
7. There shall be a private treatment room on the unit for patient examinations and specialized diagnostic and therapeutic procedures.

Personnel

1. There shall be appointed a physician medical director of the unit. This physician shall have the following responsibilities, inclusive, but not limited to:
   (a) The development of written by-laws, policies, and procedures governing patient admissions, treatment, and care modalities; and standards of care to facilitate quality and therapeutic outcomes.
   (b) A mechanism to define physician qualifications and privileges for the primary treatment of eating disorders.
   (c) The development of admission criteria, guidelines for medical documentation, and standards of outcome for the evaluation of care.
   (d) The establishment of policies and procedures for the integration of medical education and clinical research on the unit adhering to the protection of patients' rights and confidentiality.
   (e) The development of a comprehensive and on-going medical quality assurance program focusing on the evaluation of therapeutic outcomes of care.
2. There shall be appointed a unit nurse manager who shall have the responsibility for the overall planning, direction, control, and evaluation of the nursing staff and the delivery of care. Responsibilities shall include 24 hour accountability for the operational management of the unit.
3. There shall be an established, reliable, and valid patient classification/acuity system for the qualification and quantification of patient care needs on a shift-to-shift basis.
4. There shall be a sufficient number of professional registered nurses along with supportive and technical nursing personnel to provide comprehensive nursing care on all shifts. Quantification of personnel shall be determined by, but not limited to, a developed patient care classification system.

5. There shall be a planned, ongoing continuing education program for the nursing staff focusing on the care of patients with eating disorders. Instruction shall be provided by qualified physicians, psychologists, nurse specialists, and other health care professionals trained in the care and treatment of eating disorders.
6. The following professional staff shall be available at all times for patient consultation and care as deemed appropriate by the primary physician or unit medical director:
   (a) staff psychologist(s)
   (b) medical or psychiatric social worker
   (c) occupational therapist
   (d) registered dietitian
   (e) psychiatric nurse specialist
   (f) activities therapist
   (g) registered pharmacist
   (h) registered physical therapist

Therapeutics and Treatment

1. There shall be a mechanism to include the patient's family or significant other(s) in the overall treatment plan and process as deemed appropriate by the medical and professional staff.[9]
2. There shall be developed on admission and continually updated a comprehensive nursing care plan, individualized and focused on the overall nursing and ancillary support care needs of the patient. There shall be a mechanism to actively include the patient in the development of the nursing care plan.
3. The nursing care plan will be developed utilizing a multidisciplinary approach to patient care inclusive of all involved medial and ancillary support services.[10]
4. There shall be held minimally once a week, a multidisciplinary patient care conference for each admitted patient. The care conference will include representatives of the medical staff, nursing staff, and all other professional and paraprofessional services involved in the care of the patient. When deemed appropriate, the patient will actively participate in the conference. The conference will focus on the establishment of short- and long-term treatment goals as well as evaluation of outcomes realized.
5. There shall be a medical plan of care developed by the primary or specialist physician addressing the overall health care needs of the patient as well as a multidiscipinary care plan.
6. There shall be provided on a daily basis planned unit activities that enhance patient socialization.[11]
7. There shall be provided planned, comprehensive, patient centered teaching programs and sessions focusing on understanding, acceptance, and therapeutic strategies for living with eating disorders.[12]

8. All patients shall have an all-inclusive dietary assessment completed by a registered dietitian. An individualized nutritional treatment plan shall be developed and evaluated daily with the patient.[13]
9. All patients shall have a psychological evaluation within 24 hours of admission, preformed by a qualified psychiatrist or psychologist in the area of eating disorders. Recommendations for interventions shall be included in the multidisciplinary plan of care.

Documentation

1. There shall be an all-inclusive and comprehensive medical record for each patient.
2. There shall be documented upon admission a comprehensive physical, psychosocial nursing assessment, as well as the assessment of the patient's self-perception.[14]
3. The following shall be the minimally required scope of documentation in the medical record:
   (a) Daily patient weights
   (b) Daily vital signs.
   (c) Daily nursing assessments to include physical and psychosocial assessments.
   (d) The nursing care plan, including goals for patient outcomes.
   (e) The medical plan of care including daily progress and patient evaluation.
   (f) The psychological assessment and plan of care.
   (g) Social services consultations.
   (h) Dietary plan of care, including daily evaluations.
   (i) Specific planned medical and nursing interventions.
   (j) Patient response, evaluation, and outcomes.
   (k) Interdisciplinary team conference reports and plans.
   (l) Daily evaluations of socialization progress and response to planned activities.
   (m) Evaluations of the plan of care from the patient's perspective.
   (n) Daily documentation of the patient's eating patterns.
   (o) Documentation of counseling sessions, including patient response.
   (p) A written plan by the physician for discharge and ongoing therapeutic interventions.
   (q) At the time of patient discharge there shall be documented:
      (1) self-perception assessment
      (2) evaluation of established patient goals
      (3) dietary plan for discharge
      (4) long-term goals for treatment and outcomes.

Quality Control

1. There shall be developed a unit-specific mission statement and patient care philosophy.

2. Unit goals and objectives shall be developed from the mission and philosophy.
3. A comprehensive unit-based quality assurance plan encompassing a multidisciplinary approach to total patient care will be developed.
4. A structured, ongoing quality assurance program will assess process, structure, and outcomes.[15]
5. The quality assurance program shall focus on evaluation of patient care outcomes and correction of problems and/or deficiencies in the delivery of care.
6. The unit quality assurance plan shall be reviewed and updated annually.
7. Unit quality assurance activities will be reported to the hospital-wide quality assurance committee or program.

Conclusion

The administration and management of a hospital inpatient eating disorder unit is both complex and challenging. Little has been published to guide health care executives in this domain. Because of a lack of established and accepted criteria and standards, such development remains in its birth phase. Health care executives must take the lead and work collaboratively with physicians and nurses specializing in eating disorders to create appropriate standards, guidelines, and processes for patient care and unit management.

A quality health care service can be developed that leads to cost effective, quality outcomes in patient care. Experiencing the pitfalls and promises of managing eating disorder units will provide for greater analysis and decision making in the future development and management of such units. Health care executives must take the lead in designing eating disorder units and facilitating an agenda for quality management.

References

1. American Psychiatric Association. Diagnostic and Statistical Manual of Mental Disorders (third edition). Washington, DC, American Psychiatric Association, 1987; 65–70.
2. LaRocca F (ed). Eating Disorders, New Directions for Mental Health Services. San Francisco, Jossey-Bass, Inc, 1986.
3. LaRocca F. A Public Primer on Eating Disorders. St. Louis, BASH, Inc, 1988.
4. LaRocca F (ed). Eating Disorders: Effective Care and Treatment. St. Louis, Ishiyaku EuroAmerica, Inc, 1986.
5. Yates A. Current perspectives on the eating disorders: II. Treatment, outcome, and research directions. *J Am Acad Child Adolesc Psychiatry* 1990; 29(1):1–9.
6. Miller NS, Giannini AJ, Gold MS, Philomena JA. Drug testing: Medical, legal and ethical issues. *J Substance Abuse Treatment* 1990; 7:239–244.

7. Flarey D. A methodology for costing nursing services. *Nursing Administration Quarterly* Spring, 1990; 14(3):41–51.
8. Carroll J. Patient Care Audit Criteria, Standards for Hospital Quality Assurance (fourth edition). Illinois, Dow Jones-Irwin, 1983; 173–174.
9. Herzog D. Eating disorders. In Nicholi A (ed): The New Harvard Guide to Psychiatry. Cambridge, The Belknap Press of Harvard University Press, 1988.
10. Geary M. A review of treatment models for eating disorders: Toward a holistic nursing model. *Holistic Nursing Practice* 1988; 3(1):39–45.
11. Staples N, Schwartz M. Anorexia nervosa support group: Providing transitional support. *J Psychosocial Nursing* 1990; 28(2):6–10.
12. Flood M. Addictive eating disorders. *Nursing Clin NA* 1989; 24(1):45–53.
13. Krey S, Palmer K, Porcelli K. Eating disorders: The clinical dietitian's changing role. *J Am Dietetic Assoc* 1989; 89(1):41–42.
14. Plehn K. Anorexia nervosa and bulimia: Incidence and diagnosis. *Nurse Practitioner* 1990; 15(4):22–31.
15. Ente B. Stimulating improved patient care: The Joint Commission's Agenda for Change. *Top Hosp Pharm Manage* 1990; 10(2):22–30.

23 Literary Resources

A. JAMES GIANNINI

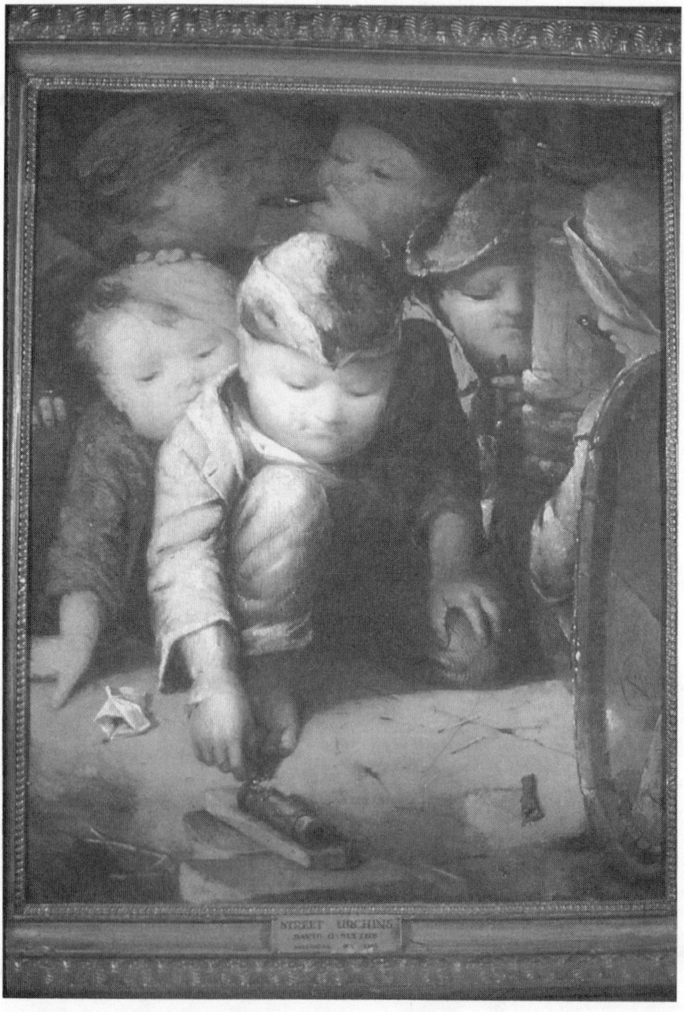

Blythe, David G.—*Street Urchins*—(Butler Institute of American Art, Youngstown, Ohio)

As the reader has now learned, the anorectic, the bulimic, or the obese person is more than a compounded result of psychiatric motivations, hormonal secretions, sociological impulses, and cultural influences. The traditional scientific paper is a necessary part in the transmission of medical knowledge. It reproduces faithfully the elements of diagnosis and treatment. It however fails to encapsulate the essence of confronting the patient with an eating disorder. While short on accurate detail, the novel, short story, movie, and play faithfully reproduce the sweat and fire generated in treating these patients. To assist in capturing the intuitive "feel" of this process, the following literary resources are recommended.

Birth of the Modern (Paul Johnson)

According to this historian, the modern diet began in the years following Waterloo. The ensuing explosion of general prosperity produced "a superabundance of animal food in wealthy and advanced societies and their excesses of sauces, spices and stimulants." Physicians however began to advise their patients to eat less; white meats, vegetables, and whole grains were now emphasized in medical and cook books. No longer was the stout trenchman considered a paragon. It was at this time that the conflict between material abundance and good health arose. Obesity began to emerge as a disease of the lower classes with their emphasis on starches and their sudden access to a supply of red meat. Doctors now began to notice a relationship between dietary excess and certain medical disorders.

Bonfire of the Vanities (Tom Wolfe)

It was in Wolfe's book that the materialistic and the superficial, the twin icons of Yuppiedom were roasted. The concept of the "social X-ray," the emaciated and cadaverous husk of an anorectic socialite, was born on these pages.

Bread and Chocolate (Francis Brusati)

This Italian film is a fresh variation on the theme of food-choice as an emblem and metaphor for class-driven identification and isolation. Overconsumption is used to shield from rejection. Those who underconsume food also restrict themselves from other needs.

Decameron (Giovanni Bocaccio)

This anthology of 100 tales was written in Florence, Italy during the time of the Black Death. In the stories, we find a recurring attitude towards food: obesity is seen as a substitute for sex; anorexia as a weapon against it.

Dinner at Eight (George S. Kaufman/Edna Ferber)

This 1930s play focuses on the use of food and eating as a method of social control. The ritual of class and the ritual of the tablecloth are nicely interwoven.

Dinner for Adele (Oldrich Lipsky)

This 1978 Czech detective movie investigates the murders by a carnivorous plant who is distorted by her isolated existence. The special pain of those who substitute food for the more risky human relationship is satirized in this turn-of-the-century melodrama.

English Wayfaring Life in the Middle Ages (J.J. Jessread)

This 1899 historical work reviews in many chapters the Medieval antecedants of contemporary views towards eating and the disorders that accompany it. The medical and sociological predilections and results of obesity and anorexia are described.

Fatso (Anne Bancroft)

This 1980 film veers between comedy and pathos as a man discovers that being fat is the only true sin in America. The motivations for overeating and binge dieting are lampooned. The medical consequences of obesity are elaborated upon in black comedic fashion.

Georgy Girl (Silvio Narizzino)

A "small" British movie and international success, this was presented as an adult satire of 1960s morality. The focus is on a wealthy man's obese mistress who loses weight and, as Cinderella transformed, becomes his wife.

Good Fellows (Martin Scorcese)

This 1990 film was based upon the Henry Hill-Nicholas Pileggi novel *Wiseguys*. Food, in all its forms and guises, is presented as both subsitution and cohesion for social intercourse.

Le Morte D'Arthur (Sir Thomas Mallory)

At the end of the Age of Chivalry, Mallory published a compilation of tales of the Round Table. In it, we find denial of food described as part Christian denial of bodily pleasure and part desire for self-perfection. The impossibly ethereal bodies of the women and the emaciated yet sinewy bodies of the knights helped create an unreachable ideal towards which men and women still strive. The Holy Grail is then buried within each of our bodies, to be found only when the layers of flesh are burned away on ascetic impulses.

Metamorphosis (Franz Kafka)

In this short story, a man is turned into a cockroach. No longer able to buy the love of his dependent and ungrateful family, he starves himself to death. As he slowly wastes away, his family is able to grow.

Nina's Book (Eugene Burdick)

In this novel of the coming of age of the Americans between the wars, the full triad of eating disorders is found. Anorexia is used as a means of control as well as a badge of social status in the upwardly mobile. Bulimia is seen as purging of both food and self. Obesity is described as a mark of rejection as well as a seductive ploy to maintain the attention of the always attentive medical profession.

Pantagruel (Francois Rabelais)

It is ironic that this physician's name is associated with dietary excess ("Rabelasian"). This work and other similar novels are seething attacks on the follies of contemporary France.

Satyricon (Titus Petronius Arbiter)

This satire of Imperial Rome was written by a contemporary sybarite who indulged in its pleasures. Though the emperor Nero ordered all copies destroyed, fragments were found in Renaissance Florence and the Paris of King Louis XIV. This novelist used bulimia and obesity as the metaphor for the depravity and decadence that he felt were destroying his city. The association between food and sex, depression and male hegemony was first explored in this book.

Sermons (Bernard of Clairvaux)

This Burgundian abbot was one of the most influential men of the Medieval Era. He was afflicted by an atrophy of his sense of taste. This served him as tool for developing renunciation as a tool for self-perfection. Though arising from a unique motivation, his anorexia was as much an emblem of self-ordained worldly and spiritual perfection as that of the "social X-rays" of the 1980s. [See Bonfire of the Vanities.]

The Physiology of Taste (Jean-Anthelme Brillat-Savarin)

This French lawyer did almost say "you are what you eat" in the 8-volume work that first appeared in 1825. It deals with anecdotes based upon persons who use and misuse the pleasures of the table.

Voss (Theodore White)

The barrenness of the Australian outback and the deprivations of the flesh are variations on a theme of Christian renunciation of worldly desire. This Nobel-prize winning author reprises the Medieval theme of asceticism and anorexia as virtues in a quest for a perfect self.

Index